The Worlds of Public Health

To all those who work to ensure that
unnamed truths are spoken and faceless voices heard

The Worlds of Public Health

Anthropological Excursions

Lectures at the Collège de France (2020–2021)

Didier Fassin

Translated by Rachel Gomme

polity

Polity Press
65 Bridge Street
Cambridge CB2 1UR, UK

Polity Press
111 River Street
Hoboken, NJ 07030, USA

ISBN-13: 978-1-5095-5827-8
ISBN-13: 978-1-5095-5828-5(pb)

A catalogue record for this book is available from the British Library.

Library of Congress Control Number: 2022948491

Typeset in 10.5 on 12 pt Times New Roman by
Cheshire Typesetting Ltd, Cuddington, Cheshire
Printed and bound in Great Britain by TJ Books Ltd, Padstow, Cornwall

The publisher has used its best endeavours to ensure that the URLs for external websites referred to in this book are correct and active at the time of going to press. However, the publisher has no responsibility for the websites and can make no guarantee that a site will remain live or that the content is or will remain appropriate.

Every effort has been made to trace all copyright holders, but if any have been overlooked the publisher will be pleased to include any necessary credits in any subsequent reprint or edition.

For further information on Polity, visit our website:
politybooks.com

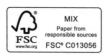

MIX
Paper from
responsible sources
FSC® C013056

Contents

Acknowledgments

This course of lectures was prepared during my tenure of the Annual Chair in Public Health at the Collège de France, to which I was elected in 2019. These lectures, and the resulting book, offered me an opportunity to immerse myself in a field I had moved away from – public health – and to revisit it on the basis of research conducted several years ago, while also drawing on material that was new to me. Words cannot express my debt to all those I met, with whom I worked, and among whom I sometimes lived, in Ecuador, South Africa, the United States, and of course France, and to those with whom I studied, and then for a time practiced and taught, public health, before moving into social science. I am grateful to Sandrine Nikel and Julie Clarini for having supported the project at Le Seuil, and to John Thompson for having manifested from the outset his interest in its English version. It has once more been a pleasure to collaborate with Rachel Gomme on the translation and to work with Munirah Bishop for the final steps. I also thank Sarah Dancy for her attentive copyediting. For obvious reasons, this exploration has a particular significance, since it took place during a time when the world faced a major health crisis. A substantial proportion of the lectures was actually written when I was confined alone in an environment highly favorable to reflection and writing, the Institute for Advanced Study in Princeton.

Introduction
Problematization

*Problematization does not mean the representation of a pre-existing object,
nor the creation by discourse of an object that does not exist. It is the set of
discursive or non-discursive practices that introduces something into the play of
true and false and constitutes it as an object for thought.*
Michel Foucault, "The concern for truth," 1988

Public health erupted into the world's consciousness early in 2020. In
the case of France, the moment can even be precisely dated: 17 March,
the first day when the majority of the population was confined to their
homes. For what is unique about the Covid[1] epidemic is not the nature
of the infection, which is of course serious, though less contagious than
measles and not as lethal as AIDS, but the way societies reacted to its
emergence. The pandemic, and the responses to it on every continent,
generated a worldwide upheaval in human activity. In many other
countries, lockdown was an experience without precedent, apart from
its echoes of some aspects of the response to outbreaks of plague in the
late Middle Ages and cholera in the early nineteenth century. Health
policing, with its arsenal of prohibitions, requirements, checks, and
sanctions, was the most widespread manifestation of public health,
even once people began to be vaccinated. But it took many other
forms: social distancing, the wearing of masks, the practice of testing,
the isolation of patients, the tracing of contacts, the recurrent and
swiftly refuted announcement of treatments, fierce and often unequal
competition in the search for a vaccine, daily public counts of cases and
deaths, intrusive and ineffective surveillance measures, not to mention
the exceptional provision for both economic and social support aimed
at preventing business failures, limiting lay-offs and mitigating the consequences of the abrupt destitution of many families. The implementation of these policies was accompanied by hesitations and reversals,

debates and controversies, martial declarations and contradictory assertions, flagrant lies and lethal obstructions. In much of the world, everything that keeps societies in motion suddenly began to revolve around questions of health. Public health, which for many until then had been no more than an abstraction, an obscure administrative matter, a rather unappealing field of expertise, became the principle for the government of lives – a "government of living beings," as Foucault puts it.[2] His phrase should, however, be taken literally – more so than he himself does – considering it as the government of human beings inasmuch as they are living beings who must, "at all costs," as the French president articulated it, remain alive.

It so happened that, a few months before the first cases of Covid were diagnosed, I was elected to the Annual Chair in Public Health at the Collège de France. My course was due to begin on 29 April, six weeks after lockdown was imposed. It was therefore postponed and took place a year later, albeit in almost identical conditions owing to both a new wave of the epidemic despite the beginning of vaccination, and a renewed, although less draconian, lockdown. For, contrary to the hopes of many and the predictions of some, the infection still loomed in the present. In the interval, however, my course had gained a new significance. Its subject, public health, hitherto barely recognized, had become the central topic of conversation and concern, insinuating itself into the everyday lives of each and every one, and equally into national politics and international relations. But it raised the question of how to tackle this topic that had suddenly invaded both public and private space to the extent that it absorbed almost all the attention of the media, politicians and citizens. Should I refocus my analysis purely around the pandemic, which lent itself to an anthropological reading on many levels, but would mean letting go of the richness of this multifaceted, diverse field? Such an approach risked giving in to the lure of presentism, forgetting that public health has a long history that could inform present anxieties. It would also mean consenting to a form of ethnocentrism, losing sight of the fact that many societies were struggling with other, more serious health issues. I therefore decided to take an alternative approach. I started from a banal and little-known scene illustrating various aspects of public health which I analyzed through a number of case studies over the course of the lectures, and I ultimately showed how each of these aspects sheds a different light on the Covid pandemic.

The scene in question is the emergence in France of the epidemic of childhood lead poisoning in the late 1980s. It can be considered both in terms of social production, the result of harsher immigration policies and a slowdown in housing policy, and in terms of social construction, through the fumbling, digressions and resistances of the actors involved. As a linking thread through the lectures, this investigation enables me to explore some seemingly unusual but nevertheless fundamental dimensions of public health: the power of positivism, the boundaries of disease, conspiracy theories, morality tests, and finally the challenges posed by the health of migrants and prisoners. The exploration transports readers from France, which has the highest level of prison suicides in Europe, to South Africa, the country that has been the worst affected worldwide by the AIDS epidemic, and Ecuador, which announced that it had the highest official maternal mortality rate in Latin America; from the scientific controversies of the "worm wars" in Kenya to confrontations between physicians and patients around Gulf War syndrome in the USA; from exotic pathologies at the Institut Pasteur to colonial psychiatry at the École d'Alger; from the origins of psychic trauma in World War I to the enumeration of deaths during the 2003 heatwave in France. The journey ends with an examination of the Covid pandemic in light of each of the dimensions explored in the preceding lectures in order to propose a new reading of it – revisiting it from an anthropological point of view.

Anthropology, as I understand it, is a way of looking at the world otherwise, of reflecting, like Ulrich, Robert Musil's "man without qualities," that "it might just as well have turned out differently."[3] It is an exercise in intellectual dishabituation. In order to accomplish this, it can draw on more than a century of research by anthropologists who have explored multiple facets of human activities and relations in diverse places around the world, from the Nuer of South Sudan to the Nambikwara of Brazil, as well as among various groups in their own societies, from the anti-witches of the Mayenne Bocage region in western France to the Canadian experts in Alzheimer's disease, and have thus learned that everything that seems self-evident in one context may appear completely differently in others.[4] But this cultural relativism does not lead them to become hunters of the exotic: quite the opposite. As Jean Bazin emphasizes, when faced with alterity they strive to reduce it by familiarizing themselves with the social worlds in which they conduct their research, whether geographically remote or close to home.[5] This practice helps to make intelligible phenomena that experts have defined as imaginary, such as chronic Lyme disease, by showing that they result from the impossible confrontation between the authenticity of patients' suffering and the authority of doctors' knowledge. It also contributes to the explanation of phenomena that arouse anger or derision, such as paranoid beliefs around AIDS, which can be shown to have a heuristic value as they provide clues to interpret lines of cognitive fracture in contemporary societies. But it also leads the anthropologists to defamiliarize themselves with their own social world, making what is taken for granted less self-evident. For example, it can prompt them to wonder about the belief in the single, neutral truth of numbers in describing health, when the validity of randomized trials is contested or when disputes arise around the interpretation of mortality statistics, or to question the existence of a separate field of migrant health, as if exiles presented specific pathologies when in fact their poor health is a product of the way they are treated by the so-called host society. Thus, the anthropologists know, through their own experience and from that of those who have preceded them, that there are many ways of being in the world, and that the one that has long seemed the only right way is not necessarily more right than others.

It is such a shift of gaze with regard to public health that I have proposed in this book. Hence the subtitle "anthropological excursions." An excursion, the dictionary tells us, is "the action of traversing a region to explore or visit it." The word, which first appeared in both English and French during the sixteenth century but only became common much later, derives from the Latin *excursio*, meaning "journey," "incursion," and, in the figurative sense, "ramble" or "digression."[6] This idea of exploration, freedom, and adventurous investigation points to the method of my inquiry. It explains my frequent preference for a narrative form, after the manner of what could be the tale recounted by a traveler in the "worlds of public health."[7] Here I speak of worlds not in the sense of particular geographies or specific activities, but rather as sets of questions that arise for society in the language of public health, and which to a certain degree revolve around common stakes – the desire to quantify, the legitimization of knowledge, the meaning of conspiracy theories, the rationales of immorality, and disparities in the treatment of exiles and detainees.[8] The word "stakes" is important. And it should be understood more broadly than it usually is, in the sense of what is socially at stake, of what is being staked in and for society. The corresponding issues are not predetermined or set once and for all. On the one hand, they are subject to negotiations, debates, and arguments, struggles to bring them to light or conversely to conceal them, among the agents and institutions involved. On the other, the researcher who analyzes them is himself part of constituting and recognizing them. In the studies I present, I shall consider the stakes from this dual viewpoint, internal and external, whereby public health emerges simultaneously as a mirror held up to society and the reflection society returns to that mirror.

This methodological and theoretical choice to enter into the subject via the stakes is thus a matter of both using a prism that refracts public health into a series of images and, conversely, understanding how broader questions can be grasped through the images thus refracted. "The Truth in Numbers" invites reflection on how the work of quantification claims to represent social and health facts. "Epistemic Boundaries" examines the clash between lay and scientific conceptions of illness that are based on competing legitimacies. "Conspiracy Theories" reveals reactions of distrust of authorized knowledge and official power. "Ethical Crises" exposes mechanisms of violation of rights and diversion of public goods for the benefit of private interests. The studies on "Precarious Exiles" and "Carceral Ordeals" open a way to understand the genealogy and sociology of government of groups subject to various forms of state surveillance and repression, through two categories that have become central to thinking contemporary societies: migrants and prisoners. The refraction of public health into these multiple stakes thus offers a new approach to understanding it, without exhausting the spectrum. It is always an open reading.

This approach differs substantially from those that have dominated social science studies of public health. The most traditional considers public health as a set of knowledge and practices around collective management of disease, and its emergence and development can be traced back through time to Greco-Roman antiquity.[9] But most of the research that takes this approach is limited to shorter time periods and more precise topics, whether they be epidemics, specific methods such as statistics, or particular institutions such as psychiatric asylums. Their contribution to knowledge in this domain is invaluable. Working through a genealogical reading, Foucault broke with this approach in two ways.[10] On the one hand, he placed public health within a larger context of management of populations. What he names biopolitics comprises the work of both knowledge and action that is legitimized by the very concept of population, notably the science of demographics that makes it possible to count births, deaths, life expectancy, individual mobility, and practices of governmentality such as family planning, social security, and control of migration. On the other hand, he established a discontinuity in the traditional, more-or-less linear account of public health. This is the shift from sovereignty as the right to kill to biopower as the duty to make live, which arose during the eighteenth century as a signature of modernity. Nevertheless, despite their manifest differences, the historical and genealogical approaches, each in their own way, tend to confer a degree of unity and even coherence on their subject: public health in the first case, biopolitics in the second.

What I am trying to do here is different. I propose neither a homogeneous representation of public health nor a consistent theory of biopolitics. Rather, I break down this amorphous matter into a range of stakes that I aim to identify, so that the different pieces gradually brought together sketch an image of public health like an incompletely assembled jigsaw puzzle. The argument is that public health is, no more than science or religion, a coherent ensemble, and rather than trying to give it an artificial unity, which always comes down to a catalogue of missions or, symmetrically, to a paradigm erasing its discrepancies, it is more heuristic to explore what is at play through its various dimensions. Indeed, each stake unveils games of power and knowledge involved – in the production of biostatistics, the legitimation of diseases, the imaginary of conspiracies, the emergence of crises, and more specifically the treatment of migrants and prisoners.

The Covid pandemic represents a life-size experimentation of this approach as each fragment I have proposed to study finds its place in the composite image presented in the final lecture, shedding a distinct light on the pandemic. The fetishization of numbers is put to the test by the contradiction of those produced. Epistemic borders are drawn between recognized and invalidated clinical trials. Conspiracy theories flourishing everywhere reveal a loss of trust not so much in science as in government. Ethical crises occur around the uneven distribution of resources. Migrants and prisoners are made more vulnerable and, paradoxically, more at risk for being confined at the very moment when the rest of the population is under lockdown. Finally, while the debate has been mostly around health versus wealth, or between the critique of the measures adopted for their effects on the economy or for their consequences for democracy, it is more urgent to address the considerable inequalities in morbidity and mortality that have been established, and perhaps even more those to come in terms of lives lost and lives ruined.

At this point I have to acknowledge the dilemma I was presented with when I found myself writing in the context of the pandemic – in other words, just as a major public health event was emerging. On the one hand, if I waited for the circumstances to "cool down" before rendering an account of them, I risked exposing myself to the criticism often addressed to the social sciences, particularly anthropology, of never being there when history is being made before researchers' very eyes. But on the other, if I offered analyses "in the heat of the moment," there was a danger of running after a present that was changing almost daily, where one day's assurances might be contradicted the next, without giving myself time to take the distance appropriate for scientific reflection. By linking my final study to those presented in the preceding lectures, I felt it was possible to present a reflection free of both the rush to act, which tends to become an invitation to avoid thinking, and the urge to condemn that ultimately neutralizes any possibility of genuine critique. Having written most of the first seven lectures before the start of the pandemic, I therefore retained their form and their theses,[11] reserving my reflections on the health crisis for the final lecture – "untimely meditations" on current events, which made it possible, I hope, to read these events otherwise.

The Birth of Public Health
14 April 2021

*Expert knowledge and social sciences. – Refusal of a theory of public health.
– The exploration of what is at stake in public health as a way to understand
contemporary societies. – A paradigmatic case study. – From a rare disease to
a silent epidemic. – Two approaches, two languages, two policies. – Discovery
and invention. – Work and workers. – Ignorance, negligence, and resistance. – A
public secret. – Culturalist variations. – Political economy and moral economy. –
Social construction and social production of public health.*

This course has a curious history, caught up as it has been by history
itself. Taking public health as its subject, it was brought up short
last year by the advent of a public health crisis on an unprecedented
scale. The Covid pandemic made it impossible to present the lectures and of course, more broadly, paralyzed the economic, cultural,
and social life of France as of most other countries in the world. It
thus revealed all the more starkly the pertinence, and indeed urgency,
of studying the hitherto somewhat indeterminate domain of public
health. Epidemiologists and statisticians, biologists and doctors,
economists and political scientists have engaged with it, sometimes
as counselors to princes and sometimes criticizing their decisions,
expressing themselves with caution or with confidence, warning of disaster or promising panaceas, exhorting the populace to adopt rules of
good conduct, and influencing, through their analyses and opinions,
decisions that could have considerable impact on the lives of millions
of people.

In this concert of experts, what role could be played by historians,
sociologists, anthropologists – those represented as social scientists
though they by no means account for the entirety of this field? They are
certainly not experts, and what they engage with is perhaps precisely
that which resists expert knowledge. It is not that they contest its

importance in managing a crisis as serious as the one that is currently convulsing the world, and whose aftershocks will continue to be felt for years to come. But through their research and their reflections, they maintain that, in order to contend with such an event, a society needs something more than just expert knowledge. Another realm of knowledge is possible, perhaps more distanced, or rather engaged in a different way, seeking less to tell people what must be done than to understand what is at stake, in the belief that such an understanding has political as well as ethical implications. In response to the pandemic, the interruption of the normal activities of businesses, schools, universities, theaters, festivals, entertainment complexes, sports clubs, and research institutes, the suspension of civil liberties and fundamental rights, such as moving around, meeting, protesting, the introduction of intrusive mechanisms for surveillance of behavior and repression of deviance from the norm, the ban on family members being at the side of the sick and dying, the drastic restrictions imposed on funerals – all of these elements of the response to the pandemic highlight the seriousness of the political and ethical stakes and call for an approach distinct from that of the experts. There is a need to think a world in transition, in which public health is a catalyst. Social sciences – whether history, sociology, or anthropology – offer keys to interpretation that draw on perspectives from other times and other places, the study of empirical material and a tradition of critical reflection.

It is this other gaze that is offered in this course. Do we need to begin with a definition of public health? A literature review published twenty-five years ago already listed around sixty, but the most frequently cited is Charles-Edward Winslow's classic 1920 definition: "Public Health is the science and the art of preventing disease, prolonging life, and promoting physical health and efficiency through organized community efforts for the sanitation of the environment, the control of community infections, the education of the individual in principles of personal hygiene, the organization of medical and nursing services for the early diagnosis and preventive treatment of disease, and the development of the social machinery which will ensure to every individual in the community a standard of living adequate for the maintenance of health."[1] There are of course more recent definitions that put forward more sophisticated modalities and are more democratically expressed, but none of them escapes the normative and administrative functions of a discipline that is designed to serve public action toward collective well-being in the matter of health. It is easy to understand why the British historian Dorothy Porter states, in the introduction to her reference book on the field: "For many students the idea of studying the history of public health provokes a very big yawn."[2] How, then, are we to avoid the anthropology of public health provoking the same bored reaction? How do we spare readers a discussion of the definition of the field of public health, its ideology, its procedures, and its politics, with the ultimate aim of proposing a general theory of it?

In his lecture "The birth of biopolitics," which is in truth an inquiry into the origins of liberalism rather than the birth of biopolitics – as he himself recognizes in the summary he wrote at the end of that year's course – Michel Foucault, who wanted to show how liberalism was constructed in opposition to the state, or at least on the basis of a limitation of its prerogatives, imagines his interlocutors reproaching him for doing "without a theory of the state," and he responds: "Yes, I do, I want to, I must do without a theory of the state, as one can and must forgo an indigestible meal."[3] I think that if anyone ventured to construct one, a theory of public health would risk precisely resembling an indigestible meal: the list of its activities is to be sure a copious menu but hardly enticing, mingling as it does public hygiene, health education, epidemiological monitoring, the fight against infections, disease prevention, the protection of the environment, the control of medicine, care for people with disabilities, the inspection of working conditions, the administration of the medical and paramedical professions, and much more.

But Foucault's ironic remark should not be misunderstood. Refusing to make a theory of state does not mean refusing to think the state, or more precisely the practices involved in its activity. What Foucault intends is rather to reject the idea that there can be "an essence of the state," that it is possible to begin by asking the question of what is this "political universal" called the state. For, according to Foucault, the "state is nothing else but the mobile effect of a regime of multiple governmentalities," and what merits study are its practices. Following a similar approach, what I propose in this course is to address public health not as a total social fact, to use Marcel Mauss's famous formula, but via a range of partial social facts in which it is or has been engaged. The question I shall attempt to answer is not "What is public health?" but, rather, "What are the stakes – theoretical and epistemological, political and moral – that can be illuminated by problems deemed to be concerns of public health, and how do they contribute at the same time to constructing the field of public health?" More broadly, what can they contribute to the understanding of contemporary societies?

To begin at the beginning: the birth of public health. Birth here should not be understood as the origin of the discipline or field that is called public health. I undertook that genealogical enterprise in an earlier work going back to Roman, Inca, and even precolonial African societies.[4] My aim now is rather to grasp the moment when, in specific circumstances, it emerged as a new reality in the social world, the moment when it was recognized. Here I return to a historical and sociological inquiry I undertook in the early 2000s, in Paris and the Seine-Saint-Denis department, into an epidemic undoubtedly singular in that it involved not a microbe but a heavy metal – lead. I shall focus more particularly on lead poisoning in children.[5] This study will form a guiding thread through this series of lectures. As historian of medicine Elizabeth Fee writes, "childhood lead paint poisoning is ... a classic public health problem, reaching beyond science into politics, economics, education and race."[6] To this list, I would readily add morality and ethics.

As a classic problem, then, childhood lead poisoning has been one of the most comprehensively studied public health issues for more than a century, and has given rise to an entire scientific industry, particularly in the United States. However, it is the little-known tale of its history in France that I intend to relate. I shall do so in a way that takes account of two aspects that are manifested in any health issue. On one side, there is its social construction by agents, human or nonhuman, physicians, and experts, as well as bioassays and statistical tests that led to the recognition of its existence, its seriousness, and its causes; on the other, there is its social production via structural phenomena woven from the combination of history, economics, law, population distribution and housing policies, that resulted in the risk to the lives of young children owing to the presence of lead in their environment. Because childhood lead poisoning is a genuinely paradigmatic case, I shall address it with a degree of detail that I feel is necessary in order to unpack its multiple dimensions.

In 1987, the main French pediatric journal, the *Revue de pédiatrie*, published a seven-page article entitled "L'intoxication par le plomb chez l'enfant. Un problème toujours actuel" ["Lead poisoning in children: A problem that has not gone away"].[7] The author reports three clinical cases observed in a Paris hospital, the most tragic of which concerns "the child Sylla B., aged two years and three months, brought to the emergency room on 7 March 1986 in a deep coma." His parents are described as being "of Malian origin." A year earlier the child had been treated for iron-deficiency anemia, and it was noted then that his growth was severely retarded. In the days before his hospitalization he was suffering from "abdominal pain" and "uncontrollable vomiting." All tests, including a lumbar puncture and toxicology screening, were normal, but the scanner showed a "diffuse cerebral edema," for which antiviral treatment was started in the hypothesis that this was a case of herpes simplex encephalitis. The child, whose condition did not improve, was transferred to intensive care where, for a month, pediatricians were still unable to establish a diagnosis of his severely impaired consciousness. Finally, almost by chance, an abdominal X-ray revealed "micro-opacities in the rectum" that pointed to the possibility of lead ingestion. When questioned, the parents admitted that the child "consumes flakes of paint from a window in the apartment" in which the family was living. Analysis of lead blood levels indicated a level of 3,720 μg/l – more than ten times the maximum level deemed safe at that time. Despite treatment with chelating agents, which bind in the blood with heavy metals to form compounds that can be excreted in the urine, it was too late and the child died only a few hours after administration of the medication began. As if to justify the difficulty in establishing a diagnosis, Cohen observes: "Lead poisoning has been known for a long time. In France, it is rare in children." It is true that a literature search conducted four years earlier found only ten cases in a quarter of a century in the French pediatric literature. In order to facilitate the recognition of lead poisoning in children, Cohen therefore formulates recommendations, stressing the need to remember the possibility of this pathology when presented with certain symptoms, since it is easily diagnosed from a simple blood test as long as the practitioner has it in mind. And Cohen even gives a list of "products containing lead that could cause poisoning in children," in which he includes, haphazardly lumped in together, "newspapers and printed materials," "enameled artisan pottery," "smoke and ash from burning metal shelving," "ball-point pen casings, lead from red, yellow and orange colored pencils," "metal packaging like that on toothpaste tubes," "eye shadow from Africa or Asia." Remarkably, "paint" arrives only at the bottom of the list with the note that, although banned "since the beginning of the century," lead can still be found in paint in "pre-1940 dwellings." This is how childhood lead poisoning was seen in 1987, as a rare condition caused by the ingestion of a variety of more or less out-of-the-way products, giving rise to serious neurological manifestations and seen in hospitals by pediatricians.

In 1999, an eighty-page report entitled *Plomb dans l'environnement. Quels risques pour la santé?* [*Lead in the Environment: What are the Health Risks?*] was published by the National Institute for Health and Medical Research (Inserm, Institut national de la santé et de la recherche médicale).[8] The outcome of a "collective expert assessment," it was put together by twelve specialists in epidemiology, bio-statistics, economics, toxicology, neuropharmacology, biochemistry, genetics, pediatrics, occupational medicine, and public health. The authors focus particularly on the effects of lead on children's cognitive functions, discussing around forty studies from all over the world that almost all show negative statistical correlation between the presence of lead in the blood, even at levels substantially lower than those then authorized, and the results of psychomotor tests, educational achievement, and behavior in class. In addition, meta-analyses, which gather and synthesize series of studies using similar methods, confirm that, even at very low levels, the presence of lead in the blood is associated with a reduction in children's IQ. Furthermore, a survey of 3,445 children aged from 1 to 6 years old, extrapolated to the whole of the population on the basis of census data, estimates that in France 85,500 children in this age bracket present "saturnine impregnation" at levels considered to be toxic. As far as the origin of the contamination is concerned, the experts emphasize that "paint is considered to be the principal cause of childhood lead poisoning," derived "largely from the ingestion of toxic flakes and dust." In order to combat childhood lead poisoning, it is therefore recommended that children affected be identified and removed from their unhealthy environment. Two "strategies" are proposed, within the framework of a national program of "surveillance," to identify contaminated children. The first, ecological, involves identifying a "risk environment," such as dilapidated buildings, and then measuring the blood lead levels of those who live there; the second, clinical, is based on identifying "children at risk" when they come for a medical appointment, by asking parents how old their housing is. Depending on the strategy adopted, there are two possible interventions. The first, collective, consists in identifying all housing constructed before 1948 and in serious disrepair, and carrying out the necessary remedial work. The second, individualized, consists in identifying the children who have been contaminated among those exposed, and offering the families rehousing or the refurbishment of their apartment. The cost of the operation is between 1.7 and 3 billion euros if the issue is approached through substandard housing, and only between 0.4 and 0.8 billion if it is tackled on the basis of screening children, because in the latter case only the housing in which cases have been detected need to be dealt with. This is how childhood lead poisoning was viewed in 1999: a common problem, the consequence of exposure to paint in old housing, manifested in a statistical risk of cognitive disorders, which should be the focus of nationwide screening for both dilapidated housing and contaminated children, and requires urgent action to renovate the housing in question.

Only twelve years separate the hospital pediatrician's article from the expert committee's report, but what they discuss and the way they discuss it seem to belong to two entirely different worlds. From being a rare pathology of which a few cases have been observed, childhood lead poisoning has become what some are already calling a silent epidemic, presented as a national priority. In pediatrics, little Sylla's illness was the subject of a tragic narrative that followed the protocol for presentation of clinical cases in medicine, from his hospitalization to his death, passing through the long diagnostic quest through progressive elimination of possible causes of impaired consciousness, with that which led to the child's death finally being suggested and recognized too late. In the expert assessment, estimates of lead contamination in populations of children are derived from statistical studies which, on the one hand, reveal that even low levels of lead in the blood increase the probability of learning difficulties, even when the children concerned show no symptoms, and, on the other, establish on the basis of a random sample an estimate of the number of children contaminated in the country. A story on one side, figures on the other. A single case for the former, a population for the latter. An extremely serious disease for physicians, a quantified risk in the view of epidemiologists. A tragic anecdote in one case, a statistical calculation in the other. Pediatricians emphasized the importance of signs such as anemia, abdominal pain, and neurological disorder, and focused their questions to parents on tracking down the absorption of paint flakes. The experts look for absorption even in the absence of any discernible manifestation, and select children by asking parents how old their housing is. The former used biological and radiological examinations; the latter drew on maps of dilapidated old housing. The ones spoke of diagnosis, the other of strategies. Two procedures, two languages, two policies.

But two realities too. How are we to understand that childhood lead poisoning moved from an incidence of ten cases in twenty-five years (incidence measures new cases) to a prevalence of 85,500 cases a few years later (prevalence indicates the cases existing at a given moment)? There is of course a difference in the mode of calculation as incidence corresponds to cases actually observed (the ten children were seen in the hospital), whereas prevalence refers to estimated cases (the figure of 85,500 children is an extrapolation based on a sample). Does this spectacular rise in little over a decade indicate a sudden increase in exposure of children to lead, as has sometimes been observed at specific sites following a change in water supply or close to highly polluting factories? Were there new sources of contamination via air, water, or soil? Were there more disadvantaged families forced to live in dilapidated buildings whose internal fixtures were coated in old paint? Surely not. All the studies indicate on the contrary that, during that period, the banning of lead in gasoline had significantly reduced the presence of lead particulates in the air. Moreover, the old lead pipes that had been used in water storage and supply were being gradually replaced. And the most rundown housing in large cities was increasingly subject to demolition and development projects, easily organized because it was often in the city center where real estate prices were highest. And while there was no cause for triumphalism, the blood lead level of the general population was steadily falling.[9] How then is this inflation in lead poisoning, from 10 to 85,500 cases in twelve years, to be explained? This remarkable development is in fact due to the existence of two totally different approaches. The passive approach, of receiving children usually suffering from serious manifestations in the hospital, was replaced by an active approach, based on identifying children who were exposed, precisely before they presented such a disturbing clinical picture. The former is the approach of clinical medicine, the latter that of public health. But it should be noted that public health derives here from two quite distinct processes, whose results converge: on the one hand, the discovery of unrecognized cases, and, on the other, the invention of new cases.

Indeed, a systematic effort was initially made to identify children who had been contaminated, through targeted surveys either of dilapidated housing (the ecological method) or in healthcare facilities (the clinical method). An example of the first is a 1985 study of fifty-two individuals living in two blocks where cases of lead poisoning had been diagnosed at the hospital: four of the seven children under the age of 6 had high blood lead levels, and core sampling of the walls revealed the presence of lead at disturbingly high levels. An illustration of the second method is a 1986 survey of eighty-two children who were seen at a mother and child clinic, whose parents were asked how old their housing was: 9 percent of these children presented severe lead poisoning.[10] The process at work in these two studies can be described as one of discovery. Children who presented abnormally high blood lead levels, at a time when the threshold was fixed at 250 μg/l, had their contamination identified; some even presented clinical or radiological signs that had hitherto gone unnoticed. They were, as it were, sick without knowing it, or without being diagnosed by medicine, but were recognized as such by the study. The coordinated effort of a few health professionals thus made it possible to identify 1,500 new cases of symptomatic poisoning in five years in the Île-de-France region alone. This was 150 times the number of observations French pediatricians had reported over a quarter of a century, but still less than 2 percent of the estimate established by the expert committee a few years later. How is this persistent disparity to be accounted for?

What is at play in this saturnine inflation is an entirely different process, arising out of a redefinition of lead poisoning. In the late 1970s a study of the general population conducted in the state of Massachusetts revealed a negative statistical association between levels of lead observed in children's teeth, on the one hand, and various cognitive functions, on the other. This was the start of a series of studies conducted in different countries which established that, even at very low levels of saturnine impregnation, when the children concerned did not present any symptom or sign of disease, there was a statistical risk of reduced IQ, poorer test performance, lower school results, and attention deficit observed by teachers.[11] Pediatricians had already reduced the maximum permissible blood lead level from 350 to 250 μg/l a few years earlier. On the basis of these epidemiological studies, the internationally accepted threshold was then set at 100 μg/l. It is arithmetically self-evident that the lower the threshold, the higher the number of children whose blood lead level is considered excessive. The high figure given by the expert committee's report is largely a consequence of the modification of this threshold. But this modification has considerable effects on the very definition of childhood lead poisoning. In pediatric manuals, it was described as a disease, with its digestive symptoms, neurological complications, radiological signs, its often-difficult diagnosis, its sometimes-gloomy prognosis, and its disputed treatment using chelating agents. In the epidemiological literature, it now appeared in the form of the probability of IQ points lost, higher average scores on mood evaluation scales, higher school absence rates, more frequently reported inappropriate behavior in class. Some, admittedly controversial, studies even identified a statistical association between lead poisoning in childhood and deviant acts in adolescence, which was explained in terms of aggressive tendencies that were alleged to result from damaged neuronal function; this led some in the United States to attribute the high level of delinquency and criminality observed among poor families to the presence of lead in their environment.[12] But is this still the domain of pathology? Is the problem now not more social than medical? However that may be, a second process was emerging: the invention of a new reality that was no longer within the clinical field, but related rather to what is known as biostatistics, or, perhaps more correctly in this case, sociostatistics. No longer a disease diagnosed by pediatricians, but a problem identified by epidemiologists.

It is thus this twofold process of discovery, revealing hitherto unrecognized cases, and invention, redefining the nature of the problem itself, that explains the rise from ten to 85,500 affected by childhood lead poisoning in little over a decade. But these 85,500 children cited by the epidemiological approach substantially differ from the ten treated by medicine. They have in fact nothing in common in terms of pathological manifestations and prognosis. The most remarkable paradox of this development is that the more the number of children presenting with high blood lead levels rose, the more the number suffering from lead poisoning disease fell. While at the beginning of the twenty-first century the former numbered several tens of thousands, the latter had practically disappeared from hospitals. It would be tempting to say that pediatricians are now justified in asserting that childhood lead poisoning is a rare disease, at the very moment when experts state, on the contrary, that it is a priority issue. In fact, the development of a national monitoring system has made it possible both to identify many more children with high blood lead levels than before, and moreover much earlier, and in principle at least to remove them from their harmful environment. In short, and curiously, there are many more cases, and far fewer sick children. And it is now no longer children who are being treated, but housing. This dissociation between cases and patients demonstrates the work that has been done by public health. This work comprises both the extension of the domain of childhood lead poisoning, via the dual process of discovery and invention, and the management of the problem, through identification of children exposed and intervention in housing. A combined transformation, then, of knowledge and practices.

But for there to be work, there have to be workers. This is where the testimony of those involved is particularly interesting. In the collective memory of health professionals, everything began in August 1985 when the 2-year-old daughter of a Malian couple was admitted to a Paris hospital, this time with chronic anemia, retarded growth, and abdominal pain. Until that point the rare cases of childhood lead poisoning seen by pediatricians in France had been treated medically. Then, when children had recovered, they would return home with their parents, who would be advised not to let the child eat paint flakes, and would be seen a few months later to confirm that they continued to improve. No one seemed to be concerned that returning home implied more exposure to lead. The clinical case would be, as it were, closed without any social follow-up. Sometimes later appointments revealed renewed contamination, or new pathologies among brothers and sisters, without any preventative measures being taken, which could lead to grave consequences. But in the case of the little Malian girl, things turned out differently.

The young pediatrician, who had worked in sub-Saharan Africa, knew that iron-deficiency anemia can be caused by geophagy, a habit that involves ingesting soil and, by extension, mineral substances – a habit that is frequent in children from this part of the world. She therefore questioned the parents, who stated they had noticed that their little girl was eating paint flakes. To the surprise of the medical team, a blood lead-level test then confirmed the diagnosis of lead poisoning. But this time the pediatrician was not satisfied with medical treatment alone: convinced that dilapidated housing was the cause, she asked for a housing inspection. Unusually for hospital practice, the social worker asked for and obtained authorization to visit the parents, in the 11th arrondissement of Paris. Once there, she discovered a scene she would never have imagined in the heart of the capital: in the inner courtyard of a crumbling apartment complex, a first building where the walls were supported by shaky beams and the floor of the second story had partially collapsed, then a second, smaller building in an equally disturbing state of disrepair. Several African families were living in this squat, with young children among whom new cases of lead poisoning were discovered. The social worker contacted the district's mother and child protection unit, asking them to take over aftercare of the children and rehousing the residents of this slum. However, the physician at the clinic was initially reluctant: she was unaware of this pathology and thought it was unlikely that housing played a role. But when she was told of other cases in a block close to the first, she became interested, though she thought that the source of contamination was probably the tap water. At the time, only lead poisoning from contaminated water was taught in medical schools.[13] Even the teams at the City of Paris Health Laboratory who had been called in were circumspect: childhood lead poisoning did not form part of their body of knowledge, less so paint toxicity. The disease was seen as a curiosity, and lead in buildings had disappeared, it was thought, when lead white was banned. It would be several years before the seriousness of the problem and the role played by housing were recognized. But a link had been established between the worlds of the clinical medicine and public health, thanks to the intuition of a hospital pediatrician and the perseverance of a social worker.

Epidemiological studies were undertaken. Their methods were basic, but their results were conclusive. The two studies mentioned above, of the fifty-two members of families in the first squat identified and the eighty-two children seen at the mother and child clinic, correspond to what is called descriptive epidemiology. Other studies sought to identify the source of the lead poisoning, for example by comparing forty children seen at the mother and child clinic and living in unhealthy conditions with forty children seen for health checks who were deemed to represent the general child population. This study showed that only the former presented high blood lead levels, and it corresponds to what is designated as analytical epidemiology. But in both cases, this is a quite rudimentary form of epidemiology given that, at the same time in the United States and Australia, studies of several thousand subjects were being conducted using sophisticated tests and statistical regressions that made it possible to take into account each of the variables under consideration.

Be that as it may, it might be imagined, in view of the French studies, that the growing number of contaminated children being identified through efficient screening by childcare workers and social workers, and the increasingly evident link with old paint found in samples taken in housing, would be enough to prove that they were dealing with a worrying situation with a well-understood mechanism. There would be all the more reason to think so because there was then a substantial body of scientific literature in English, dating back to the early twentieth century but rapidly growing at that time, thanks to a renewed interest in childhood lead poisoning when it was shown that lead was toxic at levels much lower than had been imagined, and to the proliferation of preventative initiatives.[14] Such was not the case.

There were indeed many levels of resistance, on the part of both municipal authorities and medical bodies. On one side, the City of Paris housing directorate faced a shortage of social housing in the capital. Rehousing families was especially difficult, first, because it was the public lessors who made the final decision, and, second, because these were immigrant families who were subject to diversity quotas – which no one dared to call ethno-racial diversity – that could not be exceeded. There was little interest in restoring the dilapidated housing, both because it was thought that refurbishing and repainting it was a matter for tenants or landlords, since it was private property, and because such an initiative would involve substantial budgets which, in a context of growing xenophobia, the city's elected officials were not inclined to devote to foreigners, especially from African countries. In this situation, the municipal authorities attempted to downplay the importance of the problem and contest the reality of the source, in order to avoid Paris being associated with an image of unhealthiness, and their intervention arousing hostile reactions among their electorate. On the other side, the General Directorate of Health showed a mixture of incredulity, faced with this alleged epidemic of an unknown disease, and condescension with regard to the local practitioners who had sounded the alarm but had little scientific legitimacy. Lead poisoning, and the islands of dilapidated housing inhabited by poverty-stricken communities, seemed like a vestige of the nineteenth century, at a time when the health authorities were beginning to have to deal with emerging diseases that were of much greater concern to public opinion, primary among them AIDS. As for the High Committee on Public Health, the body responsible for analysis and recommendations, its environment committee was chaired by a toxicologist with links to the paint industry, who was the first listed author of an article asserting that cases of childhood lead poisoning were rare and observed only among children of African families, suggesting their way of life as the culprit. The denial of the toxicity of lead paint by the industry and its lobbyists might seem surprising, given that these paints were banned in 1948; four decades later, revealing the risk should not have affected this sector of the economy. In reality, however, the sale and use of lead-based paints continued long after the 1948 regulation, which only concerned professionals, at least until 1993 when they were completely and definitively banned. In other words, for forty-five years the recognized toxicity of these paints, which had led to them being banned for professional decorators, had not resulted in any measure governing non-professional use.

The combined efforts of a range of actors, from both the academic world and the voluntary sector, were therefore required to finally overcome these resistances. The Department of Public Health at the Bichat Faculty of Medicine worked in collaboration with the mother and child clinic to organize screening that resulted, in 1990, in the identification of the 1,500 cases cited above: the epidemic of lead poisoning was now indisputable. Members of two nongovernmental organizations, Médecins sans frontières (Doctors Without Borders) and Migrations santé (Migration and Health) took a research trip to the United States to study policies for combating childhood lead poisoning. On their return, also in 1990, they organized workshops at which researchers from North America spoke about their experience of prevention. The responsibility of paint was finally recognized.[15] Over the subsequent period, a national program was introduced and, eight years later, the law against exclusion was passed, with one section devoted to combating childhood lead poisoning.

After decades of ignorance or negligence, and despite the resistance of public authorities and industry, it thus took only a few years for the rare disease responsible for serious and sometimes lethal neurological manifestations to become a national public health priority concerning tens of thousands of children at risk of learning problems and behavioral disorders. What changed during these years was the way lead poisoning is viewed, just as the way disorders of the nervous system were viewed changed from the mid-eighteenth to the early nineteenth century, as Foucault suggests in his arresting preface to *The Birth of the Clinic*.[16] It is this shift of gaze that leads me in my turn to speak of the birth of public health on a more modest scale. Indeed, this is not a birth in the sense of the origin of the discipline, but a birth around a specific problem that is particularly illuminating. What it offers is a possibility to understand on the basis of a simple subject – the impregnation of the body with a heavy metal – the transmutation of a clinical medicine gaze into a public health gaze. A transmutation that operates a shift from diagnostic reasoning to probabilistic rationality, from individual to population, from biology to epidemiology, from the curative to the preventative, from treatment of patients to treatment of buildings. A transmutation that creates a new entity, derived from a risk of cognitive and behavioral disorders that can only by identified by statistical regression tests that control for socioeconomic variables. A transmutation that involves the efforts of a range of actors, pediatricians, toxicologists, environmental health specialists, childcare workers, social workers, health administrators, city planners, university professors, humanitarian workers, and human rights activists. A transmutation, finally, that brings into play opposing social forces of all kinds – political forces for whom the problem is posed in terms of budgeting, image, and electorate, bureaucratic forces whose routines and certainties are shaken up, economic forces that see their interests threatened. A transmutation, then, that calls for a new language, new methods, new mechanisms, new agents, new stakes.

Is this history of childhood lead poisoning particular to France? Until the 1980s its protagonists thought so. All the scientific publications emphasized that, unlike the United States, where lead represented a serious problem for children, France was fortunately not faced with a major challenge. No pediatrician wondered whether unhealthy housing in France might not be responsible for the same kind of contamination as unhealthy housing in the United States, despite the fact that lead-based paint had been equally widely used until not long before. Yet there was much to be learned from the experience of the United States, and the French experience proved to be an astonishing rerun of it several decades later.[17] In the United States too, with the exception of the city of Baltimore which had developed a screening and prevention program as early as 1931, childhood lead poisoning had long remained for physicians an acute encephalopathy encountered in its late stages in the hospital.[18] It was only in the 1960s that things began to change. First, it was realized that the gravity of the cases observed in pediatrics was due to the fact that the pathological threshold was set too high (it had been set at 600 or even 800 μg/l, twelve to sixteen times the level today) and that diagnosis was too passive (screening was therefore initiated). Then, reducing the threshold to 400 μg/l resulted in the discovery of a large number of cases through surveys of millions of children, and helped to establish the link with paint in dilapidated housing. But thinking still remained in the framework of disease. It was only when the harmful effects of lead at levels as low as 100 μg/l were revealed that the focus shifted from symptom to risk, and from curative practices to preventative programs. Complex protocols had been necessary to demonstrate these effects, in order to show not only that social environment was not sufficient to explain poorer educational performance in contaminated children, but also to refute the argument that behavioral disorders were the reason children in poor households ingested paint flakes. Nevertheless, in parallel with this evolution in the understanding of childhood lead poisoning, resistance was being organized, on the part of both the authorities in the cities concerned, who took a dim view of a costly urban restoration that would primarily benefit poor Black families, and the lead industry with its offshoots in the paint, furniture, toy, and automotive sectors, which were threatened by any prohibitive regulation. The former minimized the seriousness of the problem, the latter the toxicity of the metal.[19] For French pediatricians, the history of the disease in the United States ought to have been replete with lessons in many respects, and spared them digressions and delay in addressing it.

One point in particular would have merited their full attention. In the United States, childhood lead poisoning, especially in its most serious forms, mainly affected Black populations. This was also the case in France. In the French pediatric journals, the rare cases reported all concerned children of African origin, but this point was never taken up. In the epidemiological studies, almost all the children identified in clinics had two African parents, and this too prompted little remark. Yet it is hard to imagine that, in both cases, the fact went unnoticed. In a major survey of nearly 2,000 children seen in the late 1980s at Paris mother and child clinics, 99 percent of those presenting serious lead poisoning were of African origin, 85 percent of them from sub-Saharan Africa.[20] But in order to explain this considerable disproportion, physicians pointed to selection bias for, they explained, the public clinics where most of the cases were detected were often used by families of African origin. Yet their study showed that in the control group of children from the mother and child clinic, those of sub-Saharan African origin represented only a quarter of the consultations. In other words, there were proportionately three times more of them among the children with lead poisoning. In addition to this erroneous interpretation, which was openly put forward, there was another that remained unspoken. Acknowledging that the children suffering from childhood lead poisoning were mainly of sub-Saharan African origin would risk stigmatizing them, and calling them Black would obviously mean racializing them. Indeed, French society is particularly sensitive, not to say hostile, to any reference to race, or even more generally to anything that can lead to differentiating people on the basis of their origin.[21] This has been the case since the late nineteenth century, and even though distinctions have continued to be recreated since then by research and by governments – on the basis of legal status in the colonial period, of religion under the Vichy regime, and subsequently of naturalization – for a long time these disparities did not prompt people to question whether the principle of the supposed equality of all was genuinely being applied. Until the mid-1990s discrimination was barely discussed in France, as if the problem did not exist, and when it was spoken of it was never described as racial, which led to obscuring its reality.[22] Those who proposed evaluating racial discrimination were even accused of helping to establish the idea that races exist in the minds of French people. The inverse effect of this accusation was to deny the existence of racial discrimination, to the point where mentioning it in relation to an institution known by everyone to practice it – the police – exposed one to the risk of being prosecuted for defamation.[23] Thus, the fact that almost all the children contaminated with lead were Black and of African origin remained for a long time, among physicians and experts, a public secret.

This overrepresentation nevertheless continued to intrigue researchers. Some saw it simply as a manifestation of the inequality to which these children were subject, asserting that it was not because they were of sub-Saharan origin that they were contaminated, but because they belonged to the working class, without acknowledging the massive overrepresentation of African families in this disadvantaged section of society. It was all about class, not race. Alongside this neo-Marxist reading, culturalist interpretations also developed. Many found these particularly satisfactory because they drew on a well-worn stock of exotic representations and shifted blame for the contamination to the families. This can be described as practical culturalism, a very common way of thinking when individuals' behavior is being interpreted on the basis of their alterity. It has two main characteristics.[24] First, it essentializes culture, presuming that it can be identified as a set of beliefs and characteristics that constitute the unity of a group defined on a genealogical or territorial basis – whereas in reality each individual locates himself or herself in relation to a multiplicity of cultural references that vary with context. Second, it makes culture the ultimate explanation, a way of accounting for a set of facts that pose a problem. Such culturalism dismisses other more plausible interpretations, external to individuals and their cultural attributes. Thus, this practical culturalism is a defensive ideology often used by public health agents when they need to account for the failure of programs in societies or groups with which they are not familiar. In the case of childhood lead poisoning, it became the dominant mode of analysis of the epidemic for approximately a decade. This history was divided into two phases. To begin with, culturalist explanations contributed to denying the part played by paints. Subsequently, they recognized this source, but gave a strictly culturalist reading of it.

The denial, by local housing authorities and national health authorities, was initially based on allegations of idiosyncratic practices. A rumor that a number of the fathers of contaminated children were traditional healers or practicing Muslims led some in the municipal and ministerial corridors to talk of "marabout's disease" in reference to the name of religious healers in popular Islam. It was suggested that the ink used to write on Qur'anic tablets might be the cause, because, once the suras have been transcribed, the ink that has been used is diluted in water and given to an individual in need of protection to drink. But tests on the suspected ink were inconclusive. It was then thought that the kohl women used as make-up contained the harmful metal. Here again, test results eliminated this as a possible source of contamination. A more realistic hypothesis focused on the utensils in which food was prepared, since it was known that the glaze of traditional pottery often contains lead and it was supposed that African women were cooking their food in these receptacles. But it was discovered that, much more prosaically, they used cheap aluminum cooking pots. The facts had to be faced. The lead was not coming from products or objects associated with unusual practices. The source was indeed the old house paint in poor condition in which very high concentrations of lead were found. But why then, people wondered, were only African children exposed to this source in such large numbers?

Attempts were then made to account for what was described as a particular craving these children had for paint flakes. Researchers had long since described a cultural practice known as geophagy, apparently common in a number of traditional societies, sometimes as a way of controlling hunger, and sometimes for the taste. Physicians had reported various cases of a psychological disorder known as pica, from the Latin name for the magpie, characterized by the consumption of substances not normally considered edible such as paper, plastic, and particularly soil. Although geophagy is seen as a cultural practice and pica as a pathological behavior, the distinction between the two is not self-evident; moreover, among children aged between six months and two years, whose tendency to put anything their hands encounter into their mouth is considered normal, neither can be assumed. But since African children were affected, the two interpretations appeared obvious: pediatricians often mentioned pica in their observations, while public health agents favored the possibility of geophagy. A psychological reading of geophagy also led them to wonder whether, lacking stimulation and supervision from their parents, these children, left to themselves, were abnormally intensifying these common but harmful behaviors, and thus developing a form of pica, blurring a little more the boundary between the two interpretations.

In order to better understand this phenomenon, the public authorities called on two specialists in ethnomedicine, who conducted a survey of ten Malian families living mostly in the same insanitary squat in Paris, each with at least one child with excessive blood lead levels, and eventually turned to "sociocultural factors." They pointed out that geophagy is an ancestral practice in West Africa, particularly among women and above all when they are pregnant. They suck clay or kaolin, which are both reputed to have therapeutic and nutritional benefits, and even sometimes give it to their nursing infant to hasten weaning. These practices were supposedly resumed when these mothers were transplanted to France, with paint flakes substituting for traditional substances among the children. Consequently, the researchers wrote, "the active consumption of fragments of wall coatings in the Paris region should be associated with indigenous norms of geophagy as an acceptable practice," affirming that, among African women, "there is a very particular tolerance of a child sucking on fragments of wall coatings."[25] This explanation immediately persuaded some hospital pediatricians, who found it satisfactory in view of their exotic conceptions of African societies, and particularly some public officials, for whom it represented a new way of blaming the disease on the families. To be sure, dilapidated apartment blocks exposed children living there to lead, but educating mothers could offer an inexpensive alternative to rehousing the families or refurbishing the apartments. One official went so far as to state at a meeting that even if the walls were replastered the children would scratch them so that they could eat the paint behind the plaster. Some local authorities implemented this kind of alternative solution, teaching women to cut their children's nails and wash their hands, to take them to the city's parks, and to do their housework with a wet mop.

However, for those who had resolutely committed to the fight against childhood lead poisoning, this analysis was unacceptable. First, for logical reasons: how was it that those primarily affected in the United States were African American communities, many of whom had lived there for more than ten generations, while in the United Kingdom they were Caribbean and South Asian communities whose culture was obviously different from that of Malian and Senegalese women in France, all of them nevertheless sharing the same poor housing conditions? Second, for political reasons: how could the cultural argument be used to evade local and national authorities' responsibilities toward the children of immigrant families contaminated by lead? As it happened, new research had shown that lead poisoning in children was due as much to passive inhalation of dust from peeling walls as it was to active ingestion of paint flakes. There was therefore no longer any call for talk of geophagy or pica. The problem lay not with the behavior of children but with the disrepair of housing. The campaigning work of these public health activists, supported by not-for-profit organizations and academics, eventually won out over the culturalist argument. Indeed, a few years later several of them held senior administrative posts in the ministries of health and housing, and were then involved in drawing up the chapter on childhood lead poisoning in the law against exclusion that was passed in 1998.

Once the culturalist explanation had been ruled out, the question remained of why children from sub-Saharan Africa were so disproportionately the face of childhood lead poisoning in France. It is tempting to suggest that the reason for their considerable overrepresentation in lead poisoning, particularly its more serious forms, was due simply to the considerable overrepresentation of their families in the most dilapidated urban housing. In order to account for this situation, it is necessary to look at the history of immigration policy and housing policy over the past fifty years. On the one hand, after several decades of recruiting labor from the African continent to help rebuild the French economy, the shutdown of labor immigration in the mid-1970s, the tightening of rules on reuniting families ten years later, and finally the generalization of restrictive practices with regard to all migrants, including asylum seekers, led to an increase in the number of undocumented foreigners from the global South. This was particularly because residence permits were less frequently being renewed, even for those who had long been settled in France. In the final decades of the twentieth century, the most vulnerable sector of the immigrant population, whether or not they held valid documents, therefore consisted of people from sub-Saharan Africa, mainly West Africa, who had few educational and professional qualifications, in a climate where industry, formerly a major employer especially in the automotive sector, was being restructured. On the other hand, the so-called oil crisis of the 1970s had been accompanied by a rise in unemployment and precarity, to which the immigrant population was highly vulnerable, helping to intensify the concentration of these communities in social housing, since, unlike French people, they were unable to buy their own modest homes. During this period, construction of social housing fell far short of need, and the requirements for ethno-racial diversity imposed by public lessors made access increasingly difficult for African households. All that was left for these families was the lower level of private-sector housing, consisting of apartments in poor condition on dilapidated blocks, squatted or rented by unscrupulous landlords whose practices went virtually unregulated.

It is, then, the combination of restrictive immigration policy and selective social housing policy, exacerbated by discriminatory employment practices that were only belatedly subjected to scrutiny, that explains the confinement of African families in substandard housing and hence the exposure of their children to contamination with lead. The culturalist reading therefore needs to be replaced by a political economy of childhood lead poisoning, weaving together both the colonial genealogy of France, since the immigrant populations who were first recruited to contribute to the national effort of postwar reconstruction, and then rejected and marginalized, almost all came from former French colonies, and the country's ethno-racial ecology, which reveals the socio-spatial distribution of minorities of African origin.[26] This colonial past and this ethno-racial distribution are among the most hidden and most contentious subjects in France, in public spaces and even in scientific circles. By ignoring them, one condemns oneself to not addressing its most severe consequences. This explains why childhood lead poisoning was so difficult to recognize, and why, once it had been recognized, it was so difficult to interpret: blindness to the matter accounts for the silence and, in the end, the apathy.

But this political economy gives only a partial picture of the question if we fail to take into account what could be called the moral economy of childhood lead poisoning – in other words, the production, circulation, and appropriation of affects and values around this problem.[27] For as those involved in the fight against childhood lead poisoning immediately noted when they discovered the places in which the majority of the families concerned were living, the problem could not be limited to the existence of a disease that had to be prevented, however serious it was. What was at stake were the appalling conditions to which the most economically and legally vulnerable immigrant families were reduced. Until this epidemiological situation was revealed, indifference had been the rule and the apparent ignorance of the public authorities resulted from a wish not to know, as their subsequent efforts to deny or minimize the problem once they had been alerted to it testify. It is therefore remarkable that the exposure of a public health problem was the impetus for the hitherto unthinkable recognition of a social reality that was intolerable, and yet tolerated. We may hypothesize that it was the suffering of bodies, rather than the infringement of dignity, particularly when young children were concerned, that triggered the reaction. It was possible to be blind to the flouting of the basic rights of immigrant men and women abandoned in degrading conditions, but the sickness of their children, seen as innocent victims, was finally enough to arouse a feeling of compassion and a demand for justice. Thus, public health became the final vector for the expression of affect and the defense of values, both of which had become difficult to express and defend in relation to groups that were regarded as both undesirable and illegitimate. The fight against childhood lead poisoning can thus be seen as the illustration of a more general phenomenon I have analyzed through other case studies.[28] And indeed, this language of the suffering body and of life under threat is tending to become the most socially audible and politically acceptable way of talking about inequality. While it is deaf to the indignity of the most vulnerable sectors of the immigrant population, both in housing and in other areas of their lives, society can still be moved by and react to their physical ordeals, especially when children are involved. The history of childhood lead poisoning thus reveals a moral economy in which biological life prevails over other forms of life – those forms whereby the person is recognized as such.

At the end of this journey, analysis of the birth of public health, or more precisely of the birth of a public health problem, reveals two sides of the phenomenon, which can be termed social construction and social production. On the one hand, I have shown that it was the reformulation of the definition of childhood lead poisoning, shifting from a disease to a risk, the modification of the blood lead level threshold to take account of the new epidemiological reality, the mobilization of individuals, professions, methods, and discourses to raise the awareness of the public authorities, and the rejection of culturalist hypotheses, replacing them with a political economy and a moral economy, that led to this problem becoming a public health priority: this, then, was construction by social agents. On the other hand, I have made clear how the reason why childhood lead poisoning not only existed, but also disproportionately affected children originating from the African continent, derived from the combined effects of immigration, housing, and employment policies. The first position takes a constructivist approach; the second is a specific type of realist approach. Both are critical, since the first shows that a public health problem does not exist per se, but has to be constructed in order to be grasped as such, while the second shows that a public health problem is not simply a matter of nature and biology, but results from human actions, power relations, the play of forces, and value systems. Both interpretations are necessary to the understanding of a problem. To speak only of social construction is to risk derealizing it and ignoring its seriousness. To speak only of social production is to risk ignoring the way it has come to be recognized in the form in which it is known. Through the following lectures, I shall show that these two concepts of social construction and social production are essential, and that the case of childhood lead poisoning is indeed paradigmatic in this respect.

The Truth in Numbers
5 May 2021

*A threshold disappears. – The regime of veridiction of numbers. – The encounter
between statistics and probabilities. – A working definition of positivism. – The
advent of analytical social sciences. – Evidence-based public health. – The empire
of biostatistics. – Three pitfalls of randomized trials and their implications. – The
worm wars. – Lessons of a dispute between economists and epidemiologists.
– Quantification as narrative. – Manipulation of maternal mortality data. –
Statistical cacophony around deaths linked to a heatwave. – Controversial
interpretation of the causes of death at the end of apartheid. – Positivism beaten
at its own game.*

We have seen how, in only twelve years, the approach to childhood
lead poisoning in France evolved from a situation where, in 1987,
pediatricians in university hospitals asserted that it was a rare disease
with only ten known published cases in twenty-five years, to one where,
in 1999, experts from the National Institute for Health and Medical
Research (Inserm) estimated the number of children affected to be
85,500. Yet the spectacular inflation of this pathology, which led some
to speak of a silent epidemic, was not due to an environmental accident
causing mass lead contamination. It reflected a change of perspective
on the problem, which had led to a shift from a clinical medicine
approach to a public health approach, from an interpretation of symptoms to a calculation of risk, from diagnostic reasoning to statistical
rationality. By seeing this pathology no longer from the point of view
of a semiology based on a set of neurological manifestations ending in
coma and death but in terms of the probability of reduced IQ scores,
declining educational achievement, and an increase in the prevalence
of attentional disorders, one signaled the need to reduce the threshold
above which the level of lead in the blood was considered toxic. Thus,
the blood lead level considered safe fell within a few years from 350

to 100 μg/l and even, a little later, to 50 μg/l; by simple arithmetic, the estimated number of children contaminated was increased by all those whose levels lay between these two values. In other words, the shift in gaze brought with it a change in the threshold and an increase in cases that made it possible to assert that there was a serious situation justifying urgent measures to deal with it. The requantification of the problem led to a requalification of it, but the reverse was also true. Recognition of the silent epidemic of childhood lead poisoning is therefore not only a question of gaze, but also a matter of numbers.

However, numbers are more than just a matter of threshold. They were also involved before and after the epidemic was recognized. Before, in descriptive epidemiology studies that measured the intensity of the phenomenon in dilapidated buildings, in analytical epidemiology studies that identified the source by comparing children who were and were not exposed to old paint in crumbling housing, and above all in the large surveys where statistical regression calculations demonstrated the effect of even low concentrations of lead in the blood on cognitive function and deviant behavior, independent of social background. And afterwards, in the enumeration of dwellings in disrepair, the financial estimate of the cost of preventative intervention strategies and, later, the evaluation of the impact of the different measures implemented. Figures are therefore omnipresent, whether in the form of thresholds, numbers, frequencies, probabilities, or statistical tests, and they have decisive importance in both the definition of the problem and the modes of response. Yet these numbers do not always remain stable over time. Thresholds of acceptable blood lead levels fall; numbers of children affected rise; frequencies vary; probabilities are debated, especially around cognitive and behavioral disorders whose link with blood lead levels is questioned; and statistical tests are contested, particularly when they are considered weak because the low number of subjects leads people to assert, perhaps incorrectly, that the groups compared are not different and therefore to conclude, in some studies, that no lead toxicity is present.

On this point, the most recent and perhaps the most radical critique questions the very existence of a safe blood lead level. At a meeting organized by the French General Directorate of Health, the expert invited to give the plenary address concluded with the astonishing statement: "One point remains to be resolved: that of the threshold."[1] In fact, studies had shown that even at levels below 100 μg/l, or now 50 μg/l, blood lead level remains statistically correlated with IQ. There is therefore no longer any normal or safe level of saturnine impregnation. Any presence of lead in the blood is harmful, at least in children.

But lead will always be present in the air, water, soil, and food, and it is no more possible to eliminate lead in the blood than in the environment. All that can be hoped for is to reduce it, which has been done primarily through the ban on leaded gasoline. The threshold of 50 $\mu g/l$ set in 2015 merely corresponds to the standard value above which it must be declared. This final twist in the history of childhood lead poisoning consequently ends with the rejection of the idea of a toxicity threshold and even of numbers of children contaminated, since any presence of lead in the blood carries risks. For all that, numbers have not disappeared from the new epidemiological landscape. It is simply that the understanding is now in terms of a continuous rather than a discrete variable, a risk gradient rather than a probability of occurrence.

So, what do they say, these figures that describe childhood lead poisoning first as a rare disease, then as a widespread pathology; at one point defined by a limit, at another represented by a curve? As Judith Rainhorn notes in her history of white lead in the late nineteenth century: "Rather than the name, it was the numbers that were invested with the task of depicting 'reality' and translating the epidemic into aggregate cases."[2] This symbolic power of numbers, and their capacity to claim to depict reality, are all the more remarkable given that now as in the past they are both assertive and inconsistent, peremptory and flexible. If we may venture this parallel, the authority of numbers is like the authority of economic knowledge: invalidation or falsification of their statements in no way undermines their assurance that they are telling the truth and their faculty of persuasion. It is therefore this truth in numbers, or, more precisely, to use a concept dear to Michel Foucault, their "regimes of veridiction" – in other words the different ways they have of telling, or claiming to tell, the truth, and therefore excluding doubt and uncertainty – that I wish to discuss.[3] But I am interested in these regimes of veridiction less as "truth games" as such, in Foucault's words, than for the cognitive and above all political and moral stakes they reveal. My discussion of them will be in two parts, first analyzing the origin of some contemporary developments of positivism in public health, and then considering three case studies that I conducted on three different continents.

Let us begin, then, with a brief detour into history. It is generally recognized that it was in the nineteenth century that the science and politics of numbers were imposed as modes of knowledge and action. Analyzing how numbers govern the facts of the contemporary world, Ian Hacking observes that statistics about "sport, sex, drink, drugs, travel, sleep," and probabilities of "meltdowns, cancers, muggings, earthquakes, nuclear winters, AIDS, global greenhouses," all of this numerical apparatus, and, he goes as far as to say, this "obsession" with evaluation by counting, "descend from the forgotten annals of nineteenth-century information control."[4] He even states: "only around 1840 did the practice of measurement become fully established." He is of course aware that statistics and probability first emerged in the seventeenth century, and were then consolidated through the eighteenth century. The German statistics codified by Hermann Conring and institutionalized by August Ludwig von Schlözer produced a knowledge about territories and their inhabitants that claimed to be exhaustive, for the purposes of governing them. At the same time, English political arithmetic, initiated earlier by John Graunt and developed by William Petty, proposed methods of enumerating the population on the basis of birth and death registrations. Pascal in France and Huygens in the Netherlands developed techniques for calculating mathematical expectations in games of chance, which were later applied in the calculation of life expectancy. But, as Alain Desrosières notes, it was in the nineteenth century that the ostensibly unlikely encounter "between statistics, a set of administrative routines required to describe a state and its population, the calculation of probabilities, a subtle way of guiding choices in situations of uncertainty, and estimates of physical and astronomical constants based on disparate physical observations" occurred.[5] This encounter between administrators, mathematicians, and physicists generated the possibility of "creating entities that could be used as a basis for describing the world and acting upon it." And these quantifiable entities "could be said to be both real and constructed"; in other words, they referred to objects that were certainly present in the world but were derived from choices involving categorization, assignment, projection, and evaluation. Thus, the same combination of difference and complementarity between the realist and the constructivist perspectives that I described in relation to childhood lead poisoning is to be found around statistics and probability.

According to Hacking, the nineteenth century thus produced both "statistical laws" thanks to which it was now possible to decipher human behaviors and social facts, and "the imperialism of probabilities" that forms the basis for predicting risk for the individual, society, and even the entire planet. As he points out, the emergence of this belief in the virtues of numbers is concomitant with the appearance of Auguste Comte's positivism. He emphasizes, however, that Comte held that "statistical regularities collected by the number fetishists were contemptible" and that "the mathematics of the probabilists were 'childish speculations and erroneous principles'."[6] In other words, the intellectual association generally made today between quantification and positivism was not relevant for the founder of the doctrine. The link between the two arises out of their initial synchrony, but the fact that they were contemporaneous does not mean they should be identified with one another. The statistical laws that distribute individuals within a society on the basis of particular characteristics have nothing to do with the historical laws that govern social progress, according to an evolutionist paradigm. In fact, although he coined the term "positivism," Comte is not the best guide to grasping its meaning as it is understood today. On the one hand, the term often carries a negative and polemical connotation: few of those described as positivists would present themselves as such. On the other, the concept, if it is one, is polysemic and unstable: there are many versions of positivism that do not always have much in common.

Nevertheless, in order to investigate the relation contemporary societies have with questions of quantification, it is important to have a working definition. Fundamentally, positivism rests on the idea that facts in the world are realities external to the observer, who can therefore give an objective and neutral account of them using scientific methods independent of his or her individual position, particularly his or her moral or political position, in the social space. This idea aligns perfectly with the principle of representing the world and facts through numbers, since quantification presupposes the construction of aggregates of objects deemed to be external to the enumerating subject, whether they be deaths or births, people sick or exposed. Furthermore, quantification reinforces positivism, by confirming the regularity of social phenomena and even the regularity of their variations, as Adolphe Quetelet in 1829 and Émile Durkheim in 1897 realized in relation to the annual number of crimes and of suicides respectively: in both cases the consistency in a given place was such that it could be predicted from one year to the next. In philosophy, moreover, the influential logical positivist current, which is sometimes called neopositivism to distinguish it from its Comtian forebear, emphasizes this fundamental link. Thus Bertrand Russell writes that, for logical positivists, "questions of fact can only be decided by the empirical methods of science," and what distinguishes them from earlier empiricists is "the attention to mathematics and logic" that links them to a tradition that emerged with Plato and continued through Spinoza and Leibniz.[7] It is a version of this positivism that operates today in public health.

However, contrary to what might be imagined, this close relationship between positivism and quantification did not evolve over time in a linear fashion that would be supported by progressive refinement of methods, with numbers providing an increasingly accurate representation of the reality of the world. In the history of science, and particularly in the history of social science, it emerges in cycles, with periods of triumphant positivism, laying claim to ever more reliable quantification, alternating, as George Steinmetz has shown, with periods of retreat, when critical epistemologies and qualitative approaches were in the ascendant.[8] At the end of the twentieth century, in the United States and the countries that most mimetically follow its model, as is often the case in Latin America, the social sciences emerged from the poststructuralism and postmodernism of the 1970s and 1980s. The heritage of the latter persists only in marginal but creative enclaves within the humanities such as gender studies, race studies, and postcolonial or decolonial studies, while positivism and quantification have made their comeback through what are known as the analytical social sciences, which, following the model of economics, have taken over political science and a significant part of sociology. The director of the Institute for Quantitative Social Science at Harvard, Gary King, describes the emergence of the new knowledge in these terms: "The social sciences are undergoing a dramatic transformation from studying problems to solving them; from making do with a small number of sparse data sets to analyzing increasing quantities of diverse highly informative data; from isolated scholars toiling away on their own to larger scale, collaborative, interdisciplinary, lab-style research teams; and from a purely academic pursuit focused inward to having a major impact on public policy, commerce and industry, other academic fields, and some of the major problems that affect individuals and societies."[9] Noteworthy in this enthusiastic description is the absence of any reference to the idea of critique, particularly critique of the production of knowledge, in the tradition that runs from Hume and Kant to C. Wright Mills and Bourdieu. In the view of King and many others, what characterizes this so-called analytical revolution is the introduction of big data, the huge volumes of numerical data that digitalization makes it possible to extract from multiple, particularly commercial, sources, and that offer the potential for investigating every domain of social life, including health.

Public health is indeed not impervious to these changes, for at least two reasons. First, its origin, as what was called public hygiene, more or less coincides with that of modern statistics at the beginning of the nineteenth century. The hygiene specialists produced quantified data on a plethora of facts, from "the length of life of the rich man and the poor man" to "the average height of man in the town and the country," from "mortality in prisons" to "the influence of climate on chronic diseases," from "moral hygiene in the Netherlands" to "statistics on

lunatics in Norway," to take only a few examples drawn from articles
in the first two years of the famous *Annales d'hygiène publique et de
médecine légale* in 1829 and 1830.[10] For the first time, multiple aspects
of health and the social were being quantified together, opening the
possibility of not only knowing but also acting. Second, the pre-emi-
nent discipline behind public health was epidemiology, which, having
long been dedicated to detailed qualitative description of infectious
and parasitic diseases, and practiced mainly in the context of tropical
medicine, had changed paradigm completely, becoming an exclusively
quantitative discipline and fully adopting statistics as an application
of the latter in medicine. Whether descriptive (measuring frequencies),
analytical (researching statistical associations or correlations between
risk factors and diseases), predictive (estimating the probability of
occurrence of health events), or evaluative (assessing the results of
an intervention or program), it is a science of numbers.[11] Currently
its central pillar, it is epidemiology that has given public health its
modern status in France, far from outdated prescriptions about "cor-
poreal hygiene" and problematic guidance on "population eugenics"
that continued to be taught until the early 1980s in the great public
hygiene lectures at the School of Medicine, delivered at the Institut des
Cordeliers, where successive generations of doctors have trained.

Yet at the same time a wind of change had begun to blow, under
the influence of the practices of community health, which had come
from Canada, and primary health care, practiced in what was then
called the Third World.[12] These approaches drew on qualitative and
participatory methods, combining different disciplines, among them
social science, and made use of local human resources, including citizens. They aimed to offer a way of thinking and working less centered
on the hospital, restoring a place for patients, integrating the psychological dimension, highlighting disparities in care, and emphasizing
the role of social determinants of health. Their spread was, however,
limited in time and in space, as they were quickly submerged by a wave
of positivism coming mainly from the major research centers of the
United States, such as Harvard and Johns Hopkins. They have not
completely disappeared today, remaining present in some university
departments and some urban communities, in France and especially
in Latin America, but the current that has become dominant since the
early 2000s demands more rigorous administration of evidence in both
the analysis of health phenomena and the evaluation of the benefits of
interventions. This approach is essentially quantitative. The numbers
tell the truth about the seriousness of a problem to be addressed, the
importance of a risk to be controlled, and the efficacy of an interven-

tion, and thus establish hierarchies in the world of knowledge and priorities for action.

Evidence-based medicine, born in the early 1990s out of the concern to replace, in medical decision-making, the intuition and experience of physicians with the critical examination of medical literature, particularly in the context of clinical trials, was imported into public health in the form of evidence-based public health, which operates on the same principles. A paradigmatic example of this approach, the Cochrane Collaboration, an international network named for the Scottish epidemiologist Archie Cochrane, regularly summarizes the reliable knowledge available on treatment of disease and issues recommendations on best practice. It has created a branch, the Cochrane Public Health Group, that offers the same analysis and advice service for population-level interventions.[13] But in this domain, the question is not only whether a proposed measure produces a positive effect, but also what it costs. Evidence-based public health therefore draws not only on epidemiology but also, increasingly, on economics. It no longer talks only of the relative risk of occurrence of a pathology in relation to exposure to a pathogenic factor, but also, for the purpose of comparing various possible interventions, of cost-effectiveness and even cost-benefit analysis, which presupposes that a monetary value can be attached to the reduction in frequency of a disease or the gain in life-years of good health.

In this context, two indicators have become major factors in guiding international bodies' allocation of resources. The QALY, or quality-adjusted life year, assesses the "quality of life," indicating the gain in years of good health resulting from an intervention; it is supposed to help decide which action should be prioritized. The DALY, or disability-adjusted life year, evaluates the "disease burden," expressing the loss of years of good health by adding up those lost owing to premature death and those impaired by disability; it is supposed to help decide which pathology should be priority for action. The QALY, which measures the gain in quality of life, is more used in the countries of the global North, while the DALY, which measures a loss of quantity of life, is more used in the countries of the global South. These variables allow for comparisons between countries, based on the evaluation of different causes of disability to which coefficients are attached. Thus, for any country, the coefficient for migraine is 0.433, that for tuberculosis 0.331, that for autism 0.259, that for impotence 0.019, and that for amputation of a thumb 0.013, with no account taken of the way the experience of disability may vary in different national contexts depending on social environment, the person's job, cultural understandings, or whether there are support structures and anti-discrimination laws.[14] It is thus clear why it is difficult to draw anthropologically valid conclusions from these international comparisons, and how these measures limit appropriate decision-making about how problems are to be ranked and interventions prioritized. Nevertheless, these indicators are part of the statistical arsenal increasingly used by the World Health Organization, the World Bank, and other international organizations in deciding on their programs.

In parallel with this quantification of the health of populations, an experimental model was developed for the purpose of determining the efficacy, often coupled with the cost or benefit, of interventions in the field of health. These experiments were called randomized control trials, or RCTs. The general set-up is simple, the aim being to compare the effects of an action implemented in a population drawn at random either with the previous situation (a before–after comparison) or with the situation observed in a population deemed similar (a here–there comparison). A classic example, conducted by MIT's Abdul Latif Jameel Poverty Action Lab, compared the progress of immunization coverage in three groups of Indian villages. In the first group there was no intervention; in the second, mobile teams of well-trained health workers were sent in each month; in the third, these teams also distributed sacks of lentils and metal dishes. The study showed, unsurprisingly, that the best results were obtained in the last group.[15] These trials, which have proliferated and won international recognition since the 2000s, have become a sort of absolute reference – a "gold standard" in the field of development. Presented as a major innovation in economics, the method won its promoters, Abhijit Banerjee, Esther Duflo, and Michael Kremer, the Sveriges Riksbank Prize in Economics in Memory of Alfred Nobel in 2019.[16] In fact this inquiry method is an adaptation of a technique used in epidemiology since the 1970s, in medicine as early as the late 1940s, and in agriculture since the 1930s. In epidemiology, it has been used among other things to measure the cost-efficiency ratio of a set of care and prevention interventions integrated locally in developing countries, and was decisive in justifying the World Health Organization's introduction of its primary health care policy.[17] Rediscovered by economists at the end of the twentieth century, randomized trials thus have a long and rich history.

Whether they are used in epidemiology or economics, or indeed other disciplines, and whether they consist of measurement tools, such as QALY and DALY, or experimental techniques such as RCTs, the set of procedures and practices involved in quantification of health can all be called biostatistics.[18] The latter has become the dominant and sometimes even hegemonic mode of production of legitimate knowledge about collective health. But this approach raises various types of problems, which are particularly critical in the countries of the global South. First, at the risk of tautology, only that which is quantifiable is quantified. Yet a substantial part of what characterizes public health, and more generally human activity, whether in terms of behaviors, decisions, living conditions, or the success of an action, escapes quantification. Relying only on quantification is to risk finding oneself in the situation of the drunk man in the fable, who searches for the key he lost in the nearby park under a street lamp because it is the only place where there is light, as he explains to the police officer who has come to his aid. This bias, known as the streetlight effect, consists in studying what is easiest to study, and therefore neglecting what is not. Frequently, in discussions following the presentation of a quantitative study, when it is pointed out that an essential aspect has not been taken into account the author will respond that it is indeed the case, but that this particular aspect was not quantifiable. Conversely, the promoters of these techniques readily assert that what cannot be measured, and therefore evaluated quantitatively, is not worth implementing, despite the fact that in development the non-quantifiable processes of training health workers, community participation, and changes in social relations are often more likely to lead to improvement in the long term than the measurable results obtained in the short term. Thus, there are entire swathes of social life about which no knowledge is obtained, and potentially beneficial actions that populations are deprived of. Second, while the translation of a fact into quantitative data may fit in one place, it may not necessarily do so in another, if fit is understood as the correspondence between the fact analyzed and its representation in the form of a number that gives a correct account of it. It is also possible that this fit is not even confirmed in the original study, making it even less probable that it can be in subsequent studies. But even assuming that it is, the quantification of a concept or a practice that may be valid for a West African society is not automatically so for Indian or Mexican societies. Yet this is what is presumed when data produced using the same supposedly universal indicators are compared, or the same recipes resulting from trials deemed unaffected by contexts are applied. Third, quantification often results in limiting the responses to problems with solutions that are apparently simple and strictly technical. This is the very principle of scientific reductionism, which should of course not be challenged as such, but which may become problematic in the conclusions drawn from it and the use made of it. Measuring necessarily presupposes a work of simplification, of which the experts are aware, and results in practical responses that can be useful. But the effect of this operation, which tends to prioritize the simplicity and technicality that often go hand in hand with lower costs, is that complex analyses and structural interventions are discarded. It is easy to see why the international actors in development, who are increasingly rich philanthropists, find merit in these approaches. But it is also easy to understand that the lauded objectivity and neutrality of these approaches are merely apparent, and that, while they deny acting politically, those who promote them are doing precisely that in their own way, by ruling out the most transformative responses and thus restricting the domain of possibilities.

These three problems – bias of neglect, temptation to universalize, and praise for minimalism – have not hampered the success of quantification as a mode of veridiction, in other words, a way of telling the truth via numbers. Quite the reverse – they advance it. The place now accorded to the randomized trials developed by economists offers telling evidence of it.[19] One of the most famous examples in the field of development was the evaluation of the impact of a deworming campaign among schoolchildren in a poor region of Kenya during the 1990s, carried out under a partnership between a Christian humanitarian organization and the local directorate of the Ministry of Health.[20] This campaign, which was based on the administration of a deworming treatment every six months and an anti-bilharzia medication once a year to all schoolchildren in areas with high levels of parasite infestation, was conducted in three stages, making it possible to measure and compare the results between schools that had been treated and those yet to receive treatment. Two renowned economists, Edward Miguel and Michael Kremer, from the universities of Berkeley and Harvard respectively, were thus able to carry out a study comparable to a RCT, funded by the World Bank and a deworming research unit affiliated with Imperial College London. Published in 2004 in one of the most prestigious international economics journals, this study established first that children in treated schools were less infested than children in non-treated schools, but only with respect to two of the four parasites concerned; second, that they reported being less often sick during the previous week, yet without showing objective benefits such as increased body mass or hemoglobin level; and third, that absenteeism from class on a given day had fallen by 5–7 percent, while there was no improvement in school test scores. Despite this limited success in terms of both health tests and educational performance, the authors asserted that deworming offered a definite advantage in terms of cost-efficiency compared to other competing health programs. On the basis of a series of bold hypotheses about treatment externalities, which enabled them to include in their calculations the favorable effects of treatment on children who had not been treated, they optimistically deduced that it cost only 5 dollars per DALY, that is, per life-year with disability, saved. In their view, deworming was therefore a very profitable "investment in human capital," since a treatment costing 49 cents produced a gain of 15.9 dollars per child treated. They concluded that "the large improvement in school participation following deworming estimated in this study points to the important role that tropical diseases such as intestinal worms may play in reducing educational attainment in sub-Saharan Africa and provides microeconomic support for claims that Africa's high tropical disease burden is a causal factor contributing to its low income." A somewhat hyperbolic conclusion, in view of the modest rise in class attendance and the absence of an improvement in school results.

This research was nevertheless an immediate hit with development agencies, for reasons that are easily understood if the message was that a year of life in good health could be gained for only 5 dollars. The US organization GiveWell, which undertakes to evaluate the cost-efficiency of NGO programs in order to help private donors choose which ones to donate to, placed deworming on its list of top charities, stating on its website that "it offers donors an exceptional opportunity to do good with their donations."[21] At the time, deworming was booming in poor countries worldwide, under the impetus of the World Health Organization. But the study of Kenyan schools puzzled epidemiologists. A number of them decided to verify its results. Their analyses were published in a major international epidemiological journal. Their method was to take the data from the initial study, on the one hand, reproducing the original procedure but correcting coding errors and redoing the calculations, and, on the other hand, proposing a different statistical strategy that seemed more appropriate. In both cases, the benefits in terms of education, which formed the basis for the proclaimed importance of deworming for economic development in Africa, were not more significant and even became contestable owing to serious biases.[22] While Miguel and Kremer acknowledged some of their errors, they maintained their conclusions. There followed what have been ironically termed the "worm wars," with new randomized trials conducted by other economists, which confirmed their colleagues' results, and meta-analyses carried out by epidemiologists, from which some studies had to be excluded owing to lack of rigor. In the end, both sides stuck to their guns, dividing the worlds of science and of development into two camps, for or against the evidence for the benefits of deworming. On one side the Cochrane Library, an independent scientific body that produces peer-reviewed reports on current validated knowledge in medicine and public health, asserted that there was "now substantial evidence that this does not improve average nutritional state, hemoglobin level, cognition, school performance and survival." On the other, GiveWell, a private moral authority that classifies charitable organizations in support of effica- cious altruism, acknowledged these meta-analyses but criticized them for eliminating studies that showed favorable results on the grounds of methodological flaws, asserting that "these do not change our overall assessment of the evidence on deworming."[23] Two lessons are to be drawn from this war without victors.

First, from the perspective of the sociology of science, there is the clash between economists and epidemiologists. There are two aspects to this conflict. One, which can be described as external – relating to the field of social sciences – concerns the imperialism of economists, who have penetrated every domain of knowledge, from history to anthropology, from psychology to criminology, building on the ideal- ism of their neoclassical theory and the power of their quantitative tool.[24] This drive to take over irritates more than it persuades special- ists in these disciplines, who often see this approach as a simplifica- tion that fails to grasp the complex phenomena they are dealing with. Epidemiologists, who in their turn encountered the presence of econo- mists in their field, have the advantage of also having sophisticated statistical techniques at their disposal, without the need for a unifying theoretical model. The other aspect of this conflict is internal – relating to the so-called black box – and results precisely from this singularity.[25] It touches on the matter of science itself, and clearly in the worm wars epidemiologists were better methodologically armed to take on these complex questions than economists, who acknowledged their errors even though they were not willing to withdraw their conclusions. An opportune reminder that there is never anything lost by delving into the detail of data analysis.

Second, from the point of view of the anthropology of development, the three problems I identified earlier arise once again. The bias of neglect leads the authors to restrict their study to a minor but quantifi- able aspect while ignoring practices that have more impact in terms of both health and education. The temptation of universalization leads them to extend the conclusions of one study of seventy-five villages to an entire continent, and even to all poor countries. The praise for minimalism translates into promoting an intervention on the basis of its technical simplicity and low cost. However, even setting these three problems aside, the scientific soundness of the Kenyan study claimed by their authors is demolished and their results are weakened. Their evidence-based science is refuted by another evidence-based science. Thus, the significance of this controversy is clear: it is veridiction by quantification and its endorsement that are shaken. Or so one might think. But GiveWell's restatement of its support for deworming, even after doubt had been cast on its efficacy, shows that such is not actually the case. The draw of a low-cost measure that can be presented favorably to the public and above all to funders as a magic bullet is too powerful. A policy that has not been proven, but has the merit of being credible, therefore continues to be promoted.

But let there be no mistake. The point here is not to deny the usefulness of deworming, which is effective in doing what it is supposed to do, eliminating parasites, and is therefore both a need and a right. Neither is it to condemn randomized trials, which can, with some reservations, contribute to validating public health initiatives. It is simply to encourage caution in intellectual exercises that have practical consequences such as the generalization of results and the adoption of recipes, particularly where poor communities and developing countries, which have little say in the implementation of these programs introduced from outside, are concerned. Ultimately, no more than what economist Angus Deaton, another winner of the Sveriges Riksbank Prize in Economics in Memory of Alfred Nobel, and philosopher Nancy Cartwright say in a report for the US National Bureau of Economic Research: "RCTs would be more useful if there were more realistic expectations of them and if their pitfalls were better recognized."[26] The reason I have devoted so much attention to this famous study, which brings together major elements of positivism in public health – RCTs and DALYs, the empire of evidence and salvation through experimentation, confident assertions, and the increase in generality – is above all because it illustrates both the power of quantification and the fragility of the truth it produces. As João Biehl and Adriana Petryna phrase it, "such approaches perpetuate a limited understanding of narrowly conceptualized problems and support a rhetoric that offers only temporary control over isolated aspects of a given disease."[27] This is, in short, an invitation to critically interrogate veridiction, which is confirmed by three of my own research projects.

When I was conducting a study of maternal mortality in Ecuador in the 1990s, examining data on the death of women during pregnancy, childbirth, and the forty-two days following, which is the definition of maternal mortality, I was struck by the gap between the rates I read in the official reports of the Pan-American Health Organization and those I calculated from birth and death registration data produced by the Instituto Nacional de Estadística y Censos (National Institute of Statistics and Census). The former showed a much higher maternal mortality rate than the latter: they presented an alarming picture of Ecuador that gave it the second highest rate on the continent after Haiti. When I became more familiar with Ecuador's "reproduction policy" and had met the national director in charge of it, who was deeply marked by the death of her own mother at her birth – a fact not unrelated to her commitment to this work – I understood the reason for this gap. The reportedly poor position of the country, combined with very real work on the part of its health officials, had enabled Ecuador to take the lead in the continent-wide crusade against maternal mortality. The country had been allocated substantial international aid to carry out this program for improving women's health.

As such projects involve working toward quantified goals, the Ministry of Health had announced that it would reduce maternal mortality by 75 percent between 1990 and 2015, a formidable challenge in a country with major social inequalities and deep disparities in access to care, especially for rural Indigenous communities. When the time came to account to the funders, on the basis of public registration data on maternal deaths during this period, the demographers engaged in an unorthodox exercise of statistical correction, asserting without showing any real empirical evidence that, at the beginning of the program, there had been a substantial understatement of these deaths. The initial figure was therefore arbitrarily doubled, allowing them to present a much more unfavorable starting point. Thanks to this contrivance, the maternal mortality rate fell dramatically over the period, from 153 to 45 deaths per 100,000 live births, a drop of 71 percent. The declared objective, which was virtually unachievable given the economic and health situation in the country, had almost been reached.[28] There was thus a dual benefit in this maneuver. Reporting high maternal mortality rates served at the outset to demonstrate the urgency of the action for women's health, and at the end to prove the efficacy of the intervention. Here the truth in numbers is to be sought less in the reflection of epidemiological reality than in the expression of a political commitment. It could, indeed, be considered that this instrumentalization of statistics helped to mobilize human and material resources, and ultimately effectively to reduce maternal mortality. Where the champion of a Kantian morality, which presupposes being obliged to tell the truth, might be shocked, a consequentialist, who judges an action on the basis of its effects, might say that, after all, these little economies with the truth were to the advantage of Ecuadorian women, especially the poorest.

The Ecuadorian case is certainly not unique. In her study in Nigeria, Adeola Oni-Orisan shows how, following a World Bank study of millennium development goals, the governor of one of the states with the highest maternal mortality rates in the country was able to apply for and secure substantial international aid to improve its "reproductive health system," specifically making it possible to provide free consultations to pregnant women and children under the age of 5. Within a few years, the rate had halved, and the state had thus achieved the announced objective in record time. Yet on closer inspection, this result was based on a manipulation of the data where some deaths of women during pregnancy or in childbirth were removed from the count of maternal mortality while the program was under way. Performance therefore improved. As Oni-Orisan notes, "the numerical metrics mandated by global health funders today not only have the power to determine which interventions are successes, which are failures, which will be funded and which will not, but they also carry the political clout to determine who will get reelected to office, who will be promoted to chief medical director of a hospital and who will win a government contract."[29] The funders who intervene in the politics of health development in African countries such as Nigeria are both multilateral agencies like Unicef and powerful philanthropists like Bill Gates. Because they demand statistics, they are provided with them, even if it means massaging them to present the situation as worse than it is when requesting aid and better than it is when interventions are evaluated.

But these methods ignore what cannot be measured, and is often the most crucial from the point of view of economic development – social change, reduction of inequality, and quality of life. The success of an enterprise is judged purely on the basis of the results it is deemed to have achieved, neglecting its non-measurable benefits in terms of citizen participation, social justice, respect of rights, gender equality, consideration for minorities. Criticizing the expansion of these evaluation practices in global health programs, particularly the hegemony of statistics and the power of numbers in DALYs and RCTs, Vincanne Adams outlines an alternative. As an anthropologist, she argues for a return to storytelling, in the form of stories that can reveal the complexity of what is at stake in public health, and of accounts that can fill the spaces not covered by numbers. While recognizing the potential efficacy of this approach, I would like to explore a different path, not replacing numbers with narratives, but rather showing that the numbers themselves produce narratives or are set within narratives.[30] They tell tales that offer a certain way of reading the world.

In contrast with a positivism suggesting that data are ready to be collated to provide an objective and neutral account of the world, a reading can be provided in terms of narratives, in which statistics and probabilities, modeling and projections, tables and graphs are protagonists that influence the representation of reality and shape courses of action. These protagonists change over time, not only because facts change, and with them the numbers that represent them, but also because they compete with one another when describing these facts, with the consequence that some disappear and others appear. Depending on whether one uses one method of calculation rather than another to produce a statistic, draws on these hypotheses rather than those to support a model, displays the results on a graph with a linear or a logarithmic scale, a different reality will emerge, reassuring or disturbing, suggesting stabilization or aggravation of a phenomenon, calling for a political or a moral interpretation, or both. But pointing out this narrative component of quantification and considering how numbers tell a story does not mean ceding to a relativism that would lead us to give up measuring facts. On the contrary, it means taking it seriously. Revealing this diversity of narratives means resisting the seduction of numbers, inviting greater rigor in the analysis and interpretation of data. The heatwave of 2003 offers an illustration.

In August of that year, Europe experienced a heatwave of exceptional duration and intensity. France was hit particularly hard, seeing temperatures unprecedented in the history of modern meteorology. The worst of the heatwave lasted ten days from the 3rd to the 13th of August, the temperature beginning to fall subsequently. But this brief period was enough to generate a serious health crisis manifested in the loss of tens of thousands of human lives. A report by the European Union four years later estimated that, in sixteen countries, the number of excess deaths that summer was over 71,000, including 45,000 in the month of August alone.[31] In France, the excess mortality was 19,490, equal to 11.8 percent over the normal rate. Only Italy experienced a worse fate, with 20,089 deaths, while Spain had 15,090. By contrast, England and Wales, which were also hit by the heatwave, saw only 301 excess deaths.

Yet, at the time, these data, which have now been confirmed and acknowledged, were the subject of a real "war of numbers," as Delphine Brard notes.[32] As the Ministry of Health was delaying publishing the statistics, journalists fell back on the assessment of clinicians on the ground. On 11 August, the director of the Paris emergency medical service (Samu, Service d'aide médicale urgente) reported sixteen deaths that had occurred the previous day in Paris public hospitals, and therefore extrapolated to potentially fifty deaths in the Île-de-France region. Two days later, the hot-headed president of the Emergency Doctors' Association warned of the possibility of thousands of victims. On 13 August, the Director General for Health finally made a statement, giving an approximate figure of 3,000 deaths for the whole of the country. This was immediately amended by the minister, who suggested a range of between 1,500 and 3,000, minimized the significance by saying that the deceased were mostly sick people at the end of life, and, seeking to reassure people, asserted that hospitals were not overloaded. The same official data, still just as vague, were communicated to journalists on 18 August, when the director of the Institute for Health Monitoring had the day before suggested that a figure of 5,000 deaths was plausible. Forty-eight hours later, the Pompes funèbres générales, France's largest funeral service provider, estimated on the basis of their activity that the excess mortality for the first three weeks of August was 10,416 – an assessment that the French Red Cross however deemed exaggerated. For two weeks, the only official statistics therefore remained the approximately 3,000 deaths cited by the Director General of Health, who had in the meantime been forced to resign over the health crisis. On 19 August, the Institute of Health Monitoring announced that there had been 11,436 deaths, a figure that was corrected a month later by Inserm, which estimated that 14,800 people, 84 percent of them aged 75 and over, had died as a direct result of the heatwave between the 1st and 20th of August.[33] Throughout this period of growing anxiety and persistent uncertainty, newspaper articles and television reports proliferated. People sought to understand why France had fared worse than its neighbors. On 16 August, when the French figure was still 3,000 deaths, an article in *Le Monde* suggested some comparisons quite unfavorable to France. The journalist noted that in Italy too there was difficulty in calculating the number of victims, but reported details on Germany, where no loss of life had been recorded, Spain, where forty-five deaths, half of them from heatstroke, had been noted, Portugal, where eighteen people had died in a fire, and the United Kingdom, where only a few drownings had occurred. The subsequent European study would show that during the month of August there were in fact 15,251 excess deaths compared to previous years in France, with 9,713 in Italy, 7,295 in Germany, 6,461 in Spain, 2,196 in Portugal and 1,987 in England and Wales. These figures are far from the handful of deaths from heatstroke, fire, or drowning. To be sure, France was the country with the highest number of victims, but the excess mortality was only between 1.5 and 8 times higher than that of its neighbors, rather than the 100 times reported by *Le Monde*.

There is certainly much to say about the management of this crisis, which has generated various works of reportage and analysis.[34] I shall limit my comments to the question of numbers. How are these variations, these controversies, and these strange comparisons to be explained? One important factor, pointed out by Marc Milet, is the narrative phasing of the crisis.[35] Until 7 August, the narrative was the drought, which had continued since the month of June and was worsening with the arrival of the heatwave; there were reports of farmers in difficulty, forest fires, ozone pollution, but no one was talking about health. From the 8th to the 12th of August, the narrative was dominated by the question of electricity supplies, as an increase in the temperature of waste water from power stations had combined with a rise in electricity consumption: there was talk about the prevention of a nuclear accident and the risk of countrywide power cuts; however, the media did report the first alerts from emergency doctors. From 13 August, the date when the "emergency plan" mobilizing health professionals in the Île-de-France region was put into action, the health narrative became dominant, but this was already the end of the second week, the last day of the heatwave and, as would later become apparent, the first day after the peak of mortality: this belated account was dominated by questions and polemics around statistics. There was thus a substantial time lag that explains the delay in producing reliable figures.

But there was also a discrepancy in the method of data collection, between the practice of emergency clinicians and the measurements of demographers and epidemiologists. The former reported deaths of patients they had transported or seen at the hospital. The latter analyzed the death certificates drawn up by doctors that were sent to the National Institute of Statistics and Economic Studies (Insee, Institut national de la statistique et des études économiques) and to Inserm.[36] In the first case, the knowledge is local, partial, and immediate. In the second, it is national, quasi-exhaustive, and deferred. The emergency medical practitioners counted the patients they knew died from the effects of the heatwave, especially from hyperthermia and dehydration, but they could not do the same for patients whose death ensued several days later, whose death appeared due to another cause or, of course, for those who died at home. Demographers and epidemiologists measured the number of excess deaths compared to a normal year, and their assessment was based in practice on the difference between the number of deaths observed and the number expected, subsequently broken down by declared cause of death, allowing them to take into account, after the event, those deaths the clinicians failed to identify. It is then easy to understand, first, why the emergency medical practitioners provided figures well before demographers and epidemiologists and, second, why the figures cited by the former were much lower than those provided by the latter. Although both groups of experts were talking about mortality, these data have nothing to do with one another, since the former derive from a medical gaze and the latter from a statistical calculation. This means that the 3,000 deaths in France could not be compared with the forty-five deaths in Spain, as the journalist did on 16 August, because the method of counting was completely different. The definitive figures, moreover, show that the gaps were in fact much smaller, since the excess mortality in France was a little over twice that in Spain. As a final irony, it was the funeral directors, contradicting the health authorities, who were the first to put forward an order of magnitude that proved correct, when they asserted that the number of deaths was over 10,000.

The figures from the 2003 heatwave are thus remarkably eloquent. They speak, but the accumulation of their disparate discourses produces a cacophony rather than useful information. The multiple accounts they support produce a diffracted view of the health reality. There was the dramatic warning from the emergency clinicians, yet with modest numbers: around 50. There were the reassuring statements from the minister of health about hospital capacity, when his department was announcing high figures: 3,000 deaths. There were the comparisons of responses from countries based on data collected in such different ways that they became absurd: several thousand deaths on one side, a few people burned to death or drowned on the other. There was the minimization of the death statistics through the argument of a "harvesting effect," as it is somewhat brutally known – alleging that the only consequence of the heatwave was to hasten the anticipated deaths of old people who were already very weak: it was only when mortality data for subsequent years were available that this hypothesis could be refuted. Finally, there were the belated studies of excess mortality that provided consolidated and reliable results, but whose emotional resonance and political repercussions remained modest, as it was already well after the event. The proliferation of numbers that were inconsistent with one another thus generated what Umberto Eco calls "noise," that is a "perturbation in the nature of the signal" that makes it difficult to detect or produces a response opposite to that desired.[37] Here, the noise of the different clashing statistics makes it impossible to understand the situation and above all to make appropriate decisions. Because they are saying too much, the numbers say nothing.

While the confusion of numbers and their interpretations can only indicate the weakness of the information systems that produce them,

as is the case with the 2003 heatwave, comparing numbers with the
way they are interpreted can, by contrast, be rich in meaning, and
even become a key to reading society. A case in point is the scientific
and political controversy around mortality data in South Africa that
arose on 9 July 2000, the opening day of the thirteenth international
AIDS conference in Durban.[38] This controversy was set within the
broader context of the dispute between the world scientific community
and a small group of dissident researchers who rejected the theory of
the viral etiology of AIDS and condemned the use of antiretroviral
drugs as harmful. The most high-profile figure in this debate was the
then South African president, Thabo Mbeki, who had just triggered
an international scandal by convening a panel of scientists belonging
to the two camps, as if the heterodox scholars could be treated in the
same manner as the orthodox ones, in order to compare their points of
view and, he asserted, shed light on the cause of the epidemic. In this
atmosphere of heightened tension, the main national daily paper bore
the headline, in huge letters: "Young, Gifted and Dead." The phrase
echoed the title of Nina Simone's famous song "Young, Gifted and
Black," an anthem of the civil rights movement in the United States.
The article presented four diagrams showing mortality in relation to
age for both sexes for the years 1990 and 2000. While in 1990 the curves
of the death rate in the general population rose from 15 to 70 years,
as is the case almost everywhere in the world, in 2000 on the contrary
the peak was between 30 and 55 years for men, and between 25 and 35
years for women. In South Africa people were now dying before the
age of 50 twice as often as they had ten years earlier.

These graphs had already been presented a few days earlier, the
article reported, by biologist Malegapuru William Makgoba, director
of the Medical Research Council, to the members of the presidential
panel. "That we are at war, engaged in a major conflict: that is the only
possible explanation for the high number of young men and young
women who are dying today in our country," he declared, stating that
it was indeed AIDS that was responsible for this tragic situation, not
poverty as the president asserted. Although nothing was said about
the racial distribution of these statistics, the substitution of "dead" for
"Black" in the newspaper headline evidently suggested that those who
were dying in excess were black – in other words, that it was mostly
they who were affected by AIDS. But the association of AIDS with
"Africans," meaning Blacks in the South African racial classification,
was an explicitly racist trope of the final years of apartheid. The choice
to make an unfavorable comparison of the situation in a democratic
South Africa with that in apartheid South Africa added an additional

symbolic violence, reflecting a discourse that was fairly common in conservative circles, according to which things had only got worse since the first free elections in 1994. The headline therefore could not fail to grab people's attention, thanks to the revelations about mortality, but also the subtext that was clear to all.

The next day, the Interior Ministry made a statement correcting this information.[39] Its services are in charge of registering deaths, but not for analyzing mortality data. The ministry nevertheless contested Makgoba's interpretation, noting first that large numbers of South African adults died from accidents and violence, and the mortality profile could not therefore be imputed to AIDS alone, and second that the comparison of the two years was invalid, since, under apartheid, four of the ten Bantustans into which the government had forcibly grouped people on the basis of their supposed ethnic origin were not taken into account. This two-pronged argument, which was taken up by a number of high-profile figures, including Mbeki himself, in the following days, aimed to re-establish two historical truths. First, deaths from other than natural causes, in particular homicide, are the legacy of the regime which, after dispossessing the Black population of their land, segregated them in homelands (in the rural areas) and townships (in the cities), where most subsisted in poverty and where the powerless and corrupt administrations failed to maintain law and order. The violence and criminality inherited from apartheid could not vanish overnight, and indeed broke out further with the introduction of democracy, which gave new mobility to people who had hitherto been constrained by "passes." Second, the exclusion and abandonment of Black people by a government rooted in the ideology of white supremacy were manifested, among other things, in a lack of interest in epidemiological and demographic data on Black populations, with very incomplete registration of births and deaths. Thus, during the 1970s, information was collected on fewer than a third of Blacks, and one-fifth of the death records indicate unknown causes; during the 1980s information on all rural areas was incomplete, or even entirely non-existent, for almost half the Bantustans. Thus, because they did not count in the eyes of the white South African authorities, Blacks were not included in the nation's counts. The two sides of statistics are evident here, in that they correspond to a reality, that of the violence of apartheid, and that they are constructed, in this case by discounting part of the population.

A year later, the main South African demographic research center published a document putting forward an analysis of mortality between 1988 and 2000, and thus offering a way to understand both the transition from apartheid to democracy and the development of the AIDS epidemic.[40] This was no longer the sonorous pronouncements of sensationalist journalism. The analysis of the data and their limits is rigorous and austere. The incompleteness of the death statistics was confirmed, since between 1990 and 2000 statistical coverage rose from 54 percent to 89 percent. The increase in mortality during the period was also established, since the corrected number of deaths had increased from 237,000 to 412,000, with a considerable bias toward adults aged 15 to 49, in both sexes. People were therefore dying younger and younger. Moreover, the authors estimated cautiously, on the basis of an international model, that mortality from AIDS among adults represented around a quarter of deaths in 2000. But they also demonstrated that mortality from external causes was responsible for between one-third and half the deaths of young men. It is therefore tempting to suggest that, objectively, both camps that were at loggerheads a few months earlier were partly right – first because mortality had certainly increased, but the data were not strictly comparable, and second because AIDS was responsible for a substantial proportion of the worrying increase in deaths, while violent and accidental deaths, although lower than in the years following liberation from apartheid, remained a major cause of mortality among young men. But the two camps were not to be reconciled.

For the question as to who was right was perhaps not the most crucial point. What the controversy revealed was how the interpretation of statistics reawakened the pain of the past, how it divided the nation along fault lines inherited from a century of racial segregation, and how pointing to AIDS or violence as the explanation for the number of deaths was not simply a question of scientific discussion, but a manifestation of a political disagreement with profound implications. Not that it was impossible to look at the data objectively, but the analysis of them sensitized the wounded subjectivities of a history whose traces remained omnipresent. The two accounts that the mortality data produced thus performed two veridiction operations: one apparently neutral, and yet saturated with racial connotations and insinuations; the other, full of noise and fury, but asserting facts that were as incontestable as they were concealed. Nevertheless, these operations of veridiction cannot be reduced to the articulation of contradictory truths about mortality statistics. They also reveal the buried historical truths of South African society.

In sum, if, as Alain Supiot argues, contemporary societies are increasingly governed by numbers, the declared triumph of positivism, heralded by the celebration of big data, the success of QALYs,

DALYs, and RCTs, and advances in artificial intelligence and machine learning, certainly calls for critical appraisal.[41] Whether they relate to the benefits of deworming in Africa or maternal mortality in Ecuador, the heatwave in France or AIDS in South Africa, statistics are never simply describing reality. They construct it, interpret it, manipulate it. They narrate it. Far from the objectivity they claim, they manifest prejudices about what is interesting and what is not, what is to be shown and what is to be concealed. The truth in numbers is therefore not a single truth. It is multiple and contradictory.

At the inaugural lecture of his course in Leuven in 1981, Michel Foucault proposed not to oppose positivism, but rather to produce a "counter-positivism" that would be the "counterpoint" to positivism, characterized by "astonishment before the very ancient multiplication and proliferation of truth-telling, and the dispersal of regimes of veridiction."[42] As Foucault so often does, he avoids going into detail about what he intended by this phrase, leaving his audience free to imagine its meaning. The reflection I have put forward here on the truth in numbers in a sense extends this ellipsis. It reveals both the diversity of and the competition between positivist claims to state the truth in numbers. Economists and epidemiologists draw different conclusions about the efficacy of a public health measure, despite the fact that they are looking at the same survey data. Ecuadorian experts overstate maternal mortality rates, while Nigerian doctors minimize them in order to justify funding either before or after the fact. French emergency clinicians and demographers produce very different data on deaths due to a heatwave, by using different counting methods. South African researchers interpret an excess of deaths in contradictory ways, some referring to an epidemic in the present, others pointing to a violent past.

Positivism finds itself as it were beaten at its own game – that of the truth in numbers. For there is not one, there are many numbers, and there is not one, but many truths. But we need to go beyond the relativism that these variations and instrumentalizations suggest. These uncertain numbers invite exploration of richer, deeper, and more unstable truths about the contemporary world than those positivism claims to make them say. They speak of practices of development and methods of evaluation, the relation to time and the value of lives. They speak, in short, of morality and of politics.

Epistemic Boundaries
12 May 2021

A nosographic anomaly. – What normal means. – Transient mental illnesses. – The possibility of ecological niches. – A conflict of legitimacy over the after-effects of military operations. – The avatars of chronic fatigue failing to gain recognition. – The authenticity of suffering versus the authority of science. – A partial victory for patients and a partial defeat for experts. – Reversing the moral valence of psychic trauma. – Populations forgotten in the epidemiology of wars. – Public health at a loss when confronted by diseases without patients and patients without diseases.

Returning to the guiding thread of the history of childhood lead poisoning that I mapped out in my first lecture, what stood out was the remarkable transmutation that occurred over a little less than a decade, from a serious condition with neurological complications potentially leading to coma and even death, with precisely identified clinical and radiological signs and a medical treatment whose success could not be guaranteed – a condition observed so rarely in pediatric hospital departments that it was often only diagnosed too late – to a completely asymptomatic state that is manifested today in a statistical risk of lower IQ, poorer school results, more frequent attentional disorders, and perhaps even, in adolescence, an increased probability of criminal behavior. This is a state that now prompts preventative interventions in housing, either by rehousing the families concerned or by refurbishing unfit apartments, because the primary mechanism of contamination is ingestion of flakes and inhalation of dust from old and crumbling paint with a high lead content. Until the 1980s, there were a very small number of sick children. By the late 1990s, there were many children apparently in good health but who might develop cognitive and behavioral problems. A shift had occurred, from a potentially lethal pathology to an environmental hazard, from a clinical picture to a statistical evaluation of risk. In two decades, childhood lead poisoning had become a disease without patients. During the same period, a shift had occurred from medicine to public health.

But are we even sure that childhood lead poisoning can still be considered a disease? Does the mathematically calculated possibility of the loss of a few points in psychometric tests, of a higher rate of absence from school and a higher proportion of children showing inappropriate behavior in class amount to an entity that can be classified in a nosography, or classification of diseases, on the same level as tuberculosis, rheumatoid arthritis, or laryngeal cancer? The fact that the same signs may be observed in children from disadvantaged families even when they are not exposed to lead gives all the more reason to question the nature of this entity. It is therefore not the combination of these features that is sufficient to identify a pathological condition, but the higher probability of their occurrence at higher blood lead levels. And this relationship persists when social environment and economic conditions are taken into account, something that can only be established by statistical regression calculations that make it possible to analyze this relationship on the basis of "all things being equal." This entity, which is no longer clinically objectifiable but statistically constituted, therefore forces us to rethink our frame of reference for disease – for what is a disease without symptoms or signs, a disease defined solely in terms of the excessive but invisible presence of a heavy metal in the organism and the higher frequency of certain cognitive and behavioral markers? Moreover, the definition of this entity has become increasingly vague, since the blood lead level that determined the boundary between normal and pathological, having been progressively lowered from 350 μg/l to 50 μg/l to take into account the results of epidemiological studies that showed lead to be toxic at low levels, is ultimately disappearing: even below the latter threshold, the probability of disorder continues to rise, and any presence of lead, however low, is now considered pathological.

The redefinition of lead poisoning that took place in the late twentieth century thus seems to run counter to Georges Canguilhem's well-known theory of the normal and the pathological in what he calls the "second problem": can there be "sciences of the normal and the pathological"?[1] Before responding to this question, Canguilhem drew a distinction between two meanings of the word "norm." The first is statistical: the normal is the average, it is the norm in the arithmetical sense. The second is therapeutic: the normal is what is understood as good, in relation to a norm in the evaluative sense. The first is a matter of measurement, the second of judgment. Taking up André Lalande's observation in his *Vocabulaire technique et critique de la philosophie*, Canguilhem remarks that in French the noun "anomaly" [*anomalie*] has no adjective attached to it, and that the adjective "abnormal" [*anormal*] has no corresponding noun, leading to them being coupled as if "anomaly" was the substantive of the adjective "abnormal."[2] But the words have different etymologies, since the word "anomaly" comes from the Greek *anomalia*, meaning "irregularity," in opposition to that which is uniform, equal, and smooth, while the word "abnormal" comes from the Latin *norma*, meaning "square," becoming a rule of conduct in the figurative sense. An anomaly is therefore a departure from the norm in the sense of what is most frequent, whereas abnormal refers to a failure to meet the norm, in the sense of what ought to be. And Canguilhem argues that the semantic confusion which leads to the blurring of the two meanings is both a philosophical and a practical problem, for it leads to the idea that it is possible to "reduce the norm to an objective concept determinable by scientific methods." And this is not the case. "It is not an objective method that leads to a given biological phenomenon being qualified as pathological. It is always the relation to the individual patient through the intermediary of clinical practice, which justifies the qualification of pathological," for it is not possible for the "pathologist" to treat "his object" as if it was "matter without subjectivity." The case of childhood lead poisoning – other examples of the extension of the powers of what, in a previous lecture, I proposed to call biostatistics could be cited – appears to operate in the opposite direction to this recommendation, since the vast majority of the children now deemed to be affected by lead contamination do not suffer from any symptoms or present any signs. It is not therefore the "relation to the individual patient through the intermediary of clinical practice" that defines the pathological in this case. It is the combination of a bioassay and a probabilistic calculation that leads to them being identified as patients, or rather, in the most recent revision of the criteria for definition of childhood lead poisoning, that situates them on a curve of increasing pathology.

But I do not mean to suggest that Canguilhem's analysis is outdated, or "history," as he writes in his foreword, and indeed I intend to show how relevant it remains today for conditions claimed by patients and denied by physicians. Nor do I mean to assert that the reasoning and the strategy employed by the experts in lead poisoning are inappropriate because they do not take into account that the children appear to be in good health – for there is no doubt that the new policies for combating childhood lead poisoning, when they are genuinely applied,

lead to measurable improvements in the present and better future prospects for the children concerned. My aim is rather to show the extent
to which the refinement of the science of numbers is changing not only
the domain of public health, but also, more fundamentally, the relation
to the normal and the pathological in contemporary societies. In this
sense, biostatistics extends and deepens what Foucault calls biopolitics.[3] But in the case of childhood lead poisoning, the aim is not so
much to control or regulate the population as to recognize and protect
the most vulnerable within it.

What are the theoretical implications of this observation? The order
of diseases is customarily thought of as a discrete set, comprising
clearly defined pathologies – albeit expressed in a variety of ways –
that are markedly distinct from normality, even if the early forms may
be difficult to diagnose. The study of childhood lead poisoning shows
that this dual distinction may prove tenuous when symptoms and signs
are replaced by probabilities, when the division between normal and
pathological is removed, and indeed when the biological becomes difficult to separate from the social domain, given that poverty and mar-
ginalization have effects similar to those of lead contamination. This
case thus serves as a starting point for a reflection on what might be
called epistemic boundaries – in other words, the liminal zones where
diseases are redefined, where they are contested, or indeed where they
overturn medical certainty.

A reading of treatises on pathology from the last few centuries
would, of course, show that nomenclature and classification change
continually with time. Thus phthisis, dropsy, apoplexy, and neurasthenia belong to the medical language of the nineteenth century. Today
they have disappeared, surviving only in the works of romantic or
naturalistic writers. But I am interested in other epistemic boundaries –
boundaries that emerge not from diagnostic advances but rather from
semantic restructuring and semiological challenges. They owe less to
the work of physicians than to the mobilization of other actors, particularly patients. They concern not only individuals, but entire populations. In this sense, we can talk about the epistemic boundaries of
public health. They reveal societal stakes that incorporate, to varying
degrees, cognitive, political, and moral dimensions. In exploring these
issues, I shall draw on case studies that illustrate, first, the disputed
emergence of new conditions that manifest differences of opinion
between clinicians and patients, such as Gulf War syndrome; second,
the interpretation of disorders that have no simple explanation, such
as chronic Lyme disease; and, third, the reconfiguration of known
entities, which may extend to inverting their meaning, as in the case of

psychological trauma. In each case, the cognitive dimension relates to management of uncertainty and ignorance around health problems of unconfirmed status; the political dimension relates to the question of who holds the legitimacy and authority to define what is pathological; finally, the moral dimension relates to the positive or negative value assigned to both the disease and the patient.

In his pioneering work on what he calls "transient mental illnesses," Ian Hacking offers a productive starting point.[4] The adjective "transient" is to be understood not in terms of the history of the individual, but of society. These pathologies are ephemeral not in the sense that people suffer from them only briefly, but in the sense that their social existence is limited in time and space. The conditions concerned appeared at a particular moment; cases proliferated over a certain period, often a few decades, and in a particular place, sometimes migrating to other spaces; they fascinated psychiatrists, psychologists, psychoanalysts, and commentators, giving rise to diagnoses and debate; they eventually disappeared, dying a natural death and leaving barely a trace except in the medical archives, and occasionally in a few novels or films. The example Hacking cites is the condition of the "mad travelers," who apparently emerged in large numbers in the late nineteenth century. Although the phenomenon of fugue has probably always existed, Hacking asserts that it only entered psychiatric taxonomy in 1887 with the case of Albert, a 26-year-old man hospitalized in Bordeaux for his compulsive tendency to take to the road, leaving behind family and work, walking several dozen kilometers each day for weeks or months, and covering substantial distances toward destinations as far away as Moscow, Constantinople, and Algiers. Over the following two decades other observations were published, first in France, then in Italy, and especially, a little later, in Germany, but rarely in Britain or the United States, where the diagnosis of multiple personality was more usually used to account for such episodes of wandering. In each place, debate arose among psychiatrists in relation to this condition, which, depending on the country, was termed *automatisme ambulatoire*, *determinismo ambulatorio*, or *Wandertrieb*, or even (following a widespread custom in medicine of creating neologisms from Greek roots) poriomania, from *poreia*, walking. In the view of Jean-Martin Charcot, pathological fugue was related to epilepsy and would benefit from bromide treatment; Fulgence Raymond, Charcot's student, believed, rather, that it was a symptom of hysteria and should be treated by hypnosis; later, Eugen Bleuler, another of Charcot's students, saw it as an expression of schizophrenia. Perhaps more significant than these nosographic discussions is the social context in which this new mental disorder emerged. In France, the medicalization of fugue correlates with a period of stigmatization of vagrancy and a political drive to get rid of such nomads. In Germany, it arose in the context of conscription, with the problem of defections from the army and hence of deserters, which explains why the disease was identified primarily by army doctors. The appropriation and redefinition of the condition by psychiatrists did not help the runaways escape the repression of vagrancy or punishment for desertion, but it was part of the psychiatric reconfiguration of behavioral disorders characteristic of that period. However, shortly before World War I, mad travelers disappeared from scientific discussion and their pathology ceased to interest psychiatrists. For Hacking, this disappearance, which occurred earlier in France than in Germany, can be precisely dated to 1909, when a conference of alienists and neurologists relegated hysterical and epileptic fugues to the old-fashioned ideas of the preceding century, at a time when French psychiatry held sway. From then on, German psychiatry would take up the baton. A new nosographic order prevailed.

How, then, is fugue compulsion's brief moment in the limelight to be explained? How are we to tell the difference between the emergence of a new mental illness suffered by certain patients, and a condition merely dreamed up suddenly by psychiatrists? In other words, should we take a realist or a constructivist view? As I have already noted in relation to the history of childhood lead poisoning and the rise of biostatistics, the two are not mutually exclusive and often, indeed, gain from being brought together. This is also how Hacking addresses the problem, effectively by reversing the question. Ultimately, he points out, "wandering driven by irresistible impulses seems, when you come to think of it, such a natural way to be insane," and we should, rather, "wonder why, in the course of human history, has not compulsive traveling without purpose more often, and in more places, been thought to be a kind of madness." In order to understand how the possibility of such a framing arose, he proposes the novel concept of an "ecological niche." In Hacking's view, there are four conditions essential to the appearance of a transient mental illness. First, a "medical taxonomy" is required: the two possible diagnoses of hysteria and epilepsy, making it theoretically interesting for psychiatrists to ascribe the condition to one or the other. Second, a "cultural polarity" is necessary, with a spectrum ranging from positive to negative: here, from tourist trip to criminal vagrancy, the pathological fugueur lacking the resources of the former but seeking to be differentiated from the image of the latter. Third, the entity needs "observability" in order to be rendered visible: in this case, via the identity documents that had to be presented to police or customs officers. Fourth, the mental disorder must provide "release" from an experience of constriction and confinement, from which the socially maladjusted can thus escape. These four vectors were present, in different forms, in France and Germany at the very end of the nineteenth century. However, in Britain and the United States, both cultural polarity and observability were absent: the former because tourism had not become an industry and vagrancy was not a serious problem, the latter because there was no requirement for possession of identity documents.

The model of the ecological niche thus essentially unites two perspectives – that of physicians and that of patients – within a specific context. The physicians are involved at the level of taxonomy. The patients benefit from release. The context combines a moral dimension, in the cultural polarity with respect to stigma, with a political dimension, the observability associated with surveillance. According to Hacking, if all these elements are present the mental disorder can emerge, whereas if some are missing it cannot.

But I would like to reflect on other, more complex configurations. Sometimes, in fact, it happens that physicians and patients disagree on the emergence of a new clinical picture. This is particularly the case when the symptoms lie at the interface between the physical and the psychological, with patients expressing physical suffering and physicians interpreting it in a psychological register, the former arguing from their subjectivity and the latter rejecting this in the name of objectivity. What, then, is the nature of the power relation between these two protagonists? How is the conflict resolved, if it is? Can the concept of the ecological niche account for these situations? These are the questions I would like to try to answer through three case studies, starting with what has been called Gulf War syndrome.

On 17 January 1991, a coalition of thirty-five countries led by the United States launched the military operation Desert Storm against Iraq, which had invaded and annexed Kuwait a few months earlier. While the official justification for the intervention was the violation of the territorial integrity of an allied country, public opinion in the United States was rallied following the revelation, by a young woman in tears, that premature babies in Kuwaiti hospitals had been pulled out of incubators and thrown to the ground. This fueled a wave of anger against the alleged barbarism of the Iraqi army and compassion for the poor children thus sacrificed, until it was discovered shortly afterwards that the testimony was actually a fake put together by a Kuwait-funded public relations company, and that the tearful young woman was in fact the daughter of the Kuwaiti ambassador. In the meantime, the military campaign had begun, with the carpet-bombing of the Iraqi troops that also hit the civilian population. While admitting that the data are very uncertain, the Pentagon estimates that during this lightning six-week war approximately 100,000 Iraqis were killed and 300,000 injured, while, of the 697,000 US soldiers, the very precise figures showed 148 dead and 458 wounded; Iraqi casualties were thus 700 times higher.[5] But the price paid by the US army did not stop there. In the months following the soldiers' return home, a growing number of them complained of symptoms that physicians could not ascribe to a known pathology: fatigue, insomnia, muscular weakness, joint pain, skin rashes, digestive problems, headaches, impaired memory, difficulty in concentrating, mood swings. With the aid of political and media attention, this clinical picture garnered the popular epithet "Gulf War syndrome." It was the subject of numerous epidemiological studies, gave rise to the creation of parliamentary commissions of inquiry, and fed the press with testimonies from veterans describing their suffering.

But the results of these various investigations were disappointing.[6] Biochemical and radiological examinations revealed no significant, reproducible anomaly among the returned soldiers presenting with these disorders. Statistical comparisons did show that soldiers deployed in the field were two to four times more likely to suffer from each of these symptoms than others, but they did not seem to be more frequently affected by cancer or to have a higher mortality rate. Nor was any increase observed in congenital malformations among the children of soldiers from the contingent sent to the Middle East. On one level these observations, which were confirmed, bar a few details, by long-term follow-up of several cohorts of tens of thousands of participants, could seem reassuring, since medical investigations and statistical tests identified no known pathology. But on another level, their negative conclusions increased confusion and unease. For what were these veterans suffering from? Was it more legitimate to speak of Gulf War syndrome, as it was dubbed by the media, a term suggesting a clearly identified set of symptoms, or of Gulf War illness, as physicians named it, indicating that it was an illness perceived by individuals rather than a disease recognized as such by experts?[7] The soldiers presenting these disorders, which were atypical but incapacitating, suspected the government and health services of concealing the truth about the weapons and substances used during the war. The physicians remained undecided as to the reality of the pathology, many taking the view that it reflected the consequences of stress rather than a true organic disorder, in other words one inscribed in the body. As a consequence of this discordance between what the sick soldiers and their families experienced and the conclusions of the majority of physicians, the US government refuted the existence of a pathology linked to deployment in the Gulf War, and the federal Department of Veterans Affairs refused to compensate, or sometimes even to provide care for the individuals concerned. The latter became aware of this when they went to military hospitals, as they were told by staff that their disease did not exist and that they were suffering from psychological problems. The government's denial was thus passed down in the challenging or even contemptuous attitude of care professionals in veterans' services, who had received training in which they were repeatedly told that there was no evidence for the existence of this syndrome and were even instructed under no circumstances to refer to it by its name in front of their patients.

Was there, then, nothing to suggest that the symptoms of which soldiers deployed in the Persian Gulf complained might be due to the conditions in which the war was waged? Although initially denied or minimized by the US military, exposure to multiple substances was eventually acknowledged, but it was difficult to evaluate the consequences both because knowledge about the pathogenic effects of some of them was limited and because it was hard to determine the level of potential contamination of soldiers.[8] Neurotoxic chemicals, such as the sarin gas released by the bombing of some Iraqi munitions depots, were blamed, but the massive use of pyridostigmine bromide, which was supposed to protect US soldiers against the effects of these chemicals, also paradoxically proved dangerous. The multiple vaccinations administered, usually without informing the recipients what they were for, were also suspected, as was immunization against anthrax. In addition, the paints used to protect vehicles against chemical and biological weapons were investigated, as were the pesticides and insecticides widely applied to avoid contamination and infection. Finally, the risks from dispersal of smoke and particles from burning oil wells were pointed out. By contrast, little was said about the consequences of the use, for the first time, of depleted uranium bombs and missiles, of which 944,000 were launched during the conflict.

Given the accumulation of these substances in the theater of conflict and the knowledge gained from studies of their toxicity, and even if serious doubts remain about the effects of particular substances and the level of exposure of the soldiers, it is nevertheless remarkable that institutions and experts were so disinclined to give credence to the hypothesis that Gulf War syndrome was real. It is all the more surprising given that after the Vietnam War the Veterans Administration had acknowledged that Agent Orange, which had been used as a defoliant, could cause more than a dozen conditions, including leukemia, myeloma, prostate cancer, type 2 diabetes, coronary heart disease, and Parkinson's disease. In the case of the Gulf War, by contrast, the official position remained, for more than a decade, that there was no objective evidence such as changes in blood count, erythrocyte sedimentation rate, nerve conduction velocity, or other factors, although it should be noted that only potential effects were being measured with very basic tests, while the presence of toxic substances was impossible to detect so long after exposure. In this reading of the condition, only subjective elements were observed, symptoms that were, to be sure, troublesome but nothing out of the ordinary. The picture was therefore filed under the broad category of psychosomatic disorders. It was also pointed out that each great conflict in which the US has been engaged throughout its history had been associated with a specific clinical picture. During the Civil War it was "irritable heart syndrome," with palpitations, chest pain, shortness of breath, and, in some, a disorder described as "nostalgia"; during World War I, "effort syndrome," also called "neurocirculatory asthenia" and manifested in physical and psychological weakness, as well as "shell shock"; during World War II, "combat stress reaction," sometimes known as "battle neurosis," with panic attacks and signs of anxiety; following the Vietnam War, "post-traumatic stress syndrome," which was officially recognized in 1980.[9] Notwithstanding the diversity of designations and the various combinations of symptoms, wars were thus deemed to produce common forms of somatization of psychological origin, with the variation in manifestations being mainly due to the circumstances of the conflict and the available vocabulary.

Thus, during the decade following the return from the Gulf War and beyond, two main readings of this mysterious clinical picture faced off against each another. The first version was that of the patients who experienced serious bodily disorders they had never presented before being deployed to the Middle East, and which they attributed to their presence on the battlefield. Yet, they did not make this connection immediately. Interviews with them show that it was when they talked with other veterans that they began to become aware of the significance of their symptoms, and it was when they heard of the existence of a Gulf War syndrome through the media that they identified the disorders they were suffering from with the descriptions of this condition.[10] But it was difficult to get this intuition validated, since they came up against not only the denial of federal services but also their indifference, which they suspected of being deliberately cultivated when they realized, for example, that their case file had been lost or that certain information was being kept from them. The mixture of denial and dissimulation demoralized and embittered the veterans, but also led them to seek the information they needed to understand their situation from sources other than the official ones. This was how they gradually learned of the environmental risks to which they had been exposed, began to think again about the vaccinations they had been subjected to and the products they had been forced to take, understood they had breathed toxic gases and absorbed harmful particles, and eventually came to the conclusion that the authorities were conducting a concerted campaign to prevent them from knowing the truth. The second version of the clinical picture was that of the experts, who sought to establish links or statistical correlations between clinical, biochemical, and radiological data and levels of exposure to particular risks. Essentially, these studies showed considerable differences in the symptoms reported by soldiers deployed in the field compared to those who were not, but apparently no more biochemical or radiological anomalies than disparities in known pathologies or premature death.[11] They concluded that they were dealing with an imaginary pathology. According to Jeffrey Sartin, a former military doctor with the US Air Force, "Gulf War syndrome is, first and foremost, a media creation," since the "various illnesses that have been identified in Gulf War veterans with complaints represent normative illnesses for any large cohort." This was backed up by Bill Durodié, a political scientist from the Defence Academy of the United Kingdom, who stated in relation to British soldiers that, "when everything around them suggests that war will make them ill, it is not surprising that claims of post-conflict illness are on the rise," especially given that, with "a growing absence of any sense of what it is that they are being asked to fight for, pain and illness are less likely to be accepted and endured." Comparing the positions of the patients and the experts, it might seem paradoxical that the realist approach of the former, who assert that the disease actually exists, is based on subjective elements (the perception of symptoms), whereas the constructivist approach of the latter, who contest the existence of the disease, is based conversely on objective factors (the absence of empirical evidence). But this is often the case at epistemic boundaries. When they present clinical pictures that cannot be linked to any known pathology, and whose existence physicians therefore tend to deny, patients can draw only on the language of subjectivity to assert the reality of their problems, whereas the experts reply in the language of objectivity, regarding these pictures as socially constructed by the media and advocacy organizations. Dialogue is hence impossible.

The law governing epistemic boundaries is thus that of authority: it presupposes that certain people have the authority to say that a disease exists, and others do not. This is the law that arbitrates in the conflict of legitimacy between patients and experts. In principle, only the knowledge of experts is legitimate, or rather, their legitimacy derives from their presumed knowledge. Conversely, patients are not deemed to have any true knowledge; at most, the authenticity of their experience is recognized. Knowledge sits on the side of objectivity, experience on the side of subjectivity. The administration recognizes the former and at best humors the latter. In such circumstances, those suffering from unrecognized pathologies are forced to forge their own legitimacy, a process that involves campaigning and alliances. On the one hand, campaigning can help them to win another kind of legitimacy, usually political, both through the media attention they are able to arouse and through the electoral influence they are credited with. On the other, alliances can also win them legitimacy in the scientific arena when they manage to recruit researchers or physicians to their cause, even if these are often specialists who occupy – or whose commitment consigns them to – the margins of expert opinion.

In the case of Gulf War veterans, it was such persevering campaigns and tactical alliances that ultimately led, after more than a decade, to recognition, following the belated establishment of scientific evidence. One of the deciding factors was the detection of anomalies thanks to the increased sophistication of neuroimaging techniques and the development of animal models of exposure to toxins.[12] A reduction in grey matter and white matter was observed in the brains of soldiers who had been close to the site where an Iraqi munitions depot was blown up and sarin gas was released, and they also showed an increase in brain cancers; the latter phenomenon was also observed among those exposed to smoke from burning oil wells. Soldiers affected by the usual symptoms of Gulf War syndrome were, moreover, shown to have altered blood cortisol levels, EEG anomalies, and atrophy of the hippocampus, an area of the brain involved in memory. The animal experiments confirmed the existence of harmful effects not only on the brain but also on the cardiovascular system and mitochondrial functioning. In 2016, the Research Advisory Committee on Gulf War Veterans' Illnesses, set up by the US Congress, therefore concluded its review of the scientific literature by affirming that the symptoms presented by persons suffering from Gulf War syndrome "are consistent with those seen in chemically induced toxic injuries and residual encephalopathies and are associated with a range of objectively measured biological alterations."[13] Having long served to discredit the subjective expression of illness, the objective description of the highly contested syndrome thus became what now vouched for it. But this reversal simply confirms the pre-eminence of the objectivity of experts over the subjectivity of patients. Given the convergence of evidence, the Department of Veterans Affairs was forced to recognize what it nevertheless continued to describe as "presumptive illnesses" associated with the deployment of soldiers in what it called South-West Asia, and specifically what it described, in inverted commas, as "medically unexplained illnesses popularly known as 'Gulf War syndrome'."[14] According to official statistics, 44 percent of the nearly 700,000 soldiers deployed at the front suffer from the syndrome, and, following the new ruling, these veterans are entitled, under certain conditions, to a disability pension, professional training, and medical care.

The history of Gulf War syndrome, which the experts renamed "chronic multisymptom illness," an extremely vague and all-encompassing term where the choice of the word "illness" rather than "disease" suggests its subjective dimension, is exemplary in that it shares many features with the history of other conditions situated on the epistemic boundaries of public health.[15] These include chronic fatigue syndrome, myalgic encephalomyelitis, fibromyalgia, and multiple chemical hypersensitivity.[16] The first three of these conditions are deemed by the Department of Veterans Affairs to entitle soldiers from the "South-West Asia theater of military operations" (in other words, effectively the two Gulf wars) to medical care and financial support, while the fourth by definition includes the specific circumstance of having been exposed to the numerous toxic substances used during the conflict.[17] But these syndromes are by no means limited to this conflict, having been identified, contentiously, before it broke out, following long struggles for recognition.[18] Their definitions remain vague and their cause unknown. However, two of them are sufficiently similar for them to have been combined under the single designation ME/CFS (myalgic encephalomyelitis/chronic fatigue syndrome) since the early 2000s.

Myalgic encephalomyelitis was the first to be identified, in 1955 in England when a virulent epidemic occurred in a number of departments of the Royal Free Hospital in London.[19] Clinicians likened this cluster outbreak to an illness initially confused with acute poliomyelitis that had been observed in England and elsewhere during the preceding two decades. However, the progression was more favorable than in the case of the latter dangerous infection, since there was neither death nor permanent paralysis. The muscle pain led to the encephalomyelitis being characterized as myalgic, and because it did not lead to death it was termed benign. However, this description was quickly withdrawn when it became clear that in the London epidemic, as in other sporadic cases observed subsequently, its delayed effects were serious and incapacitating. Yet not all experts were convinced of the existence of this pathology. In 1970, two psychiatrists produced a report based on the study of fifteen outbreaks. They concluded that they were dealing with psychosocial phenomena caused by either mass hysteria among patients or distorted perception on the part of doctors. Their report sparked controversy and responses insisted that the condition was real and serious, but doubt had been sown and health professionals would long remain suspicious about this clinical picture, which interested psychiatrists more than other physicians.

Chronic fatigue syndrome appeared under that name in the United States in 1987, at a meeting of a working group in the Division of Viral Diseases at the Centers for Disease Control in Atlanta.[20] According to this group, it manifested, as its name implies, in intense fatigue that was not relieved by rest, increased after effort, and substantially limited simple everyday activities, thereby making it difficult or completely impossible to pursue normal working and family life. However, this diagnosis could only be confirmed once a range of pathologies that could cause these symptoms, and often required specific treatment, had been eliminated, including malignant disease, autoimmune conditions, endocrine disorders, infections such as tuberculosis or AIDS, myasthenia, psychosis – the list is long. Other symptoms, described as minor, might be present: mild fever, dysphagia, sensitive swollen glands, muscular weakness, joint pain, headache, and insomnia. Remarkably, this expert committee study was conducted in a department of virology. To understand why, we need to go back a few years.

In late 1984, an epidemic occurred near Lake Tahoe in the Sierra Nevada. More than 100 people, two-thirds of them women, many relatively young, presented a clinical picture that looked like flu followed by a state of intense fatigue. Two local doctors conducted antibody tests for Epstein–Barr virus, which causes infectious mononucleosis, an acute and almost always benign condition that mainly affects children and adolescents, but in rare cases is associated with an aggressive form of lymphoma; these tests were positive for the majority of the patients.[21] The case quickly became a national media story, and the formula "chronic active Epstein–Barr virus disease" entered everyday language throughout the country, as many other people suffering from incapacitating asthenia found in this viral causality an explanation of their symptoms, which those around them and also their physicians suspected of being due to simulation or hysteria. Patients who tested positive for antibodies to the virus mobilized, and laboratories producing tests mounted an aggressive marketing campaign, the former in the hope of gaining recognition for the source of their suffering, the latter for frankly commercial reasons. Very soon, however, studies cast doubt on the reliability and significance of the blood tests, and the link between the virus and these manifestations of fatigue was therefore qualified somewhat skeptically as sporadic.[22] In the view of the experts, if epidemic there was, it was an epidemic of diagnosis.

But although the syndrome that names it is recent, chronic fatigue is not a new condition.[23] In the United States, one probable variant became widely known under the name "neurasthenia," a term invented by the neurologist George Miller Beard in 1869 to denote a pathology whose dominant symptoms were anxiety, muscular pain, depressive mood, headache, and a form of lethargy, which he attributed to the stresses exerted on subjects by modern life, in particular by the accelerated rhythm of everyday activities. This medically recognized clinical picture was linked to changes in US culture, and the term "Americanitis" was coined, a term erroneously attributed to William James who himself suffered from the condition, as did his sister.[24] But neurasthenia was more widely popularized, reaching its peak in the early twentieth century. With the revival of interest in theories of the psyche, particularly psychoanalysis, it declined and ultimately disappeared after World War I. But subsequently advances in microbiology led to psychological interpretations being replaced by hypotheses of infection.[25] Thus chronic brucellosis had its moment of glory in the 1940s: a disease of cattle, the infection was transmitted through unpasteurized dairy products, and even after bacteriological traces had disappeared persistent problems were attributed to it. Chronic candidiasis was briefly put forward as an explanation in the early 1980s, with antibiotic treatment being accused of deregulating the intestinal flora and favoring the development of harmful microorganisms. Epstein–Barr virus was, then, just one of the multiple avatars of infectious agents to which chronic fatigue has been attributed, and was not, moreover, the candidate most recently proposed for an infectious etiology. In 2009, an article in the prestigious journal *Science* reported a link between chronic fatigue syndrome and the XMRV retrovirus, or xenotropic murine leukemia virus-related virus.[26] Two years later, the editors, having noted that this discovery had not been reproduced by other researchers and was probably due to contamination in the laboratory, announced that the article had been retracted. Bereft of causality, chronic fatigue therefore remains a syndrome.

But this lack of a proven etiology has not prevented interpretations which, for lack of a physical foundation, have swung between two hypotheses, according to which chronic fatigue syndrome is either a psychosomatic or a cultural condition. In the first case, it is described as a psychiatric disorder manifested in physical symptoms. In the second, it is seen as a clinical picture that reflects a particular moment in a society. But these two explanations are not mutually exclusive. Psychiatrist Simon Wessely, for example, argues that this syndrome is "a twentieth-century illness" resulting from a "somatization" in the context of a "rejection of psychiatry": patients refuse psychiatric diagnoses because, by placing them in the psychological register, they fail to validate the organic origin of their symptoms.[27] For those presenting these disorders, both the psychiatric interpretation and the cultural explanation essentially fail to recognize their suffering as "real," that is physical, and even hold them responsible if not for their fatigue, at least for "exaggerating" it, and for not making an effort to resolve it, as Norma Ware describes on the basis of patient interviews.[28] Their experience is thereby both delegitimized and stigmatized, leading either to a social withdrawal that helps to exacerbate their situation, or, conversely, to vehement protests.

However, in the early 2000s, thanks mainly to campaigns by patients and media attention to their illness, there was a change on both sides of the Atlantic. In parallel moves, the British Chief Medical Officer and the Centers for Disease Control and Prevention, the principal US public health agency, decided to confer official status on chronic fatigue syndrome.[29] It was, they stated, a genuine and indeed a serious disease that required the full attention of health services. It was estimated that between 800,000 and 2,500,000 people were suffering from it in the United States, 90 percent of whom had not been diagnosed because they had not been taken seriously by doctors. The Institute of Medicine, set up by the National Academy of Sciences to advise the federal government on health issues, even proposed to rename this entity "systemic exertion intolerance disease," in an effort to consolidate its place in the nosography.[30] Each word counts in this designation: it is indeed a disease, not a syndrome; it is systemic, as it can affect all organs; it is an intolerance of exertion, implying that the patient cannot be held responsible for it. All in all, a remarkable evolution. Previously suspicious, the health and scientific authorities now assert that a disease can exist without its cause being known, its mechanism being understood, or even any marker being detected. These missing elements do not condemn it to being relegated to the stigmatizing typology of mental disorders. The change is remarkable. Alongside physical diseases, for which clinicians identified an organic source, and mental illnesses, which psychiatrists determined on the basis of empirical observation, there is now a new class of diseases that affect both physical condition without leaving any specific trace, and mental state without having any precise semiology. Most importantly, these diseases are defined by patients themselves, who have secured recognition of the condition through their campaigns and their alliances.

The most controversial entity in this new class was chronic Lyme disease. Described for the first time in 1975, acute *Borrelia burgdorferi* is caused by a tick bite in zones where it is endemic, such as the east coast of the United States. In France, the health authorities estimate the number of cases at 50,000 each year, 800 of whom have to be hospitalized.[31] The disease manifests in a suggestive skin rash sometimes accompanied by fever and joint pain, and occasionally neurological signs. Treatment is based on antibiotics with no known bacterial resistance. Without treatment, and even with it, more serious cutaneous, articular, and neurological manifestations may occur. This is the clinical picture on which almost all the medical community agrees. Then there is chronic Lyme disease.[32] A growing number of individuals complain of symptoms reminiscent of those of chronic fatigue syndrome: profound asthenia, muscle and joint pain, impaired memory and concentration, and various other incapacitating problems. They attribute these symptoms to tick bites, even though they may not remember being bitten. But most experts refute the existence of a link between the two, given the absence of past or present signs of acute infection and the lack of biological evidence in many cases. This is the position taken by the Infectious Diseases Society of America and the French Society of Infectious Diseases (Société de pathologie infectieuse), the official authorities on infectiology on either side of the Atlantic. However, some physicians take the opposite view, criticizing their colleagues for denying reality, and treat their patients with long courses of antibiotics. These practitioners gather in the United States in the International Lyme and Associated Diseases Society, and in France as the French Federation Against Tick-Borne Diseases (Fédération française contre les maladies vectorielles à tiques). For a long time, vehement debate raged between the two camps, for and against the existence of chronic Lyme disease; it was fueled by patients who also formed their own organizations, and were not slow to accuse orthodox clinicians and the authorities of culpable complicity.[33] Nevertheless, as in the case of myalgic encephalomyelitis and chronic fatigue syndrome, the condition eventually found some legitimacy with the health authorities, although this did not win the adherence of infectiologists or fully reassure patients. In the United States, the National Institute of Allergy and Infectious Disease now uses the expression "post-treatment Lyme disease syndrome," while in France the High Authority for Health (Haute Autorité de santé) refers to "persistent polymorphous symptomatology/syndrome, possibly consequent on tick bite."[34] While recognizing the existence of a hitherto contested pathology, these obscure designations also express the disagreements that persist within the scientific community and particularly the continuing reservations as to the link between infection and condition, since they refer to a chronology subsequent in one case to treatment, and in the other to a possible tick bite. According to these new designations, it is therefore possible to develop the disease without having presented proven borreliosis, and even without being certain of having been bitten by a tick. The presumption of one or the other is sufficient. For patients, this was a partial victory. The authenticity of their suffering, and even of their condition, was acknowledged, but no definite link to Lyme disease was recognized.

There is, then, a series of clinical pictures located on the epistemic boundaries of public health. Their dominant symptoms are incapacity caused by persistent fatigue, diffuse pain, and cognitive disorders. Their cause is uncertain or highly disputed, and their treatment therefore cannot be based on etiology. Those affected number hundreds of thousands, if not millions. These boundaries of the medical episteme are the site of conflict between two incommensurable types of legitimacy, resting on radically different foundations: on one side the authenticity of suffering, and on the other the authority of science. The former appears confined to the restricted space of individual experience, where patients are alone with their symptoms, the anxiety they generate, and the stigma they arouse, but are able to express themselves in public space thanks to the work of advocacy organizations and through the media. The latter is embedded in the space of scientific expertise, where it benefits from the authority of the community of colleagues, but beyond this enjoys recognition in the institutional space, where decisions are made about care and the allocation of resources. The legitimacy of physicians is certainly greater than that of patients, and suffering carries little weight compared to knowledge. At least, such was the case until the beginning of the twenty-first century.

Indeed, the incredulity, indifference, and irony of the experts who, unable to determine a diagnosis, reject the reality of the disease or seek psychological mechanisms or cultural reasons for it, are now challenged by two distinct logics. The first emerges from the extension of knowledge that leads to recognition of the problems experienced: this is the case with Gulf War syndrome, where results from neuroimaging and animal experiments appear to confirm its toxic origin. The second derives from recognition of the experience of patients even when it is not corroborated by medical evidence: this is the case with chronic fatigue syndrome, where the perseverance of patients and media attention seems to have won out over the experts' reticence. In both cases, history thus seems to confirm Canguilhem's assertion that it is not scientific method but the relation to the sick individual that justifies the identification of a pathology. In other words, subjective experience should prevail over objective knowledge. On the epistemic boundaries I have described, the community of experts long held the upper hand over the community of patients, but the relationship may be in the process of turning around, with the official introduction – albeit with some hesitation and ambiguity – of these various syndromes into the nosography.

The configuration that takes shape in the account of how these syndromes emerged is quite different from Hacking's ecological niche. Until recently, there was no pre-existing taxonomy, but a classification that had to be built from scratch; no cultural polarity, even if the suspicion of malingering undermined claims to truth; no indisputable observability, for the very notion of a syndrome as a coherent set of symptoms was rejected; finally, no release for patients, since, on the contrary, the skepticism and disapproval they face confined them in stigma. The consensus between physicians and patients illustrated by the ecological niches of mad travelers' pathological fugue, of multiple personality, or of hysteria contrasts with the conflict between experts and patients, and the former's contestation of the latter's condition. The history of Gulf War syndrome, like that of chronic fatigue syndrome and chronic Lyme disease, is not a long quiet river: it is the struggle between two regimes of truth. The peaceable metaphor of the ecological niche therefore needs to be replaced with that of epistemic conflict. The difference is not only that the former relates to abnormal behaviors that are the domain of psychiatry and the latter to unexplained symptoms contested by medicine. It is also that in one case the condition concerns a few individuals, and in the other the epidemic affects hundreds of thousands, or even millions. It therefore becomes a matter of public health and thereby much more explicitly raises not only cognitive issues, but also economic, political, and moral stakes.

Gulf War syndrome is telling in this respect. In the United States, because the reference population is made up of nearly 700,000 soldiers deployed under operation Desert Storm, the Department of Veterans Affairs, a federal body, faces potentially substantial financial implications in light of the compensation, invalidity pensions, and long-term care the consequences of the conflict are likely to entail. The 18 million veterans represent more than one-tenth of the country's adult population, and the portion of the federal budget allocated to them rises to 243 billion dollars. Above all, however, recognition of the condition implies recognition of its causes, that is the multiple toxic agents liberally released on the battlefield and the various accidents caused by the bombing of munitions depots and oil wells – all risks to which the US army exposed its soldiers, and those of the other coalition countries, without apparently being overconcerned about the secondary effects of these substances. For the most bellicose country in the world, whose history since its birth is an uninterrupted succession of wars and which takes every opportunity to celebrate its troops with fulsome deployment of the national anthem and emotional tributes, admitting the indifference or the negligence evidenced by the fact that these risks were not anticipated or, worse, were ignored, means revealing the contempt of the leadership for the troops. This adds a political and moral stake to the economic dimension of Gulf War syndrome, for what is at issue is respect for the lives of those who are sent to the front for the declared purpose of defending the nation – even when, as in this case, it involves protecting an allied oil monarchy.

Yet the difficulty in achieving recognition for the existence of Gulf War syndrome arose in a very particular context in this regard. Eleven years before Operation Desert Storm, the American Psychiatric Association had introduced a new entity into the third edition of its classification of mental illnesses, the *DSM-III* – post-traumatic stress disorder, or PTSD.[35] This is a psychological disorder linked to exposure to a terrible event in the context of war, violence, or disaster. It manifests in insomnia and nightmares, flashbacks where the individual relives the event, and avoidance reactions that may go as far as amnesia about it. As Allan Young has shown, trauma first appeared in the medical literature in the late nineteenth century, initially as the physical expression of the sequelae of railroad accidents, and then as a psychological manifestation emerging some time after events that had been buried in the memory.[36] World War I marked a crucial turning point, with the appearance of shell shock following bombardment in the trenches, and manifested in multifaceted neuropsychiatric pictures in which the dominant symptom was a state of profound shock. Traumatic neurosis, the contemporaneous term for a set of poorly defined syndromes, gave rise to heated debates in German, British, and French psychiatry as to whether the soldiers concerned were malingerers or hysterics – in other words, whether they were consciously faking in order to avoid returning to the front and receive financial compensation, or whether they were unconsciously seeking secondary benefits that could keep them away from danger. Supporters of the malingering theory did not hesitate to use electric shocks to unmask and discourage the alleged impostors. Adherents of the hysteria theory favored suggestion or hypnosis to help the patient relive the painful experience. But whatever the interpretation of the psychological mechanism, war neurosis brought a mixture of suspicion and disapproval down on those affected. The neurotic was either weak or a scrounger; he was either afraid of returning to battle or wanted to benefit dishonestly from compensation. After the war, this distrust and discredit were transposed onto two figures: the "Muslim native," as he was called at the time, who had fought bravely and loyally under the French flag during World War I but who was portrayed as cowardly and duplicitous; and the injured worker, whose accident drew suspicion of an attempt to prolong sick leave and gain compensation for his incapacity. The former was a concern of colonial psychiatry, the latter of forensic psychiatry, and it is clear that the racial ascription in one case and the social status in the other contributed to the denigration of them.

With Richard Rechtman, I have retraced the long road that led from this rejection of the suffering of soldiers who had often either participated in or witnessed terrible or terrifying scenes to its reclassification sixty years later under the henceforth legitimate form of post-traumatic stress: we called this transformation the moral economy of trauma.[37] Indeed, with *DSM-III*, trauma moved from the shadows of suspicion and stigma into the light of recognition and compensation. It is noteworthy that the identification of this condition resulted from the concurrent, albeit separate, work of Vietnam veterans' associations seeking compensation, feminist movements condemning the denial of sexual violence, and reforming psychiatrists who had just succeeded in getting homosexuality removed from the list of mental illnesses. The reversal in the moral valence of trauma derived above all from the revision of a psychiatric dogma, since rather than being considered pathological, post-traumatic stress was now defined as a normal response to an abnormal event. In other words, the suffering individual was not sick: it was the circumstances that were aberrant. The semantic change in some sense exonerated the patients, paving the way to their recognition as victims. The US soldiers returning from Vietnam not only had legitimate reason to be traumatized by what they had experienced, been subjected to, or even subjected others to; they could thereby accede to the status of victim. Yet as we have seen, only a decade later soldiers returning from the front in the Middle East were unable to win this status. The incapacitating symptoms from which they were suffering were not recognized. Like the Vietnam veterans before them, they had once more to do battle with the experts and the administration.

But this fight, which ended in partial victory, left another aspect of the Gulf War completely overlooked – the conditions suffered by the local, mainly Iraqi, population, both military and civilian. For if half of the coalition soldiers exposed to the toxins used or released by the US army presented with disorders, what was the situation of those who continued to live in these regions contaminated with substances which sometimes have a half-life numbered in billions of years? How many Iraqis presented unexplained symptoms such as extreme fatigue, joint pain, cognitive disorders, insomnia, depression, similar to those of which the soldiers of the alliance complained, and for which the latter received compensation? Which research institutes, epidemiologists, toxicologists, or psychiatrists even inquired as to the existence of this suffering? Studies concerning the civilian population of Iraq are as few and cursory as those on Gulf War syndrome among US veterans are numerous and rigorous. Has anyone even heard this diagnosis applied to them? The only studies available are limited and controversial surveys of the effects of depleted uranium, which US army experts claim is not harmful, without offering empirical evidence from studies of populations directly exposed. However the full-scale experiment represented by the massive use of them in theater has shown a substantial increase in cancers and congenital malformations, compatible with studies of animal models.[38] Just as the number of Iraqi dead from this war cannot be counted with any greater accuracy than in the tens of thousands, no precise data is available on the consequences of the massive use of radioactive munitions among Iraqi civilian and military populations. Observing such disparities in knowledge gives a measure of the depth of the inequality of lives.

Let us conclude. In addressing epistemic boundaries, I have sought to examine the ill-defined outlines of the domains of public health. I started from one case, illustrated by childhood lead poisoning, where medicine, or, more precisely, biostatistics, produced a disease without patients, when mathematical calculation revealed the increase of certain risks among subjects who presented neither signs nor symptoms. I then inverted this reasoning to examine cases of patients without a disease, the richest example being the Gulf War syndrome, since in this case patients did not know what name or cause to ascribe to their suffering, while clinicians faced the limits of their knowledge and their imagination, with the potentially generative uncertainty of new horizons often giving way to unproductive rigidity owing to the considerable vested interests. These two configurations only appear to be symmetrical. A disease without patients, as defined by biostatistics, presents a situation that is all in all reassuring, since the estimate of risk allows for stabilization of knowledge and even a potential for action. But patients without a disease, facing the incredulity of experts, find themselves in a difficult situation, since, even when a name is put to their suffering, the context remains vague, the cause often unknown, and treatment rarely possible. To return to Canguilhem's distinction, it is clear that public health has to deal, on the one hand, with objective identification without subjectivity, that is diagnosis without suffering, and, on the other, with subjectivity without objective identification, that is suffering without a diagnosis, patients without a disease. Public health certainly has a better command of the cognitive issues in the first case than in the second, but in both cases, it must also take into account the social, political, and moral stakes, which it is much less successful in interpreting.

Conspiracy Theories
19 May 2021

Conspiracies of silence. – The expanding discourse on conspiracy theories. – The recurrent conflation of conspiracy theory and critical theory. – Post-truth, fake news, and conspiracies without a theory. – Neither condemning nor ridiculing, but understanding. – A parallel with witchcraft theories. – Universal and contextual factors. – The fertile soil of public health. – Ebola and some other epidemics. – Urban myths in rural areas. – Anti-vaccine campaigns, from one continent to another. – The disturbing revelations of a conspiracy theory around AIDS. – The heuristic value of conspiracy theories.

One remarkable aspect of the French history of childhood lead poisoning, my emblematic case study in public health, is the efforts made by the lead industry and public authorities to minimize the danger of paints containing the metal. But perhaps still more remarkable is the lead industry continuing to sell a product long known to be dangerous, and the public authorities' delay in taking decisions to regulate its use and sale. Indeed, in France, although a law passed in 1909, which was enforced six years later, had banned the use of lead white, a lead hydroxycarbonate used by decorators in the construction industry whose prohibition was already tardy, given that the substance had been known to be toxic for at least a century, it was 1926 before this regulation was extended to independent tradespeople, and 1948 before a revised labor code banned all professional use.[1] There is a general assumption, based on these rulings, that lead paints disappeared from the market at this point, theoretically limiting the buildings presumed to be unhealthy to run-down and dilapidated properties constructed before 1948. Yet they continued to be used for another several decades, and sale to private individuals was not banned until 1993. In other words, for nearly eighty years a product sufficiently toxic for workers to be forbidden to use it continued to be sold in France. Still more significantly, in the late 1980s, when the frequency and seriousness of childhood lead poisoning began to be recognized, the paint industry lobby did its best to minimize the risks of the metal. With the help of experts whose research it funded, the industry made the case that contamination of babies and children was probably due to the cultural practices of African families, among whom almost all the cases had been diagnosed; in the meantime, the Paris housing services and the National Directorate of Health proved reluctant to acknowledge the scale of the problem, and were even dubious concerning its existence. This was not, then, simple ignorance, but a conspiracy of silence.

There is, however, nothing unique about this situation – whether for the period, the national context, or the mode of contamination. In their history of childhood lead poisoning in the United States in the early twentieth century, Gerald Markowitz and David Rosner write: "The response by the lead industry to reports on the dangers of lead was a cynical thirty-five-year advertising campaign to convince people that lead was safe, and the most insidious part of this campaign was the industry's marketing to children."[2] During the 1920s, when the harmfulness of lead white was already well documented, the National Lead Company created the character of the Dutch Boy Painter, a cheerful boy in painter's overalls, a cap, and clogs, who lauded the merits of lead paint not only on walls and furniture, but also on toys and sports equipment. Meanwhile the Lead Industries Association was sending sales representatives all over the country to persuade school administrators to redecorate their buildings with lead white. It was only in the 1950s, as the Civil Rights Movement was winning its first victories against racial discrimination, that activists managed to get regulations passed banning the use of lead paint. Their campaign pointed to the harm it caused in poor neighborhoods and Black ghettos, going so far as to speak of a "silent epidemic in the slums." But these restrictions and bans were only gradually introduced, initially owing to the federated political and administrative structure of the United States, which meant that they were adopted at either federal, state, or city level, but subsequently and above all owing to the contrary pressures exerted on elected representatives by the lead lobby, which asserted that childhood lead poisoning resulted from the low level of education among parents in poor Black communities, and their failure to pay attention to their children. Here, then, the same pattern emerges – albeit in extreme form due to the segregationist racial history of the country, which radicalized inequality, and the way elections were funded, which encouraged corruption – the pattern of collusion of interests, duplicity of the elites, and victim-blaming that was evident a few decades later in France.

Moreover, the lead lobby did not stop at paint: it was also active with regard to gasoline. The dangers of tetraethyl lead, used as an anti-knock agent in vehicle fuels, had been known since it was discovered in the 1920s, when a number of fatal intoxication accidents occurred among workers handling it. But this did not stop General Motors linking up with Standard Oil to set up the Ethyl Gasoline Corporation, in order to continue developing the additive. These companies long held the monopoly on tetraethyl lead, which earned them substantial profits. From the mid-twentieth century, this dangerous additive gradually replaced lead white as the main source of income for the lead industry, which was beginning to suffer both from the information coming to light about the toxicity of its paints and from the regulations limiting its use. During the decades of economic expansion following World War II, sometimes known as the "golden age of capitalism," pollution of the air with metal particulates increased owing to the boom in automobile production and the parallel expansion of the road network, reaching a global annual emissions total of 380,000 tonnes. It was not until the mid-1970s that lead-based gasoline was finally banned in the United States, after the Ethyl Gasoline Corporation lost its legal action against the Environmental Protection Agency. The countries of the European Union, which then became the largest emitters of particulates, took much longer to adopt this measure. In France lead in gasoline remained legal until 1 January 2000, a full twenty-five years after the United States.

In addition to paints and fuels, lead was also present in the water pipes that supplied homes, which represented a major source of lead absorption for inhabitants of some cities, and throughout the food chain, from fruits covered in insecticides that contained the toxic metal to vegetables grown in contaminated soils – and including meat, thanks to cattle grazing polluted grass. For every contamination route, experts and politicians funded by the lead industry could be found who minimized or denied that lead was harmful to the human organism, particularly in the United States where the majority of the historical studies were carried out.[3] But if, as Markowitz and Rosner suggest, lead can rightly be considered "the paradigmatic toxin that linked industrial and environmental disease in the first two-thirds of the twentieth century," it was by no means the only dangerous chemical whose risks to health were systematically concealed, thanks to understandings between the worlds of economics, politics, and science. They show, for example, how the carcinogenic properties of polyvinyl chloride, or

PVC, a synthetic polymer widely used throughout the world, were deliberately dissimulated by the Manufacturing Chemists' Association, a lobby that was heavily invested in the promotion and defense of plastics. In these various cases, which represent just a few on a long list of products whose dangers have been concealed (the best known being tobacco and asbestos), we are dealing, according to Markowitz and Rosner, with genuine "schemes," what they call "secret agreements" made at the expense of or counter to public interest.[4] These conspiracies have been proven: the archives reveal the criminal agreements. We can, then, speak of true conspiracies conducted by unscrupulous captains of industry, corrupt politicians, and mercenary scientists whose actions are not just violations of the law but also criminal practices, because they cynically put the lives of individuals at risk. These actions should therefore be called what they are: authentic conspiracies that cause harm to public health.

But today the word "conspiracy" has lost its condemnatory power. There was no talk of conspiracies in the German automobile industry when Volkswagen falsified data on the polluting emissions of its vehicle engines, at the risk of an increase in childhood asthma; or of conspiracies in the French construction industry when construction company Eternit used asbestos to insulate buildings, despite the fact that it had been known for several decades to cause pleural cancer in those exposed.[5] Legal language terms this "fraud," which only describes the act, and everyday language uses "scandal," which refers to the consequences, but not of "conspiracy," which would point to the networks and mechanisms responsible for these frauds and scandals.

What has changed in today's parlance is the way the term "conspiracy" is used. It is invoked to criticize not those who conspire, but those who falsely assert conspiracies. To suggest a conspiracy is to risk being oneself called a conspiracy theorist, a term created precisely to discredit this designation. For the word is now pejoratively linked with the word "theory," thereby removing any sense of veracity or even any plausibility it might have. In common understanding, a conspiracy theory is a barely credible, often dishonest scaffolding that presents an erroneous picture of the world. It declares the existence of a conspiracy where there is none. It asserts that the powerful are concealing the truth of their malign intentions when this is not the case. In a sense it is a social pathology, to use a nineteenth-century expression, which some even give the psychiatric designation of paranoia.[6] There is, to be sure, no shortage of examples of such imaginaries of plots. We therefore need to start from these cases in order to understand conspiracy theories in their generality and their complexity, before addressing the many that concern public health – the domain where they have, for a long time, most proliferated.

The example most frequently cited concerns the 9/11 attacks in the United States in 2001. There are multiple conspiracy theories around this event.[7] Some believed that it was not a plane that crashed into the Pentagon in Washington, but a missile launched by elements of the US military, and that it was not the two planes that caused the Twin Towers to collapse in New York, but bombs placed inside the buildings that exploded, thus implicating enemies within in both events. Others held that the US government, or some of its intelligence agencies, or even the Israeli secret services, knew about the planned attacks or had even organized them, either to help an internally weakened US president to hold onto power, or to justify subsequent attacks on Afghanistan and Iraq, or, finally, to gain control of oil in the Middle East. Whatever the variations, all these theories have in common that they evoke a double layer of conspiracy. They assert on one level the existence of a conspiracy, that is the complicity of actors carrying out a malign plan, and on a second level the existence of a conspiracy to ensure that the existence of this conspiracy is not detected – that is, the connivance of those who have access to both the information and public space. In short, a political conspiracy and a media conspiracy. In an indication of this lexical evolution, a study of the frequency of occurrence of words and groups of words in print sources over long periods, using the Ngram Viewer software, shows that the phrase *"théorie du complot"* first appears in the French corpus in the 1970s, and sees a meteoric rise up to the 2000s. The same pattern is observed for the phrase "conspiracy theory" in the English corpus two decades earlier. Conversely, there is a decline in the use of the separate terms "complot" and "conspiracy" in the respective corpuses. Thus conspiracy theories replaced conspiracies, with the result that it has become difficult to name operations that genuinely take the form of plots against the public good.

We might indeed wonder whether there is a proliferation of conspiracy theories in the contemporary world, and perhaps even an increase in people's willingness to believe in them.[8] On the one hand, from the Great Replacement Theory that was hatched in France and rapidly spread through far-right circles in Europe and North America, and alleges that African or Muslim immigration threatens Western Christian civilization, to the theory of an international Zionist conspiracy that also circulates on the extreme right, and holds that Jewish lobbies control the governments of the world's great powers, conspiracy theories seem to be booming. However, we should not forget that the Great Replacement Theory was already present in nationalist circles in the late nineteenth and early twentieth centuries, particularly in France, with Édouard Drumont and Maurice Barrès, the difference being that, at that time, it focused primarily on Jews, and that the theory of the Zionist conspiracy reached its peak of popularity during the same period, with the anti-Semitic fake *The Protocols of the Elders of Zion* and the propaganda that followed Theodor Herzl's first Zionist Congress. But we could also go back to the Middle Ages, and the allegations of ritual murders by Jews.[9] In reality, it is difficult to measure developments in substance, and rather than tendencies, what can be observed are iterations, and above all the recurring structures of these paranoid forms. On the other hand, it would seem that very large segments of the population are increasingly receptive to conspiracy theories. In January 2018, their supposed infiltration of French society made the front page of most of France's mainstream national media, on the basis of a survey according to which eight out of ten French people gave credence to conspiracy theories. The highest rates of credulity were observed among low-income groups with low levels of education, and at either end of the political spectrum. With few exceptions, the journalists did not trouble themselves to interrogate the method, particularly the validity of paid online surveys where the fantasist and even provocative nature of some responses is well documented. Nor did they question the proportion of respondents who said they had never heard of the theories they were asked about, but were not given the option to state they had no opinion; the way a simple expression of doubt about events that might still be the subject of inquiry was assimilated to deviant belief; or the mixture of types of theory, with creationism and flat-earthism included on the same basis as the existence of secret societies that caused the French Revolution. Paradoxically, thanks to its reverberations, this survey contributed to what it claimed to condemn, the creation of a climate of conspiracy theory, by artificially amplifying the reality of the phenomenon.[10] Moreover, by disparaging low-income groups, it fed into populist arguments against elites, and by tarring two extremes with the same brush, it contributed to the frequent and pernicious confusion between critical theory and conspiracy theory. It is, then, certainly important to avoid any form of moral panic, the false or exaggerated perception of a nonconforming cultural phenomenon that is fanned by some of the media and exploited by various politicians,[11] for this has a performative effect, giving the phenomenon in question a much greater weight than it merits.

A more rigorous analysis is therefore required. And to begin with, do we actually know what a conspiracy theory is? The term was, if not coined, at least popularized by Karl Popper in *The Open Society and Its Enemies*. The book was first published in 1945 but not translated into French until 1979, and it is therefore no surprise that the phrase "conspiracy theory" emerged in the English lexical corpus in the 1950s, but that its French equivalent, "*théorie du complot*," only appears two decades later.[12] According to Popper, these theories tend to explain prejudicial social phenomena such as war, unemployment, poverty, and shortages as the result of the operation of hidden mechanisms that benefit the powerful. They combine three essential elements: the existence of an unwelcome situation, the systematic search for concealed causes, and the revelation of the play of interests and powers. According to Popper, it is essential to note that this conclusion derives from a mistaken analysis: the theory is false, and there is no conspiracy. But contrary to what might be imagined, conspiracy theories as Popper understands them are not popular beliefs: they are scientific theories, and when he talks of the "conspiracy theory of society," he is primarily targeting Marxist and neo-Marxist thought. In this thought, he writes, "the Homeric gods whose conspiracies explain the history of the Trojan war are abandoned," and "their place is filled by the monopolists, or the capitalists, or the imperialists." In other words, Popper is the first in a long line of those who confuse critical theory with conspiracy theory, or more precisely endeavor to discredit critical theory by presenting it as a conspiracy theory. But this polemical position should not come as any surprise from one who formerly held communist sympathies but had, by the time he was developing this thesis, become a fervent neoliberal, close to Friedrich Hayek and Milton Friedman, with whom he founded the influential Mont Pelerin Society in 1947.

But this confusion between conspiracy theory and critical theory is not consigned to the past. It resurfaced during the 2000s, particularly following the publication of an article titled "Why has critique run out of steam?" in which Bruno Latour asked whether, in the contemporary world, it was "really the task of the humanities to add deconstruction to destruction" through their systematic recourse to critical thinking.[13] Drawing on anecdotes, one concerning a strategist of the Republican party who stated he was unconvinced by scientific evidence of climate change, and another a neighbor in his village in the French Bourbonnais region who assured him that Mossad and the CIA were behind the 9/11 attacks, he called into question the role of researchers who, like him, had continually expressed doubt about the facts as we see them – though this was surely an optimistic evaluation of the impact social sciences have on Fox News commentators and farmers in the Allier region. Taking up Pierre Bourdieu and Michel Foucault, he asked what, ultimately, distinguishes their critical thinking from that of conspiracy theorists, since "in both cases, you have to learn to become suspicious of everything people say because of course we all know that they live in the thralls of a complete *illusio* of their real motives." Quite apart from the willed confusion between conspiracy theories and critical theory that aims to discredit the latter by assimilating it to the nebulous discourse of the former, it might be remarked that, from an analytical point of view, it is questionable whether the intellectual processes of these two authors can be amalgamated, given that they are not just very different, but almost incompatible. In fact, Bourdieu, the distant inheritor of Marxist theory, seeks to restore a hidden truth by revealing the work done by the ideology of domination, while Foucault, inspired by Nietzsche, strives to understand how truth is produced in a given context without prejudging what is true and what is not.[14] Bourdieu produces a social critique, and Foucault a genealogical one. Without lingering over this distinction, Latour's article announces the death of critical theory and advocates a return to realism. His proposal had immediate widespread impact in North America, particularly in the humanities, where people were receptive to the idea that critique had certainly gone too far; meanwhile in France, the link between conspiracy theories and critical theory resonated with a number of authors, particularly, but not only, in conservative circles.[15] In many people's view, it was time to emancipate ourselves from this way of reading the world, dubbed "the hermeneutics of suspicion," a phrase wrongly attributed to Paul Ricœur, who, on the contrary, celebrates the three "masters of suspicion," as he calls them – Marx, Nietzsche, and Freud – for the way their thinking gives access to a deeper truth.[16] There is thus an important clarification to be made: the fact that conspiracy thinking often incorporates a critical aspect does not mean that, conversely, critical thinking can be assimilated to a form of conspiratorial reasoning. The conflation of the two stems from a will to discredit any attempt to question the social order of things.

But let us return to Popper's seminal text, which many philosophers and political scientists have attempted to develop by analyzing conspiracy theories not, like Popper, in the academic sphere, but among ordinary citizens – in other words, as a societal issue. How are we to understand, if not the rise, at least the persistence and the vitality of conspiracy theories in a world where it had been imagined that rationality would triumph and transparency reign? Drawing on a study of the Oklahoma city bombing in 1995, in which a group of white supremacists detonated a truck bomb outside a federal government building, killing 168 people, Brian Keeley considers the fascination a certain section of the population held for a conspiracy theory suggesting that, in fact, those behind this attack were powerful actors belonging to the Clinton administration or the CIA and FBI.[17] This fascination, Keeley argues, is at once political because it involves opposing the official account, moral in that it claims to expose malign projects, and logical since the explanations put forward purport to shed light on allegedly shadowy aspects of the case and offer a plausible overall frame of interpretation. This threefold fascination is a feature of most conspiracy theories.

The big question, however, remains the distinction between conspiracy and conspiracy theory. This distinction is generally considered to go without saying: in the first case, there is indeed a conspiracy; in the second, the conspiracy is imaginary. But, Charles Pigden asks, are we sure things are that simple, and would it not be useful to look more closely before we reject a discourse that asserts the existence of a conspiracy by dismissing it as a conspiracy theory, and therefore presumed false?[18] We might think of the charge that Russian secret service hackers interfered in the US presidential elections in favor of a candidate over whom the Kremlin had influence – a charge depicted by that candidate, who became president, as a conspiracy theory, despite the fact that the CIA, the FBI, and six other US intelligence agencies confirmed this involvement. Or the alliances between politicians, bankers, lobbyists, and manufacturers that helped to fund election campaigns in return for tax benefits and financial deregulation and whose condemnation is derided by those involved as an imagined conspiracy despite the evidence gathered by journalists and judicial inquiries. And then, Pigden goes on, are we even sure that an actual conspiracy is a bad thing? We might point here to the attempts, successful or not, to overthrow dangerous or corrupt heads of state in Zimbabwe and Venezuela, or to oust them legally in the United States and Israel. Nevertheless, Steve Clarke observes, there are good grounds for taking a skeptical attitude to conspiracy theories on principle, because they generally involve what psychologists call "attribution error."[19] But this distrust should not prevent us from recognizing that they are to some degree useful, both because they challenge orthodox disciplines, forcing them to improve the way they offer proofs, and because they contribute to keeping society open to public debate – and even because, sometimes, they help to reveal real conspiracies.

However, this moderately optimistic reading has been seriously damaged by the normalization of a discourse that appears to take the form of conspiracy theories, particularly in the United States, where it has become a mode of government that some have called "post-truth" fed by "fake news." There was no shortage of examples during the mandate of a Twitter-happy president of the United States when, in July 2020, the *Washington Post* counted 20,000 false statements in the 1,267 days he had spent at the White House, an average of twelve per day.[20] According to Russel Muirhead and Nancy Rosenblum a new kind of conspiracy theorizing has appeared, with, for example, the discourse of the "birthers" aimed at discrediting Barack Obama by falsely claiming that he was born in Kenya and was Muslim, and Donald Trump's denunciations of a "deep state" constituted of alleged hidden forces in the intelligence services who sought to bring him down.[21] This new phenomenon corresponds, for Muirhead and Rosenblum, to conspiracies without theory, since there is no real vision of the world as there is in the conspiracy theories that have developed over time. But this new term may not really be so useful. First, from the point of view of the speaker, when a person or group knowingly makes an untrue statement, it is perhaps more accurate to describe it simply as a lie, even if we agree that in practice it may be difficult to identify as such. Second, from the point of view of the audience, not only are the alleged conspiracies often taken to be true, but they generally fit into an implicit theory, whether it is white supremacism in the case of the "birthers," or vehement anti-federalism in the case of the "deep state." The more fruitful avenue of research would then be to explore this clash between the former's lie and the latter's belief, or even simply the question of the public's adherence to conspiracy theories, whether or not those promoting them are sincere.

This is where anthropologists and sociologists differ somewhat from philosophers and political theorists. Discussions of the definition and evaluation of conspiracy theories, as propounded by the latter, certainly have their worth, but social sciences pose the questions in other terms. The issue is less to examine what conspiracy theories are, what part of truth they may contain, what deleterious impact or alternatively potential benefit for society they may have, than to seek to understand what they mean, or, to put it another way, what they tell us about the world. These theories exist, they speak of real or imaginary conspiracies and thereby also speak about contemporary societies. It is therefore important to understand them. While many commentators condemn them as dangerous or ridicule them as absurd, anthropologists and sociologists consider them as social objects to be taken seriously on the same level as religious rituals, political institutions, moral values, and scientific practices. For they are windows onto the world that can help us to see it from other points of view.

But it is important here to avoid taking a purely Western view of a series of recent phenomena while ignoring equivalents in other contexts and other times. This calls for a geographical and historical decentering: conspiracy theories are no more restricted to the contemporary period than they are to the European and North American world. A more judicious view would surely suggest that, in the long term and over a wide range of societies, there is an interpretative structure common to many of them in which the occurrence of misfortune is perceived as a persecution perpetrated by powerful beings operating in secret. The paradigmatic, and probably also the oldest and most widespread form, is witchcraft. Having studied theories of witchcraft around sickness in Senegal in the 1980s, and conspiracy theories around AIDS in South Africa in the 2000s, I am struck by the structural similarities between the two phenomena. In both cases, there is a search for a causal explanation involving malign entities acting in the shadows, and the capacity to create networks of evidence that ultimately support the establishment of an accusatory system – with the significant difference that accusations of witchcraft incriminate the vulnerable (often older people), while conspiracies implicate the powerful (in the case of AIDS in South Africa, whites, the pharmaceutical industry, or Western countries). One significant feature is that both witchcraft theories and conspiracy theories are semantically and semiotically saturated: they incorporate an excess of signifieds and signifiers. This is what makes them particularly attractive. They make sense in the context in which they are articulated. They explain, in the first case, why a misfortune has occurred and, in the second, why an agent or group is acting as they are. But they also reveal themselves through signs and symptoms to those who know how to look for them. They make it possible to decode these signs, establishing that the situation has not come about by chance, and to assemble them in a configuration that leads to the discovery of those responsible. Clearly this exposure has an ethical significance, since it supposedly unmasks harmful individuals who can then be rendered incapable of harm.

But if we confine the discussion to conspiracy theories themselves, a question arises: what makes so many people susceptible to these ideas, which often seem so implausible to outside observers? How can some people be so easily persuaded that reports of men landing on the moon were lies designed to make people believe the United States had scored a decisive victory over the Soviet Union in the space race, that climate change is an invention of environmentalist lobbies or the Chinese government aimed at weakening the oil industry and the US economy, or that senior figures in the US Democratic Party, including

Hillary Clinton, meet in a Washington pizzeria to conduct Satanic rituals and child trafficking? What is it that makes people, or at least some people, believe these ideas? There is certainly more than one answer to this question, and the scientific literature offers plentiful and widely varying explanations. Within this copious literature, we can draw a line between universal factors, which are presumed to hold for all eras and all societies, and contextual factors, which depend on the historical moment and the sociological conditions.

The factors presumed to be universal are generally cognitive, related to general epistemic and psychological mechanisms. It is posited that the human mind seeks to reduce uncertainty and contradiction by producing explanations that link facts to one another and make sense of them, as Karen Douglas and co-authors show.[22] This attitude is particularly evident among people who, first, systematically search for a meaning in events and correlations between them, and, second, overestimate their capacity to account for complex and confusing realities. Conspiracy theories have the power to connect apparently unconnected points, to detect details that have gone unnoticed and to propose seemingly coherent interpretations. They order the world, and they do so in a way that is doubly seductive. First, they stand against the authority of the generally accepted version, which is then pejoratively termed the "official" version. Second, they expose obscure machinations and thus give their supporters the feeling they are discovering the "hidden face" of things. They are therefore paradoxically valorizing and reassuring, even when they involve fearsome cartels or frightening plots. These individual logics are reinforced by collective understandings, studied by Cass Sunstein and Adrian Vermeule.[23] At the level of groups, such as political parties or social networks, there are various mechanisms that help to consolidate conspiracy theories. There are selection mechanisms, based on affinity, that lead to concentration thanks to a dual process that combines recruitment of sympathizers and exclusion of dissidents with the reinforcement of extreme positions, resulting in a polarization within groups. But whether individual or collective, these supposedly universal factors still do not explain why, at certain points in history or in certain categories of society, conspiracy theories are particularly prevalent.

Contextual factors are therefore essential to understanding, particularly with respect to the contemporary period. These factors can be roughly divided into two types, historical and sociological. First, from a historical point of view, some periods are more conducive to the hatching of conspiracy theories: a case in point would be the frenzy of McCarthyism, which led Richard Hofstadter to develop his pioneering analysis of what he called the "paranoid style" in politics.[24] In the current era, a number of factors come into play. Distrust of governments has increased thanks to the visibility of state lies, whether in France (with declarations about the cloud from Chernobyl in 1986, which was supposed to have stopped at the Franco-German border, or about police violence during the "Yellow Vest" demonstrations in 2019, which the government said had not occurred despite photographic evidence), or in China (with the Communist Party's statements contesting the emergence of SARS, the Severe Acute Respiratory Syndrome, which killed 349 people in the country, or refuting the existence of Uighur detention camps in 2018, despite the United Nations report documenting them). At the same time, news media feed paranoid ideas, with the uncovering in the United States of more and more sophisticated global surveillance systems following Edward Snowden's revelations about the National Security Agency, which is in charge of domestic intelligence, and evidence of increasingly efficient control of elections by economic and financial agents, which is now legally sanctioned following the Supreme Court's "Citizens United" ruling named for the conservative organization that won the decision that funding of electoral campaigns by private groups is unrestricted and undisclosed. More generally, the loss of trust in political institutions, the sense of an absence of transparency nourished by scandals, and the idea that truth is relative, or faked, tend to encourage belief in conspiracy theories.[25] In addition, there is a crucial technological dimension, with the development of the internet and social media networks that enable both the real-time dissemination of information and the constitution of communities around conspiracy theories. Second, from a sociological point of view, some social categories are more susceptible to these, particularly marginalized, discriminated, or ostracized social or ethnic groups, who often find in these theories explanations for their subordinate position, and confirmation of their suspicions about the dominant. In South Africa, Jean and John Comaroff show how accusations of witchcraft have proliferated among those who have lost out in the expansion of neoliberalism.[26] Compared to the study of universal epistemic or psychological factors, which seeks to decode cognitive mechanisms and group logics, analysis of contextual factors, both historical and sociological, offers much greater potential for new understandings of contemporary societies.

As an arena where conspiracy theories are particularly prevalent, public health is a rich domain in this regard. But it should be noted from the outset that this is not a new phenomenon. In the plague epidemic of 1348, Jews were blamed, and Carlo Ginzburg relates: "On 16 May, the Jewish community of La Baume, a small Provençal village, was exterminated. This event was just one link in a long chain of violence unleashed in southern France by the appearance of the Black Death, in April of that year." Indeed, "hostility toward Jews, who many believed guilty of spreading the epidemic by poisoning wells, springs and rivers, first came to a head in Toulon during Holy Week. The ghetto was attacked and men, women and children were killed."[27] During the cholera epidemic of 1830, it was the powerful who were suspected, and Jacques Piquemal notes wryly: "The hunt for the 'poisoners' began at certain crossroads, and might have raised a still restive mob, disappointed by the July Revolution, against the government. Fortunately a few members of the bourgeoisie developed cholera: the prime minister himself died, and the working-class neighborhoods quietened down."[28] Conspiracy theories thus emerge as a recurrent historical phenomenon at times of epidemics; in the face of the collective misfortune such epidemics represent, people search for culprits, on levels that vary with the context, since those incriminated may equally well be marginal or excluded groups, as in the case of the plague, or the wealthy and public figures, as in the case of the cholera outbreak.

More recently in Liberia, at the start of the Ebola epidemic in 2014, President Ellen Johnson Sirleaf was initially suspected of having invented the disease to attract international funding, and then, conversely, but by a similar logic, of having herself enlisted the country's nurses to spread the virus. Later, when President Barack Obama decided to send US troops to set up field hospitals in the country and Liberians began to see US soldiers in the streets, similar accusations emerged, for they were suspected of spreading the infection or using it for secret purposes. Rumor had it that the United States was pursuing various aims, including overthrowing the government, enriching its pharmaceutical industry by introducing a vaccine, or even preventing the population from selling Ebola-contaminated blood to Al-Qaida members who might use it in future biological warfare. Commentators and journalists did not always escape this conspiracy-theory reading of the Ebola epidemic. The well-known journalist and biologist Helen Epstein, for example, wrote an article titled "Liberia: The hidden truth about Ebola," in which she asked why international organizations, experts, and the media maintained alarmist discourses about the epidemic when the number of cases was falling, and suggested that this "disinformation" hid a desire on the part of some to damage the image of Africans, deemed as they often are to be bearers of threats to the world that they themselves are incapable of dealing with. A few weeks later she published a second article, "Ebola in Liberia: An epidemic of rumors," in which she recounted the local theories accusing the Liberian and US governments, but this time she discredited them.[29] She had thus shifted from denouncing a conspiracy to criticizing conspiracy theories.

In the early 1990s, I myself fell victim to conspiracy theories while I was conducting research, in collaboration with Anne-Claire Defossez, on disparities in maternal mortality in Ecuador. As I noted above, at that time, the WHO depicted the country as having one of the highest rates of death during pregnancy, childbirth, and the forty-two days following in the American continent.[30] In order to begin my research in Cotopaxi, a poor Andean province, I had to negotiate with the leaders of local Quechua organizations. They granted me the right to conduct my research on the condition that I provide basic medical instruction to the women in their communities, which I willingly agreed to do. At the women's request, I began with classes on contraception. A few months later, although my research and teaching were going well, I learned that I was no longer welcome in the region. This was admittedly a period of high tension nationally, following what was known as the *levantamiento indígena*, an Indian uprising that took the form of mass protests throughout the country against the oppression of the Indian population and discrimination they suffered. Two major highways were blocked, markets were no longer supplied, churches were peacefully occupied, soldiers sent to restore order were taken prisoner, and the inhabitants of cities, most of them white or mixed race, were living in fear that marches on the regional capitals would descend into violence against them.[31] In this context, I imagined that I had become undesirable because I was being likened to the city-dwellers against whom this hostility was directed. This was no doubt the case, but there was a more specific reason for my being rejected.

In my previous research I had already observed that contraception was a sensitive and complex subject around which there was both a high demand, since increasing numbers of young couples wanted to limit the number of children they had, and a great deal of distrust, revealed by a series of rumors that circulated in these communities. There was, for instance, talk of cases where women fitted with an intrauterine device still became pregnant and gave birth to children with one eye, or the cranium pierced by the device. An increase in cervical cancer was also attributed to smear tests, as it was after having them that women were informed of their pathology. Finally, people suspected that the family planning campaigns being rolled out through the country were aimed at reducing the demographic weight of Indians in the population, in order to weaken their cultural and political presence. At the time of the uprising, the criticism of the white and mixed-race majority, often subsumed under the term *gringos*, had reactivated what are generally described as "urban myths," although in this case they always emerged in rural areas. In the Andean communities where I was working the leaders had made an admittedly fairly logical link between my research, my classes on reproduction and women's health, and the rumors around contraception and cancer. Impervious to the fact that my study was focused on inequality and forgetting that the classes I was giving were in response to their request, they now saw my presence as vindication of their fear of the outside world. Individual questions about women's reproductive health became collective issues concerning the reproduction of the group. It took several weeks of negotiation and the intercession of a colleague who had worked in the region for a long time before I was able to resume my work. But this anecdote must be read from the historical viewpoint of the despoliation of Indian lands in the Andes, which continued throughout the twentieth century, of authoritarian health programs and dubious medical research, of family planning campaigns and obstetric practices that had little regard for women's dignity, modesty, or even their rights – precisely what was uncovered by our research. Significantly, the Indian uprising came two years before the celebration of the 500th anniversary of the supposed discovery of America, which activists had renamed *Quinientos años de resistencia indígena*, Five Hundred Years of Indigenous Resistance. In other words, the persecutory interpretations that had led my interlocutors to eject me were set within a genealogy of abuse that they, their parents, and their ancestors had genuinely suffered. Conspiracy theories and actual conspiracies were closely entangled.

I was once again reminded of this a few months later, with the outbreak of a cholera epidemic. When the health teams visited the Andean communities looking for people infected, the sick were taken away and hidden by their relatives so that they would not be taken to the hospital where, it was said, they would be left to die and their bodies then not returned. This belief had its roots in the draconian measures adopted and the brutal interventions conducted during previous epidemics. Cholera patients were forcibly removed from their homes, and hospitalized in unsanitary conditions. Their families were prohibited from visiting them, and, when the sick died, they were prevented from conducting funeral rites around the deceased in order to avoid further contagion. The conclusion drawn by the Quechua was that the aim of public health was to stem the disease by eliminating patients. As Charles Briggs observed when the epidemic hit Venezuela, the Warao there also interpreted it as deriving from the intention to eradicate them, but they adapted the theory to the local context. They believed that the reopening of old oil wells and the drilling of new ones by British Petroleum in the Orinoco delta where they lived had contributed to the emergence of cholera or had even caused it, going so far as to imagine that the water had been deliberately poisoned.[32] According to Briggs, these accounts combined real and imagined facts, constructing the specter of genocide on the reality of a political economy. While the Venezuelan government and the multinational corporation were not seeking to exterminate the Indians, they still found their presence inconvenient. The aggressive health practices of the former and the environmental indifference manifested by the latter had deleterious consequences for the Warao, whose suspicions of malign intent clearly resonated with their experience.

The public health interventions that arouse the greatest mistrust and generate the most conspiracy theories, in all countries and all social categories, are vaccinations. Opposition to vaccines is certainly nothing new. In 1910 William Osler, a famous Canadian doctor, ironically proposed a "challenge to the anti-vaccine campaigners," in which he would go into a smallpox epidemic accompanied by ten vaccinated and ten unvaccinated persons, specifying that the latter should consist of "three members of parliament, three anti-vaccination doctors, and four anti-vaccination propagandists." He added that when they fell sick he would look after them "like brothers" and even promised to arrange the funerals of the "four or five who are certain to die."[33] Since the 2000s, campaigns against vaccines have proliferated in the context of rumors, often fed by questionable scientific studies and generally amplified by circulation on social media. Following the publication in 1998 of a British study, which hit the headlines but was subsequently not only contradicted by a number of others, but also recognized as fraudulent and ultimately withdrawn by the journal in which it was published – the study established a link between the measles-mumps-rubella (MMR) vaccine and the onset of colitis and autism – the vaccine has been widely boycotted, leading to a resurgence of the infections targeted by this immunization. In January 2019, the governor of Washington state declared a state-wide emergency following the outbreak of a measles epidemic in one county.[34] In a similar vein, two Californian researchers sparked controversy in 1993 when they attributed the AIDS epidemic to the polio vaccine; although the theory was refuted by a series of later studies, it spread throughout the African continent, relayed by Western journalists and filmmakers, and generated a mistrust of the vaccine at the very time when the World Health Organization had embarked on a program for definitive eradication of polio throughout the world. As a direct consequence of this challenge, in 2003 Muslim authorities, both religious and medical, in Kano, Zamfara, and Kaduna states in northern Nigeria, asserted that Western powers had infected the polio vaccine with HIV and had contaminated it with substances aimed at reducing fertility. These statements led to a fall in immune coverage in the region and a resurgence of polio, of which Nigeria had 45 percent of the world's recorded cases at this time.[35] Remarkably, then, this suspicion of vaccines often has its origin in scientific studies. Given this culture of distrust of vaccination, it is easy to understand the outrage in international public health circles when it was discovered that in order to assassinate Osama bin Laden, the CIA had organized a fake immunization campaign in the village where he lived, with the help of a Pakistani doctor, in order to secure the DNA of relatives in his residence and thus confirm that this was indeed his family.[36] This precaution had been considered necessary because of the risks run by US soldiers. But once again, the conspiracy theory found confirmation in a genuine conspiracy.

The disease that has given rise to the largest number of conspiracy theories is AIDS, and the country that has seen the most striking dissemination of them is South Africa – although they have flourished throughout the world since the epidemic first arose.[37] In the early 1990s South Africa seemed so little impacted by the disease that researchers were formulating hypotheses to explain this exception. A decade later, the country had become the worst affected, with alarming statistics reporting an estimated 4.5 million people infected, representing over 10 percent of the world's total cases and more than a tenth of the South African population. A demographic projection predicted that average life expectancy would fall by twenty years within two decades – a projection that was later revised to the even more troubling prediction that this would affect only the Black population. Some were already putting forward dystopian visions of Black people, who then constituted four-fifths of South African citizens, becoming a minority in their country. At this time powerful antiretroviral treatments had already been developed, but their prohibitive cost restricted them to rich nations. No African country then had the means to take on such expenditure, and the only hope of treatment was, for a small fraction of patients, to be recruited into a randomized clinical trial – provided, of course, that they were among those benefiting from the most effective antiretrovirals. To add further complication to this tragic situation, the epidemiological crisis was accompanied by an epistemic crisis.

At the beginning of my research, in April 2008, I interviewed a friend who held a senior post in an international agency in Pretoria.

He showed me a fax he had just received. It was a copy of a confidential letter addressed by President Thabo Mbeki, who had succeeded Nelson Mandela, to a number of heads of state and the Secretary General of the United Nations. It concerned the panel of scientists the president had invited to discuss the current state of the AIDS epidemic, and expressed his outrage at the hostile reaction to his initiative as his guests included all of the world's researchers who held dissident positions on AIDS – mostly US and European scientists who asserted that the virus was not the cause of the disease and that antiretrovirals were therefore useless and even harmful. In the weeks that followed the letter being made public, the meeting of experts was held in a tense environment, but despite several months of protest from nongovernmental organizations and the biomedical community, the Thirteenth International Conference on AIDS, which had been scheduled in Africa for the first time, took place as planned in Durban. Throughout these three months Thabo Mbeki intervened in various forums to express his doubts about what almost all experts throughout the world deemed established knowledge. At the opening of the conference in Durban, he even stated that, in his view, given the rapid progress of the infection of Africa, the only possible explanation was the endemic poverty that reigned in the continent.

During this period the debate was so polarized that neither orthodox researchers, who believed in a viral cause, nor the heterodox, who supported a social etiology, could conceive that the two factors might be associated – something that had been known in the case of tuberculosis for over a century, and that was eventually recognized, a decade later, in the case of AIDS. The dual process of concentration and polarization, which, as noted above, tends to consolidate conspiracy theories, was operating more broadly through the entire public space, leading to reciprocal reinforcement of the two sides' positions. In this situation, the more researchers, advocacy organizations, and politicians hardened their criticisms of the president, the more he elaborated conspiracy theories. Exceptionally virulent charges were leveled by Mbeki, his health minister, and supporters in his party, against the pharmaceutical industry, which was accused first of setting prohibitive prices for poor countries and then of using Third World patients as guinea pigs, against white opponents, denounced for their hostility toward the democratic government and their racism against the Black population, and finally against public health, international experts, and the Western world. The denial of the authorities, then, was augmented by what most saw as a conspiracy theory.

The majority of interpretations of the contestatory, challenging stance adopted by a president whose abilities had until then been recognized, fell into one of two camps. Some saw it as the expression of a paranoid character or even mental illness, which Mbeki himself had joked about when the panel of experts was established, introducing himself as the "madman" who would tell scientists the truth they were not seeing. Others saw Mbeki's strange dissidence as a skillful tactic to divide the nation and rally his troops around simple messages, and it has to be acknowledged that if this was the case, the maneuver was undoubtedly successful, since his electoral results were even more spectacular than those of Mandela. But these two explanations, one psychiatric and the other political, fail to explain why, as opinion polls showed, a large majority of South Africans, especially Blacks, subscribed to his theories – and not only among low-income communities but also in the academic sphere. By no means all of his supporters adopted his heretical theories on AIDS, but all were sensitive to the question of social etiology, the condemnation of persistent racism, and the expression of doubts about medicine – three elements at the heart of the discourse maintained by the president and his close collaborators. It was thus possible to believe in a conspiracy without denying the role of the virus and the effectiveness of antiretrovirals. So, rather than yielding to the usual alternative between ridicule and rage that was typical of public debate around AIDS, it seemed to me that it was essential to seek to understand.

The historical heritage of public health is particularly painful in South Africa.[38] During the plague epidemic of 1900, the Public Health Amendment Act, passed in 1897, was used in cities to put in place the first official spatial segregation measures, with the construction of "native locations," the forerunners of the townships. Black residents were relegated to these areas, on the alleged grounds that they were spreading the disease, despite the fact that statistics later showed that actually fewer of them were infected than whites. In the following years, syphilis, which up to that point was not racially differentiated, was made into a marker of the "Black peril": Black women were stigmatized for their alleged inclination toward licentiousness and prostitution, and Black men for their supposed proclivity for sexual assault and rape. During the same period, tuberculosis, which had not existed among African populations prior to the end of the nineteenth century, became widespread among them: workers in the gold and diamond mines were crammed together in shacks where infection spread rapidly, and were then sent back to their villages where they infected their families. With apartheid, from 1948 on, the healthcare system was split into four separate entities for each of the four so-called racial groups, with Blacks having the least well-equipped and least effective provisions in the townships and Bantustans. When the first AIDS cases appeared in the early 1990s, the stereotypes of Black people's supposed sexual voraciousness, which informed Western researchers throughout Africa, even in countries where infection rates were low, re-emerged. The fantasy image of *Homo sexualis africanus*, to use Gilles Bibeau's ironic formula, prompted Thabo Mbeki's most virulent diatribes against whites, who saw blacks as "natural-born, promiscuous carriers of germs."[39] In low-income neighborhoods the acronym for the disease was ironically expanded to "Afrikaner Invention to Deprive us of Sex." Thus, for over a century, public health had been a tool of discrimination against, and domination of, the Black population, and was now distrusted for this reason.

This instrumentalization was set within a broader context of domination. The fantasy of eradicating the Black population hovered over apartheid, to the extent that white supremacist representatives in the corridors of parliament could gloat that AIDS might achieve what their policies had been unable to. Not that they had not tried.[40] In 1998, during the final sessions of the Truth and Reconciliation Commission, the existence of a Chemical and Biological War program was discovered, prompting the opening of a new chapter of the inquiry. The six hundred pages of the resulting report are edifying. They recount, in direct quotations from those who conducted the program themselves, how during the 1990s a secret laboratory, directed by military doctor Wouter Basson, used anthrax bacteria to eliminate political adversaries, injected cholera bacteria into wells in refugee camps in neighboring countries, imagined toxic substances presumed to act only on Black people, and had even embarked on a project to contaminate prostitutes in brothels in Black neighborhoods with the AIDS virus so that they would infect their clients – a project that was halted with the return of democracy.[41] The crimes of the man popularly known as Dr. Death were judged too serious to benefit from amnesty, and Basson was tried in the Pretoria High Court on sixty-seven charges of his responsibility for 229 murders. To the shock of many observers, the judge, Willie Hartzenberg, whose brother was leader of the Conservative Party, the white supremacist party of the apartheid years, acquitted the man a journalist had called "our country's Doctor Mengele." Thus exonerated despite the confessions of his colleagues, Basson then embarked on a new career as a cardiologist in one of the capital's main hospitals. The revelations of the trial, which the press had covered in detail over months, had nourished conspiracy theories. The acquittal only served to confirm and reinforce them.

When I was conducting my research in the townships and Bantustans of South Africa, public space and private conversations were alive with these sinister stories, which revealed the genocidal ideas of some in the white minority. Occasionally I heard people talk of macabre projects with scenarios that were partly reinvented as they were communicated from one person to another, such as the rumor that HIV was being injected into oranges to spread the disease. And often, in poor neighborhoods, the topic would resurface in interviews that those in power – yesterday white, today Black – were seeking to get rid of this surplus population of people who were of no use to the world, unproductive when they were in good health, costly to care for when they were sick. The shadow of a genocidal conspiracy was cast over the townships and former homelands – a tragic theory based on very real conspiracies.

Criticism of conspiracy theories generally mingles surprise, anger, and ridicule. Admittedly, some of them are indeed esoteric, mingling situations and characters from spy novels, science fiction, and comics. It is also true that the increasing instrumentalization of such theories in projects focused on weakening democratic institutions and destabilizing scientific knowledge can be a source of anxiety. But my suggestion, with these case studies, is that they should be taken seriously, for two main reasons. First, they sometimes contain some truth: conspiracy theories can in fact be based on genuine machinations, as in South Africa, or at least on practices that appear as such, as in Ecuador. Second, and above all, they often shed light on a deeper truth about the society that produces them: they are sources that help us to understand relations of power and inequality, the relationship between knowledge and authority, and a past that remains present, in Ecuador as in South Africa. For both these reasons, they have a heuristic value that both researcher and citizen need to be able to recognize. Ultimately, we need to put to work Clifford Geertz's famous adjunction, articulated in a different context: "Looking into dragons, not domesticating or abominating them, nor drowning them in vats of theory, is what anthropology has been all about."[42] Conspiracy theories are our dragons, and our task is to understand them.

Ethical Crises
26 May 2021

No crisis occurred. – Polluted water, corrupt government, and systemic racism. – The birth of a national health crisis. – The shared etymology of the words "crisis" and "critique." – The temporality of emergency and the reality of rupture. – Preparatory and operative conditions of felicity. – The powers of the auctor. – The opiate crisis between humanitarian liberalism and cynical capitalism. – Inverted racialization of addiction and the about-turn of moral panic. – A French tale of pharmaceutical criminality. – An ethical dispute around maternal transmission of HIV. – The treatment of vulnerable lives.

For decades in France, children of poor families living in dilapidated buildings were poisoned by dust and flakes of lead falling from the old, peeling paint on the walls of their apartments. For decades, their bodies became gradually weighed down by this metal that accumulated in their organs, especially their brains and peripheral nervous system, resulting in anemia, diarrhea, sometimes comas or even death, and, in less serious instances, in learning difficulties, behavioral disorders, and educational underachievement. For decades, the paint industry and the public authorities, despite being aware of these risks (since the risk of lead white for workers producing or using it had been identified as far back as the second half of the nineteenth century), continued to sell lead paints and allow them to be sold, and even went so far as to contest or minimize the problem when physicians and advocacy organizations began to raise the alarm. Thus we might summarize the first phase in the history of childhood lead poisoning in France, which forms the guiding thread of this course of lectures. Subsequently, thanks to the efforts of particular actors who gradually became aware of the urgency of the situation, the problem was transmuted from a rare pediatric disease to a national public health priority, and it emerged that the total number of cases of contamination in France might be as high as 85,000. Conferences were organized, reports were written, scientific articles were published, laws relating to health and housing were passed, mayors took up the issue, committing to rehousing families or rehabilitating the most dilapidated housing. This was the second phase, during which, to use the terms of political science, lead poisoning was, albeit belatedly, put on the political agenda.

One remarkable, yet little remarked, feature of this story is that at no point did this situation, critical in terms of its extent and its seriousness, prompt a genuine health crisis. It was ignored, then contested, and finally recognized, without advocacy organizations, journalists, or physicians ever escalating the problem into a crisis situation. It could even be said that the epidemic of childhood lead poisoning was kept quiet. Neither the public health experts who revealed it nor the politicians who worked to end it sought to arouse public indignation, no doubt in part because the victims were almost exclusively children of African families, sometimes without legal residence status. The public health experts were concerned about stigmatizing them; the politicians feared hostile reactions from some of their opponents or even their voters. Discretion was the order of the day. The greed of the paint industry was therefore not condemned, and the culpable negligence of the public authorities did not generate any challenge to the system that had permitted such a moral failure in the state's responsibility to protect children. Although all the necessary ingredients were present, the crisis of childhood lead poisoning did not take place.

The US version of this story is even more revealing, for the denial of both the industry and the authorities lasted longer there.[1] As early as the 1920s and 1930s, scientific articles had proliferated in pediatric journals, many emphasizing that childhood lead poisoning was probably frequent but unrecognized. Some even suggested that lead paints should be banned in toys, furniture, and interior decor, at a time when the US lead lobby was waxing ever more inventive in lauding the benefits of the metal in bright advertisements showing happy children. A number of countries, aware of the risks revealed by these studies, adopted legislation restricting use, or even completely banning lead paints, over these two decades: these included the United Kingdom, Sweden, Belgium, Greece, Poland, Tunisia, and Cuba. But in the United States the public authorities were not so eager to legislate, largely owing to the close links politicians often had with the paint industry. The industry itself relied on complaisant researchers in prestigious posts, whose research it funded, and expected scientific arguments contesting the dangers of lead in return. Until the 1940s the industry was able to ignore childhood lead poisoning even though it had to simultaneously respond to lead contamination in the professional sphere. Subsequently, faced with the proliferation of medical publications proving the harmful effects of lead on young children, it alternated between denial and minimization, sometimes going so far as intimidation by threatening the authors with lawsuits. Public health experts and their professional associations showed little interest in the question, for at this time their attention was turned away from the environmental issues of insanitary housing, and focused instead on behavioral approaches to children's geophagic practices and their psychopathological avatar, pica. It was not until 1970 that a federal law banning lead paints was passed, to almost complete indifference: the lobbies did not even try to oppose it since the sector had by then become marginal for the lead industry. For half a century, there was thus no urgency to implement measures to prevent a public health problem that affected hundreds of thousands of children, with serious neuropsychological, sometimes lethal consequences. Significantly, for the most part these children belonged to poor, often Black, families. The problem remained almost secretly confined to sites of knowledge and circles of power. It only seeped marginally into the public space. In the United States too, the acknowledged tragedy of childhood lead poisoning failed to generate a crisis.

A critical situation is thus not synonymous with a crisis. To be more precise, the former does not necessarily lead to the latter. How does one turn into the other? The case of what most journalists and observers called the "Flint water crisis," involving the poisoning of the inhabitants of the town of Flint, Michigan with lead-contaminated water during the 2010s, can help to shed light on this question.[2] Here, the critical situation gave rise to what was perceived nationwide as a major health crisis, one of the most significant the country had seen in the twenty-first century.

Flint was made famous by the 1989 documentary *Roger & Me*, by Michael Moore, who was born and grew up there. Having been the home of General Motors since 1908, the city was long linked to the automobile industry.[3] While it prospered during the 1950s and 1960s, Flint was hard hit during the 1970s by deindustrialization and the oil crisis, with the General Motors factory losing 90 percent of its workforce over thirty years; at the same time, the population halved and the city accumulated a massive budget deficit. The state governor appointed an administrator to manage the city's affairs; subsequently, as the financial situation continued to worsen, a second administrator was installed provoking a series of lawsuits brought by elected city

officials who had been divested of their power.[4] For several years, torn
between omnipotent administrators with absolute authority and local
elected officials demanding democratic accountability, the city became
ungovernable except for emergency measures taken to reduce public
spending.

It was in this extremely high-pressure situation that, in April 2014,
the authorities decided, in order to save money on the water supply
for the city's 100,000 inhabitants, not to renew the contract for the
provision of water from Lake Huron, and instead to use an old pipe
network to bring in water from the Flint River. Over the months that
followed, residents complained that their tap water tasted brackish and
smelled bad, children presented with skin rashes and various disorders,
and General Motors reported that the water was corroding its automobile components. Although they were not designed to detect the
source of such problems, microbiological tests were carried out, and
revealed the presence of bacteria. The authorities responded by increasing the amount of chlorine added to the water, and recommending
that it be boiled. Biochemical tests then identified a significant increase
in a product of the breakdown of chlorine known to be carcinogenic.
This time the public authorities chose not to inform the population,
and continued to assert that the water was safe for consumption. In
February 2015, less than a year after the new system had been introduced, the Environmental Protection Agency (EPA), to which a resident had appealed, discovered levels of lead seven times higher than
the legal maximum. The contamination was due to the failure of the
company in charge of water supply to use anti-corrosion additives
to prevent damage to lead pipes. When faced with these results, the
city council decided to return to the former source of water supply,
but the governor-appointed administrator overturned their decision.
Multiple toxicological and epidemiological studies followed. A team
from Virginia Tech, led by an environmental scientist who a few years
earlier had forced the Centers for Disease Control and Prevention to
admit that they had misled the public when they said that high lead concentration in Washington presented no danger, discovered lead levels
up to ten times higher than the legal limit in the water of the Flint River.
Physicians from the Hurley Hospital, following the initiative of a pediatrician who had taken the risk of publicizing her results before they had
been evaluated and validated by her peers, showed that the proportion
of children with lead poisoning had doubled since water had been taken
from the river, and appealed to residents to stop drinking it.[5] Residents,
especially children, were victims of poisoning whose cause the state of
Michigan refused to end for the sake of budgetary austerity.

However, in October 2015 the governor finally agreed to allocate Flint funding to return to water supply from Lake Huron, and two months later declared a city-wide state of emergency. In addition, the state of Michigan had to provide bottled water in the areas affected for a further two years. In January 2016, faced with the strong feelings aroused by the scandal of this contaminated water, Barack Obama in turn declared a state of emergency, allowing federal resources to be released, and visited Flint to meet with residents. The EPA granted the city a budget of 100 million dollars to improve its water supply infrastructure. At the same time, several class action suits were filed by thousands of residents against the state of Michigan, its governor, and a number of its officials, against the water monitoring bodies, against the city authorities, against the school districts, and against the EPA. They even targeted the federal government. These lawsuits included criminal charges against the two successive administrators of the city for prioritizing balancing the budget over residents' health, but also for diversion of emergency funds and falsifying public accounts in order to help fund construction of an alternative supply network to the one from Lake Huron. In 2016, coverage of the events moved from local to national media, with articles in the major daily newspapers and on the 24-hour news channels, reporting the experience of the residents and legal developments in the case. The city of Flint became a symbol of the "abject failure to protect public health," as one major medical journal titled its editorial, with rare vehemence.[6] "We have the knowledge required to redress this social crime," wrote its author. "We know where the lead is, how people are exposed and how it damages health. What we lack is the political will to do what should be done." With the help of researchers, physicians, and activists, it was the residents who applied themselves to this.

The history of the Flint water crisis thus comprises a number of superimposed historical and sociological strata. There is first the golden age of the automobile industry that, for half a century, attracted a labor force that quickly became segregated into poor Black neighborhoods and affluent white neighborhoods; this period was marked by memorable workers' struggles at the beginning of the US trade union movement. Then followed the hard years of deindustrialization, leading to the exodus of a large section of the white population, which halved in four decades, while the Black population became the majority. The result was a period of increasing financial difficulty for the city, which had lost almost all of its principal economic activity and most of its middle class, plunging the city budget into deep deficit. The subprime crisis of 2007, which led to many working-class residents losing their homes, made the situation worse still. The Republican governor then imposed the supervision of administrators on the Democratic city: their policy was seen as punitive, combining humiliation and subjection with austerity.

The water crisis, then, arose in a city at the end of its resources, sapped by high crime rates, where the poverty rate of 41 percent was almost three times the national average, while the average annual household income was only 26,000 dollars. The only goal of the two administrators was to reduce public spending. Changing the water supply source offered one way of doing this, and, despite the contamination with bacteria, carcinogens, and lead that the authorities were aware of, despite the evidence of the color and smell of the water, despite the symptoms presented by children, they continued to assure the population that the liquid coming out of their taps was potable. Care for residents' health, despite the risk of gastric infections and even cancer, and of lasting neuropsychic disorders for children, therefore took second place to the concern of rebalancing the budget. Two questions then arise. How did this critical situation become possible? And how did it result in a national crisis? As noted above, critical situation and crisis do not always go hand in hand, and the former may exist without the latter arising.

The critical situation that gave rise to the water crisis was linked to a long history of deindustrialization, depopulation, and pauperization combined with a municipal budget deficit that was largely due to these three processes. But it took shape at a specific point, when a political decision was made to move from a system of supplying healthy but expensive water to another supplying polluted but cheap water, the only justification being budget savings. While the evidence of a three-fold bacteriological, chemical, and physical risk accumulated within the space of a few months, and while the former contractor offered its services again on more favorable terms, the authorities persisted and signed, refusing to return to the old system. Most public health and social science researchers see the key to interpreting this move in the title of the report published by the Michigan Civil Rights Commission, which emphasized "systemic racism." What made it possible to choose to balance the budget at the cost of damaging bodies was that the population affected was majority poor and Black. The map of the distribution of high levels of water contamination and high rates of poisoning of children, and the study of the statistical correlation between racial category, socioeconomic status, and urban neighborhoods in the city leave no doubt in this regard.[7] The industrial center of Flint, where the poorest residents, most of them African American, lived, was the zone where the lead content in the water was highest, and where childhood lead poisoning was most frequent. It was not that the authorities necessarily had racist intentions, although some officials had expressed explicitly racist sentiments, but that the social structures built up over the course of the twentieth century were at issue: a mixture of segregation, discrimination, and exploitation of the poor, mainly Black, population, in which the three phenomena mutually reinforced one another. It was indeed to escape from this debate around intentionality that some spoke of "racial liberalism," a term borrowed from the philosopher Charles Mills, in reference to the way zoning policies, although non-racialized in appearance, can lead to certain minorities being concentrated in particular urban areas. Others spoke of "strategic racism," a term coined by legal scholar Ian Haney López to describe the coded language used to refer to racial groups or their attributes, and which some politicians adopt in order to appeal to voters.[8] More generally, the term "systemic racism" is used to name the structural processes that do not require a manifest expression of racism to produce effects that are racially differentiated and unequally distributed. Systemic racism is rampant in Flint, as everywhere else in the country in various degrees.

All the same, the crisis might not have occurred. The contamination of children might have gone unnoticed, the reports might have continued to be ignored, the authorities might have highlighted the savings made. Conversely, the administrator, in the light of the toxicological and epidemiological studies, could, at the request of the governor and with the agreement of the city council, have made the decision to return to the former water supply system, without residents becoming angry, without the media taking up the story, without multiple lawsuits being filed. In the first case, the critical situation would have remained invisible; in the second, it would have been silently corrected. But a crisis did occur, not only at the local but also at the national level. The city of Flint became, well beyond its borders, a symbol of the obscenity of economic logic when it is applied to the detriment of human lives. But the critical situation faced by the population only gradually gained the publicity that is a crucial element in the development of a crisis.[9] The residents' campaign was conducted in an extremely hostile context, because under the administrators' governance there was neither the financial margin for mitigating political decisions nor the democratic space to make grievances heard. The successive complaints about the color and smell of the water, the presence of bacteria and toxic substances had proved ineffectual, with the authorities continuing to assert that the water presented no danger to human health. It was the discovery of lead poisoning that altered the situation.

Initiated by the charismatic mother of the first child in whom lead poisoning was diagnosed, a local movement took form, bringing together a number of existing social, political, and religious organizations. The Flint Coalition for Clean Water made contact with lawyers, journalists, and experts at the national level, calling in the Environmental Protection Agency as well as the American Civil Liberties Union. At the same time, contact was established with scientists, including researchers at Virginia Tech, to investigate the lead levels in the water, and at Hurley Hospital, to screen children for contamination. When these toxicologists and physicians revealed a correlation between the urban zones where the water contained high levels of lead and the neighborhoods where children showed high blood lead levels, the governor and his administrators could not ignore the evidence: hence their decision, albeit belated, to return to the supply from Lake Huron. Well-known figures from the worlds of politics, show business, and sports, from Jesse Jackson to Magic Johnson, from Cher to Eminem, voiced their support. The national media seized on the story, expressing outrage at this health scandal. The transformation of a specific critical situation into a generalized national crisis was thus the product of a coalition of local forces, appeal to national celebrities, and an alliance with scientific researchers. It also translated a health crisis that might have been of interest only to specialists, since it affected marginalized communities, into an ethical crisis that was of concern to the entire population. The choice to make budget cuts, even at the cost of known risks to people's health and indeed their lives, particularly where children were involved, converted a political question into a moral issue. Public authorities are constantly making such choices. They usually go unnoticed and remain uncontested. In Flint, notwithstanding the ongoing suspension of the democratic order, residents reconnected with a history of trade unions, and more recently citizen struggles, standing up against a choice that prioritized financial reasons over health rationale. In their view, it was time for ethical considerations to be reasserted.

The development of a crisis, then, depends not only on the existence of an objectively identifiable critical situation. What happened in Flint in 2015 became known as the Flint water crisis, following the discovery of cases of lead poisoning in children, fortunately without serious consequences. But there was no talk of a housing crisis in Aubervilliers, on the outskirts of Paris, in 1985, despite the fact that one child died of complications from lead poisoning and that unhealthy, dilapidated housing was a major problem at the time. In order for a critical situation to generate a crisis, particular conditions are required. Before turning to them, however, we need to ask what constitutes a crisis. Up until now I have used the word as if it went without saying. But this is not the case – and the ubiquity of the word makes it even more problematic. Its routine use thus risks emptying it of any analytical value and making it falsely transparent, to the point where there is no longer any need to question it. Conversely, this trivialization of the word calls for investigation.

The word comes from Greek: according to the Bailly dictionary, the first meaning of the word κρίνω (*krinō*) is to separate, distinguish, or choose, and the second to judge, decide, interpret.[10] It thus comprises both an element of discrimination, particularly between persons (good and bad) or values (true and false), and an element of determination, whether in relation to a question posed (to decide it), during a trial (to sanction the accused) or in the context of a disease (to identify the crucial moment). Similarly, the noun κρίσις (*krisis*), derived from the verb, denotes, on the one hand, the action of separating, distinguishing, or choosing, and, on the other, that of judging, deciding, interpreting, and hence actions performed in particular circumstances, such as the conviction (of a guilty person), the conclusion (of a war), and the high point (of a disease). The term thus has two aspects: it is an action and it is a moment, the two being linked because, at the crucial point in a trial, a battle, or an illness, those concerned have to know how to distinguish between possible courses of action and decide which is best. This etymology is instructive. It reminds us how close the terms "crisis" and "critical" originally were. It is at the crucial point of the crisis (in its second aspect, the moment) that one must show oneself capable of resolving it by using one's critical sense (first aspect, action). The fact that, at the critical moment, the critical sense is required for action is a lesson that should not be forgotten.

Beyond this etymology, in ancient Greece the actual usage of the word "crisis," as percipiently analyzed by Reinhart Koselleck in his history of concepts, arose in three principal arenas – legal-political, religious, and medical.[11] In the legal-political domain, it refers to judgment and decision-making on subjects as varied as trials, conflicts, and elections, and is thus involved in the just order of society. In the domain of religion, more specifically Judeo-Christian religion, a link was established between judgment on earth and the Last Judgment; the way individuals act during their life determines their future in the afterlife, with the introduction of the distinction between damnation and salvation. Finally, in the medical domain, the Hippocratic Corpus confers vital importance on the moment in the disease when it may swing toward healing or death, and the physician's evaluation of the situation and the aptness of his decision are decisive. It is this last, medical usage that was to persist into the Middle Ages and even the Classical era, as the definition in the 1690 Furetière dictionary indicates: "sudden change in a disease" – though the entry also mentions a figurative sense in the context of a plot or a judicial procedure where the word means, respectively, the outcome or the judgment.[12] From the seventeenth century, the term began gradually to be extended metaphorically to other spheres, initially into politics, where in the organicist conception of society the idea could be applied to a crisis in the body politic. The word then began to be increasingly used in economic parlance, still as a parallel with disease requiring treatment, or even, in the context of trade, a parallel with epidemics, on the grounds of their international diffusion. Finally, the twentieth century saw a generalization of the metaphor to the intellectual, cultural, and moral spheres, and it was taken up by the human and social sciences too. As Koselleck writes of the contemporary period, "there is virtually no area of life that has not been examined and interpreted through this concept." But Koselleck introduces an essential theoretical question into this history of the concept of crisis. It concerns the modern relationship to time. From the end of the eighteenth century, he explains, the notion of crisis, which found its paradigmatic realization in Revolution, whether in the United States or France, implied a philosophy of history according to which the account of humanity was not linear, but passed through moments of rupture. Such ruptures marked the boundary between an old and a new world, whatever one's view of this new world, whether rich in hope (as the progressive Thomas Paine saw it), or the harbinger of disorder (as in the view of conservative Edmund Burke, for whom it heralded the destruction of the social order). However, unlike these great political crises that redefined the world, the economic crises that arose with some regularity during the nineteenth century do not fit well into this philosophy of history: they were interpreted by liberal thinkers as necessary adjustments that helped to improve the capitalist system, and by Marxist theory as failures of this system that would inevitably lead to its collapse and to socialist revolution.

What is useful to retain from this brief etymological and historical excursion, for our present inquiry? First, returning to the origin of the word, it is worth noting that a crisis is both a decisive moment demarcating two possible outcomes and an action that involves deciding immediately how to choose which is better. This dual dimension emerged in medical language, but it is clearly apt for economic, political, and indeed moral language. Second, focusing on the modern meaning of the term, it is clear that a crisis establishes both a distinction and a rupture between two states of the world, such that there is a before and an after. In this sense, the crisis is a representation of time. In the first sense – crisis as moment and as action – the temporality is that of the present, and of urgency. In the second sense – crisis as distinction and as rupture – the temporality is that of the relation between past and future. But in both these aspects, the crisis calls for critical thinking. On the one hand, critical work is what makes it possible to evaluate the crisis and resolve it. A health crisis is never just a health crisis. Alongside its medical component there are others that need to be grasped. In Flint, childhood lead poisoning revealed economic irregularities, dysfunctional politics, and environmental injustice. On the other hand, critical work is what makes it possible to recognize the crisis as such and to draw a new state of the world out of it. Naming a health crisis opens up broader concerns but also an imperative to resolve it. In Flint, transforming the supply of polluted water to the city into a crisis situation opened the way to contesting the suspension of the city's democratic functioning and the prioritization of budget savings over protection of public health. But critical work must go further. It needs to question both the temporality of emergency and the reality of the rupture. On the one hand, emergency can justify exceptional measures while at the same time avoiding dealing with structural causes. On the other, the rupture may be expressed in discourse without being translated into fact. To be sure, the Flint water crisis brought to an end the poisoning of residents, including children in the city center, but it had little effect on the problems of governance and resource allocation.

In order for the urgent decision that helps to resolve the crisis to be made, and in order for the crisis to be recognized and described, and hence for a critical sense necessary for each of these operations to be mobilized, actors are required. It is not enough that a problem exists for it to give rise to a crisis. There must also be individuals or groups to effect this transformation, and they must succeed in their efforts. In seeking to understand what turns a problem into a crisis, one can refer to J. L. Austin's theory of performativity.[13] There are, Austin argues, utterances that aim not to describe the world, but to act on it. The diagnosis of a crisis arises out of such a performative act, where to identify a crisis situation is not only to describe it but also to act on it by bringing it into existence in the public space and forcing the authorities to respond. This diagnosis normally requires two types of felicity condition: preparatory, those that characterize the critical situation, and operative, those that transform it into a crisis. The preparatory conditions imply that there is a problem (in Flint, the contamination of drinking water), that evidence of this problem is provided (levels of lead in tap water and children's blood) and that the agents establishing this evidence are legitimate (university and hospital researchers). The operative conditions require interpretation of the situation (in Flint, pollution resulted from an austerity measure with no democratic basis), more general pertinence (the situation was the product of systemic racism that persists throughout the country), the establishment of a cause to be defended (the health of children should prevail over balancing budgets), the mobilization of local actors (the individuals affected, physicians, researchers, organizations, churches), and the appeal to public figures (activists, lawyers, experts, journalists, celebrities). These preparatory and operative conditions constitute the felicity conditions that make it possible to turn the problem into a crisis.

But these conditions are not always all realized. The preparatory conditions may be present, but not the operative conditions: the problem exists but does not give rise to a crisis. For example, in 2020, on the outskirts of Calais and in the Paris suburbs, thousands of men, women and children were crammed into empty lots and public spaces in hygiene conditions that were condemned by nongovernmental organizations, at the mercy of the police who, when they intervened, would often destroy their makeshift shelters and their scanty belongings, without the situation generating a genuine crisis – though some organizations attempted to produce one by mounting spectacular stunts. Conversely, the operative conditions may be present, but not the preparatory conditions: there is a crisis, but it is not based on any critical situation. For example, in 2018, when a boat run by the humanitarian organization SOS Méditerranée, carrying more than 600 men, women, and children, was shipwrecked as it tried to reach Europe and was refused permission to dock by the Italian government, it led to not only a humanitarian crisis but also a diplomatic crisis with France, and even a political crisis within Europe, despite the fact that the claimed mass influx of migrants was corroborated by neither statistics nor observations: the number of new immigrants arriving in Lampedusa was in fact the lowest for nearly ten years. In short, not every problem inevitably issues in a state of crisis, and not all crises necessarily correspond to a real problem.

From these situations where there is no match between problem and crisis, we may conclude that a distinction needs to be made between two operations that we have already encountered several times. On the

one hand, the problem needs to be analyzed in terms of social production. The question is: how did this problem arise? In the case of Flint,
the long-term roots were deindustrialization, the exodus of the white
middle class and the impoverishment of the remaining Black population; the short-term causes were the city's bankruptcy, the imposition
of administrators and the introduction of austerity measures including sacrificing clean water. Added to these factors were the suspected
concealment of health data and falsification of public accounts. But
the crisis itself has to be analyzed in terms of its social construction.
The question is: how does a crisis emerge out of a given situation? As
noted above, felicity conditions are necessary, and they involve a series
of operations. But who brings together these conditions and performs
these operations? Who has the authority to do so, and what does
this recognition authorize? In Flint, the individuals and organizations
who first mobilized when they became aware of the water pollution
did not have the necessary authority to create a crisis situation, still
less to return to the old system; if the coalition that formed later succeeded, it was because it was supported by the threefold authority of
science (with the toxicologists and physicians), the media (journalists and celebrities), and finally politics and the courts (activists and
lawyers). The construction of the health crisis thus authorized not
only the governor's emergency decision to reactivate the former water
supply contract, but also a challenge to the nondemocratic administration of the city, the prevarication of public officials, and the historically
unfavorable treatment of poor Black minorities.

In this twofold process of production and construction of a crisis,
the crucial point is not only to ensure it is recognized, but also to
define it. Was the situation in Flint merely a health crisis? Residents
insisted that it was not. With the support of activists, they moved the
crisis into the political arena. With the lawyers, they transported it
to the world of the courts. Alongside the social science researchers
from local universities, they placed it within the legacy of structural
racism in the United States. But there is one underlying dimension of
health crises that often goes unexplored: the ethical dimension. By this
I mean the distribution of values in the social space, and the issues,
and indeed struggles, around the meaning and implications of these
values. In Flint, there was a conflict between values in the economic
sense, as understood by the administrators who sought above all to
balance the city's budget, and values in the moral sense, as they were
defended by the residents who prioritized not only their health but also
their dignity. These ethical stakes go beyond the traditional opposition
between right and wrong as ethics is usually defined. This is what I will

demonstrate through two case studies: the so-called opioid crisis in the United States, and the crisis around the prescription of antiretroviral drugs in South Africa.

On 25 October 2017, the president of the United States asked the federal Department of Health and Human Services to declare the opioid crisis a "health emergency."[14] That year, the use of drugs had caused the death of 70,723 individuals, 67.8 percent from opioids, making them the primary cause of death in people under the age of 50.[15] Between 1999 and 2017 there were 700,000 deaths from overdose, 400,000 of them from opioid overdose. During this period 130 people lost their lives through the use of these substances every day. But this epidemic was radically different from that which had struck nearly fifty years earlier. During the 1970s and 1980s drug use, mainly in the form of illegal consumption of heroin, and a few years later of cocaine, had provoked a moral panic, a fear reaction among the white majority who associated it with rising crime, the degeneration of inner cities and the desocialization of African American youth. Driven by conservative presidents, members of Congress, and governors, extremely repressive laws were passed in the name of what was called the "war on drugs," generating a huge rise in the mainly Black prison population, with up to 1 million new incarcerations each year. This policy contributed significantly to the phenomenon known as mass incarceration, with its 2.3 million prisoners, among whom Blacks outnumbered whites by five to one.[16] In contrast with the 1970s and 1980s, the later opioid crisis stemmed from the legal distribution of these products, at least initially. It was estimated that 2 million people in the country suffered from addiction to medically prescribed opioids, and the increase in overdose deaths during the 2000s and 2010s coincided with the expansion in medical prescriptions. But this was not a homogeneous phenomenon; in fact, three successive waves can be distinguished in the opioid addiction epidemic.

The first wave began in the mid-1990s, with the rapid rise in prescription of opioids for pain relief. It arose from the conjunction of two phenomena. First, the American Pain Society, a section of the International Association for the Study of Pain, incorporated the patient's assessment of pain – and hence a measure of the efficacy of treatment – into the list of vital signs, alongside temperature, heart rate, respiration rate, and blood pressure. It was supported in this initiative by the Veterans Health Administration, and evaluated by the Accreditation Commission for Health Care Organizations, whose patient satisfaction questionnaire includes questions about pain relief. What is more, the American Academy of Pain Medicine, keen to encourage physicians to prescribe opioids, played down the risks of addiction, habituation, and overdose, as well as of potential misappropriation of opioid drugs.[17] Second, the pharmaceutical company Purdue Pharma introduced a new slow-release opioid, oxycodone (sold under the name OxyContin) onto the market: this allowed for two doses a day and was recommended for the relief of chronic pain. It was aggressively marketed both to physicians, who received gifts from the laboratory to encourage them to prescribe it, and to pain treatment associations, which the company funded generously. While Purdue Pharma played a central role and its flagship product was spectacularly successful, with a 2,000 percent increase in sales over four years, it was not the only company in this market, and others quickly embarked on production of equivalent drugs in their turn. In order to overcome practitioners' reluctance to use them, experts paid by opioid manufacturers gave lectures extolling their benefits and asserting the absence of addiction, even though the long-term effects had never been studied. It was thus this collision between humanitarian liberalism (every individual should be able to escape suffering) and cynical capitalism (all money is good for the taking, whatever the price paid by those it is taken from) that led to the explosion in opioid consumption in treatment of non-cancerous chronic pain in the United States. The number of prescriptions quadrupled in fifteen years – and so did the number of deaths due to overdose.

The second wave of the epidemic began fifteen or so years after the start of the first, around 2010, and this time was centered around the return of heroin. Ease of access to OxyContin and the possibility of grinding it to a powder had made it the drug of choice for sniffing or injecting, whether it was obtained directly by medical prescription or via an exchange with an acquaintance who had been prescribed it. Misappropriation of the product thus gave rise to sustained drug misuse. Under pressure, Purdue Pharma developed a tablet that was harder to crush. This change led drug users to shift to heroin, which was now less expensive and easier to use. The number of deaths from heroin overdose rose rapidly. As evidence that this was indeed a case of a shift from one product to the other, rather than simply a new community of drug users, one study showed that eight out of ten heroin addicts had previously used prescription opioids, even if they had had no medical reason to do so.

The third wave of addiction arose in 2015, with the spread of a new illicit synthetic substance, fentanyl, which was up to 100 times stronger than morphine. It was used in anesthesia and prescribed for pain. The increase in fatal overdoses from this product was exponential, doubling each year. In 2018, nearly 47,000 people died from opioid overdose, more than 31,000 from synthetic opioids, primarily fentanyl, and 15,000 from prescription opioids. A further 15,000 people died from heroin overdose.[18] In other words, rather than succeeding one another, the three waves were overlapping and accumulated; and this development was iatrogenically driven, that is, medically induced.

No one could doubt that there was a problem with opioid prescription in the United States, given the figures on use and mortality, the age range concerned, the rise in overdoses, and the cost of related healthcare, which was estimated at 80 billion dollars annually. But this was not enough to make it a crisis. There was one factor above all others that was decisive in turning this problem into a crisis: the fact that the majority of those affected appeared to be white. This was revealed in an article by two economists, Anne Case and Angus Deaton, published in the *Proceedings of the National Academy of Sciences* in 2015, and widely reported in the media.[19] The article showed that, since 2000, there had been a substantial and steady rise in mortality among white people of both sexes aged between 45 and 54, reversing a more than fifty-year trend, that this problematic development was due principally to overdoses of opioids, and to a lesser degree to suicide and cirrhosis, that the rise in mortality from overdose, suicide, and cirrhosis was not restricted to this age bracket but extended to all adults aged between 30 and 64, and that it represented nearly 500,000 surplus deaths over fifteen years compared to what would have been the case had mortality rates continued on their downward trend. There was thus a "lost generation." These unexpected results were, however, partially corrected by a study by Steven Woolf and Heidi Schoomaker on changes in mortality and life expectancy among all age groups over the last sixty years, published in the *Journal of the American Medical Association* in 2019.[20] This study revealed that life expectancy had risen rapidly for the US population until the 1970s, had then slowed before reaching a plateau in 2011, and had been falling since 2014; that this drop was due to a sharp rise in mortality among those aged between 25 and 54 from 2010, mainly owing to addictions, with peaks in the northeastern states; and that, including all causes of death, the loss of life expectancy due to this trend was almost twice as high among Blacks as among whites. Moreover, as far as deaths specifically from opioid overdose, particularly fentanyl, were concerned, rates among Blacks, which had hitherto been much lower than those among whites, had almost caught up in the late 2010s. In other words, while for a few years the epidemic of opioid addiction and deaths from overdose of these products affected whites more, it very quickly came to affect Blacks in equal measure, and even predominantly.

But the idea that the rise in mortality affected whites primarily, illustrated by press features reporting on the distress of East Coast families after the death of a son or a daughter from overdose, had made a strong impression on society, contributing to what some anthropologists called a "re-racialization of addiction."[21] In the late twentieth century Black drug users had come to be seen as dangerous criminals. The myth of the "superpredator," a violent young African American devoid of any moral sense and threatening the social order, was used to justify harsh repression, despite the fact that statistics showed a dramatic fall in crime. Conversely, in the early twenty-first century, white drug users were seen as victims. The media often portrayed them as young men and women of the suburban middle classes, talented and full of promise, felled by the epidemic, or still alive but surviving in impoverished, marginalized rural areas, facing an uncertain future, and, in either case, as innocent victims caught in the trap of addiction. The moral panic of the Reagan and Clinton years was rooted in a fear of the other – fear of young Black people. The moral panic of the Obama and Trump years was manifested in a fear for one's own – fear for young white people. The guilty parties were the pharmaceutical corporations and the prescribing physicians who made opioids the routine choice for pain relief – rather than the dealers and drug users of the previous period. The introduction of heroin, which partially substituted for these products during the second phase, was laid at the feet of Mexican cartels – although the question of source had not helped to excuse users previously. For as long as the drug was a Black problem, it was seen as a phenomenon endogenous to their community. As soon as it affected whites, it became an exogenous reality smiting them. This exoneration of white drug users led politicians to call for less severe sanctions than those inherited from the war on drugs, and a number of states implemented penal reform introducing therapeutic rather than punitive approaches. The role of race in setting penalties is, moreover, nothing new: a law passed in 1986 punished possession of crack five times more heavily than possession of powdered cocaine, with 5 grams of the former and 500 grams of the latter being subject to the same penalty of five years' imprisonment. The toxicity of the two products was similar, but crack was the drug of poor Black neighborhoods, and cocaine that of well-off white circles.[22] A member of the New Jersey Criminal Sentencing and Disposition Commission, which has been appointed by the governor of the state to reform the penal and penitentiary system and of which I am also a member as guest advisor, told me that the consensus among Democratic and Republican representatives that legislation on the use and sale of drugs should be eased was in good part due to the fact that these practices now concerned young people from social circles closer to their own, making them more understanding. The inverse racialization of illegal drug-dealing in the late twentieth and early twenty-first centuries was thus made possible by a moral economy of addiction where judgments and affects were also inverted. While Black drug users had been convicted, white drug users were exonerated. The former faced the animosity and inflexibility of the law; the latter met with compassion and mercy from the legislators. Representatives were as sensitive to the suffering of one group as they had been aggressive toward the deviance of the other.

But in the conventional distinction between morality, as that which concerns judgments and the affects associated with them, and ethics, as that which relates to the values and principles underlying these judgments, it becomes clear that the opioid crisis incorporates not only a moral element of appraisal of drug users, but also an ethical dimension that underpins the choices made by actors. On the one hand, it is clear how the pharmaceutical industry that produced and promoted the use of oxycodone cynically suspended all ethical principles, concealing the pharmaceutical dependence created by their opioids even though they were aware of it, asserting the drugs' efficacy in relief of chronic pain when they knew that habituation rendered them ineffective, and corrupting physicians to ensure they prescribed them. Purdue Pharma, indeed, admitted this as early as 2007 when it agreed to plead guilty and was ordered to pay a fine of 634 million dollars – a sum dwarfed by the profits from OxyContin, which reached 3 billion dollars over fifteen years. The racialization and moralization of the epidemic even formed part of the strategy of the company's owners, the hugely wealthy Sackler family: aware of the high risk of addiction to OxyContin, they had chosen to target their marketing toward the white population to avoid the negative image associated with Black drug users. In this way their product could appear not to be morally contaminated. This was, then, a novel form of racial capitalism, to use the concept coined to describe the extraction of economic value based on racial differentiation, which is generally applied to the exploitation of Black populations.[23] But, on the other hand, what made this economic venture possible was developments in medicine and society with regard to pain. All of a sudden, patients no longer had to be left to suffer. Patient satisfaction in this respect indeed became an important factor in the appraisal of healthcare facilities, which depended on this evaluation for their funding. There were two aspects to the new ideology: patients should no longer suffer, and they should be given control over their pain management. It was this liberal element, making relief a right for the patient and a duty for the physician, that opened the way to the corporations' culpable activity.[24] The ambiguity of the ethical stakes of the crisis is thus clear, since a well-intentioned initiative that was certainly beneficial for some patients fostered the plans of a criminal enterprise and ultimately resulted in hundreds of thousands of deaths in less than two decades.

For a French audience, the OxyContin affair, which implicated a major pharmaceutical laboratory, Purdue Pharma, and its owners, the Sackler family, carries echoes of the Mediator, or Benfluorex affair, which also implicated a major pharmaceutical laboratory, Servier, and its owner Jacques Servier. Here again, the product was diverted from its intended use to be promoted in a much more lucrative market. Mediator is normally prescribed for high blood triglyceride levels and type 2 diabetes, but it became a drug of choice for weight loss despite being unauthorized to be sold for this purpose, and sales of it made the Servier laboratory an estimated 600 million euros. Once again, physicians were encouraged to prescribe a drug whose dangers its promoters were aware of, but had concealed from the pharmaceutical watchdogs: in this case Mediator was responsible for several tens of thousands of heart valve malfunctions, of which several thousand were probably fatal. On sale in France since 1976, but also authorized in several other European countries, this drug, which is similar to amphetamine, was the subject of warnings in 1990 in relation to both its diverted use as a slimming aid and its secondary cardiac effects. It was withdrawn from sale in Switzerland in 1997, in Italy in 2004, and gradually from most other European countries, but in France a new sale authorization was issued in 2009 for two generics, before the National Agency for Medicine Safety (Agence nationale de sécurité du medicament) finally decided to withdraw the permit. Irène Frachon, a lung specialist at the university hospital in Brest, played a key role in this affair, conducting research, alerting the pharmaceutical watchdogs and making the affair public.[25] Following a long judicial investigation, in which the final report gives the figure of 1,520–2,000 deaths, figures that obviously do not include the thousands of people suffering from serious and potentially life-threatening cardiac complications, the laboratory was convicted of "aggravated fraud" and "involuntary homicide and bodily harm" in March 2021.[26] The involvement of professors of medicine, healthcare institutions, and politicians, who received funding from the Servier laboratory, gave the Mediator affair a much broader ethical dimension and led to legislation designed to prevent conflicts of interest within the pharmaceutical industry.

An equally tragic situation and similarly high tension, although with very distinct stakes, arose around AIDS in South Africa in the early 2000s. As I have discussed, two crises came together at this point. First there was an epidemiological crisis, with a massive acceleration in the spread of the virus through the population: prevalence among pregnant women rose from 1 percent to 20 percent in ten years, and the total number of infections was estimated at more than 4 million. South Africa was the worst affected country in the world. Then there was an epistemological crisis, with the president and several of his ministers challenging the viral theory of AIDS and hence contesting the efficacy of antiretrovirals, prompting a social response in the streets, the press, and the courts. South Africa became the world epicenter of scientific dissidence. In both cases there was a genuine crisis, and the two mutually reinforced one another. Thabo Mbeki's public statements, and his summoning of an international panel for what was supposed to be a discussion between orthodox and heterodox views, but equally the dramatic campaigns by the Treatment Action Campaign and its charismatic founder, the activist Zachie Achmat, turned the biological phenomenon of the spread of the disease into an epidemiological crisis, while the intellectual face-off between theories and rules of evidence transformed it into an epistemological crisis.

Alongside these two crises, a third soon appeared, less intelligible, or rather less well understood because it was too emotionally and normatively charged: this was an ethical crisis. It was not understood because it was very quickly interpreted by most commentators in a Manichean vein, summed up as an opposition between two camps, one presumed to be attached to ethics, and the other purportedly rejecting it. In the early 2000s, as the extent of the spread of the infection in the population was becoming known, the often virulent debate crystallized primarily around prevention of transmission of the virus from mother to child. Because of the number of young women infected, this vector had everywhere in the world become both a health concern and a moral issue, since the risk involved newborns; the much-vaunted innocence of these babies left a suspicion of culpability hovering over their mothers. The risk of transmission was around one in five newborns in the absence of medical intervention, and was roughly halved if the mother took antiretrovirals during pregnancy and if they were administered to the child during the first weeks of life. Moreover, in Uganda, encouraging results had emerged in the recent clinical trial of a promising medication, nevirapine, taken in a short protocol where the product was administered to the mother before and during birth and to the child just after birth.[27] Systematic use of this simple, effective, and inexpensive prevention therefore seemed to go without saying. But the South African health minister proved reluctant to roll it out in the country, stating that clinical trials were needed in South Africa before it was introduced as a general treatment. Journalists, physicians, and activists condemned the resulting delay in the most virulent terms, some going so far as to accuse the authorities of genocide. The pages of the daily newspapers were filled with images of newborns under pathos-laden headlines such as "Babies too poor to live," and "Suffer, little children," accompanying articles suggesting that lack of treatment condemned all newborns and that treatment would save them all, whereas in reality nevirapine resulted in a more modest reduction of what was a partial transmission – from two in ten to one in ten. The conclusions seemed obvious: ethics required that the protocol be implemented without delay in order to save lives. In the view of those campaigning for it, the health chiefs, through their prevarication, were rejecting all ethical considerations. Two camps, then. The distribution of good and evil in the medical arena appeared clear.

But was it so distinct? What reasons did the ministry give for not introducing generalized prevention with nevirapine? The irrationality of some reactions, particularly at the highest levels of government, should not be underestimated, with the mixture of adherence to a sometimes exaggerated heterodoxy, mistrust of Western scientists, and resentment of white society. In particular, researchers were suspected of using African populations as guinea pigs for testing drugs before they were used on Western patients. This was not entirely groundless. Indeed, not long before, the prestigious *New England Journal of Medicine* had published an editorial by Marcia Angell, its editor-in-chief, in which she condemned the fact that fifteen of the sixteen clinical trials of prevention of mother-to-child transmission of the virus conducted in countries of the global South, almost all on the African continent, had not complied with ethical guidelines because they used a placebo to compare with tested antiretrovirals, when the efficacy of zidovudine was already known. This was a protocol that would never have been accepted in countries of the global North.[28] In addition to this controversy over the use of African populations for disguised experimental purposes, the health authorities expressed three reservations about nevirapine: the possibility of side effects that had thus far been subject to little evaluation; the risk for the mother of developing resistance to the whole family of antiretrovirals to which this one belonged; and the possibility of subsequent contamination of the child through breast-feeding. There was a further financial justification that had resulted in a clinical trial of prevention based on another antiret-roviral, zidovudine, being halted a little while earlier, on the grounds of the cost of extending it to the country as a whole and the injustice if it was only offered to a part of the population. But in 2001 the judge in the Pretoria High Court ruled on the side of the activists who had brought forward a test case on behalf of a patient, arguing on the basis of the principle of the right to life. The judge ordered the government to implement prevention of mother-to-child transmission throughout the national territory. The program was therefore launched.

Three years later, however, taking into account all the clinical trials conducted in Africa and elsewhere, the World Health Organization published revised recommendations.[29] Experts noted first the exist-ence of various complications, some serious, in both mother and child, and teratogenic effects in animals, which raised fears of a risk of fetal malformation; second, frequent resistance to antiretrovirals in up to two-thirds of mothers who had received a single dose of nevirapine, suggesting that the concern to protect children came at the cost of losing the chance of improvement in the mother's condition; and third, an increase in the rate of infection in young children when they were breast-fed in line with international recommendations, resulting in them losing nearly half the benefit of the preventive treatment adminis-tered at birth. The experts' conclusion, which largely corroborated the doubts expressed by the South African authorities a few years earlier, was therefore that monotherapies like nevirapine prescribed alone should be replaced by tritherapies, particularly in order to protect mothers. But these new protocols, which involved treatment during pregnancy and of the child after birth, were obviously much more expensive and difficult to generalize, thus once again posing the ethical problem of fair allocation of resources to the entire population.

With regard to this highly sensitive issue of contamination of newborn babies, then, what arose was not a confrontation between an ethical position (that of the activists and physicians) and a non-ethical position (that of the government), but rather ethics that on both sides could be described as impure, in that they mixed lofty intentions with murkier considerations. The physicians and biologists who argued with sincere conviction in defense of the life of newborns at the same time fell in with research practices that involved administering place-bos in their control groups, when there were treatments known to be effective, and encouraged prevention programs more concerned with saving children than with protecting their mothers. The health officials who refused to implement preventive measures that could decrease transmission of the virus to newborns by even a limited proportion might also have been acting in the name of precaution, since nothing was known about the side effects of the treatment, and of social justice, since the disparities in the healthcare system meant that the treatment could not be offered to all women. Thus the major ethical crisis that shook the country was much denser and more complex than suggested by the Manichean reduction used to describe it, which only aggravated tensions.

A crisis, clearly, can never be taken at face value. It calls for critical examination, on a number of fronts. This critical examination seeks to grasp the processes through which the crisis arises – in other words, both what produces it and how it is constructed. In the domain of public health, the social production of a crisis can be studied by looking under stones. Often, alongside the reasoning particular to the health problem concerned, economic and political issues are found, whether in relation to the polluted water in Flint, opioid overdose in the northeastern United States, or the prevention of transmission of AIDS from mother to child in South Africa. As for social construction, the question to be asked is what this language of crisis reveals, whether it is the risk of thousands of children from low-income Black neighborhoods being poisoned with lead, the risk of hundreds of thousands of adults dying from an iatrogenic cause linked to opioids, or the risk of tens of thousands of newborns being condemned to death – risks that, in some cases, were ignored for years. But we also need to ask what this language of crisis tends to relegate to the background, in terms of the deeper causes of these situations – respectively systemic racism, criminal capitalism, and the legacy of apartheid – rendered inaudible by the sense of urgency the crisis generates. These deeper causes have not only an obvious political dimension, but also a moral dimension, which, as the three situations discussed show, reveals the way that lives are treated – or rather, the way the most vulnerable lives are mistreated by governments, pharmaceutical corporations, and sometimes even biomedical teams. And this ethical aspect of health crises is often the least visible part, and perhaps the part that is hardest to articulate.

Precarious Exiles
2 June 2021

Silence surrounding a public secret. – Two centuries of immigration medicine. – Between prevention of infections and regulation of migration. – Four versions of "migrant health." – Public hygiene for border control. – Survival of tropicalism after empire. – Racial differentialism in colonial psychiatry. – Sinistrosis and Mediterranean syndrome. – The avatars of ethnopsychiatry. – The epidemiological assessment of inequality. – Healthy migrant effect and unhealthy assimilation. – A critique of the notion of migrant health. – Ages of emigration and routes of exile. – Forms of life under threat.

To return once more to the textbook example of childhood lead poisoning, which public health physicians in France gradually began to get the measure of in the late 1980s, there was one striking but little noticed feature: of the first 2,000 children diagnosed in the Paris region, 99 percent were from African families, 85 percent of them from sub-Saharan Africa. This singularity was actually twofold: first, the fact that almost all the children shared a geographical origin, a factor that had virtually no equivalent in known nosography apart from a few genetic diseases such as sickle-cell anemia; second, the apparent blindness of the pediatricians, and subsequently of the other practitioners who encountered this pathology directly, to this overrepresentation, which is astonishing, given that the ethno-racial distribution of the disease implies that almost all the children affected were Black, a fact that would be difficult to ignore. So how is this twofold singularity to be explained?

First, how is the overrepresentation of children from African families to be accounted for? As mentioned earlier, this phenomenon initially gave rise to a series of quite exotic explanations. There was talk of "marabout's children's disease," in reference to the assumed profession of the fathers, and suggestions that the ink used in their Qur'anic tablets contained lead. The kohl the women used as make-up was brought into question as well as the glaze on the pottery believed to be used by them for cooking. It was imagined that some women's habit of sucking on clay during pregnancy led them to tolerate their offspring ingesting flakes of old paint. But the facts had to be faced eventually: none of these hypotheses was empirically validated. The explanation was not cultural: it was political. With the shortage of public social housing, and decent accommodation being unaffordable in the private rental sector, the immigrant families of sub-Saharan origin whose children were suffering from lead poisoning lived in unhealthy, sub-standard housing in this sector. In a situation of both economic and legal precarity, they had to resign themselves to living in dilapidated apartments leased by unscrupulous landlords, or sometimes simply abandoned and squatted. In such conditions, inhalation of dust and ingestion of paint flakes were logically the primary sources of the contamination of children.

But this being the case, how is the apparent blindness of health professionals to the evidence of the African, and more specifically sub-Saharan, origin of almost all the sick children to be interpreted? Initially, there was no mention of the overrepresentation of African families in their articles and reports. In subsequent years, reference began to be made to it, but it was relativized with suggestions of a recruitment bias, since the screening consultations took place in mother-and-child protection units used mainly by immigrant women who could not afford to go to private obstetricians and pediatricians. But this explanation was hard to uphold, given that children of sub-Saharan origin made up only one-quarter of those consulting at these units. The proportion of them presenting with lead poisoning was in fact three times their demographic weight at these services. We need, then, to ask why it was so difficult to name and analyze this overrepresentation. France has a long tradition, inherited especially from the memory of the racialism and racism of World War II, of avoiding or even prohibiting any reference to an individual's origin, and still more any racial categorization, even when it is pointed out that such categorization is not biological but, rather, the social product of a designation, an ascription, and a discrimination. The law, the census, and statistics show the marks of this tradition. But there is also a colonial blind spot, which has led study of the key moments of French history to focus on chivalry, church spires, and the Gaulish rooster, while forgetting colonization, has brought in the best experts on immigration to ignore its continuity with the colonial past, and has resulted in naturalization ceremonies presenting a film of national history that makes no mention of the

colonial heritage.[1] Over half a century after decolonization, the subject
remains a burning issue, and merely raising it sparks heated argument.
The information that those affected by childhood lead poisoning were
almost exclusively from immigrant and, moreover, sub-Saharan or
Black families was therefore impossible to articulate, less for strictly
legal reasons than out of a form of embarrassment that mingled scientific and political concerns (so as not to appear to validate the notion
of race and not to provide a pretext for the expression of racist views)
and a form of blindness (denying the survival of a colonial past). The
price paid for this embarrassment and blindness was to leave the field
open to a denial of the problem by public authorities, and the proliferation of culturalist explanations, for years. Racial discrimination
in housing and the resulting spatial segregation, which have, since
that period, been abundantly documented, were little known at the
time. At best people were prepared to recognize lead contamination in
children as the product of socioeconomic disparities. But immigrants
from sub-Saharan Africa living in the poorest sector of private rented
housing were not just part of the working class, or even part of the sub-
proletariat; their situation was also determined by the color of their
skin and the history in which it was inscribed.

The parallel with the United States, where childhood lead poisoning
had been the focus of numerous studies and preventive programs since
the mid-twentieth century, is once again instructive. For a long time,
childhood lead poisoning in the United States was essentially a disease
of African Americans – or, more precisely, a disease of poor Black
people. There was a strong statistical correlation between blood lead
levels measured in children, manifestly disadvantaged neighborhoods,
and the presence of a Black population. This is what Robert Sampson
and Alix Winter, drawing on an epidemiological and geographical
study of the city of Chicago they had been conducting since the mid-
1990s, call "the racial ecology of lead poisoning."[2] They show that, at
the neighborhood level, neither the socioeconomic characteristics of
residents, nor air and soil pollution, nor even the age or dilapidation
of housing, entirely explained the high blood lead levels in children. A
statistical residual remained that Sampson and Winter argue can only
be interpreted in relation with the racialist and racist past. In other
words, childhood lead poisoning is the product of the history of the
segregation of Black populations, reduced to congregating in poor
neighborhoods with decrepit housing. Hispanic residents face a similar
situation, though to a lesser degree.

In the contemporary period, studies have revealed a new phenomenon, or more precisely one that had hitherto gone unnoticed: that

children of recent immigrants also present blood lead levels much higher than those of the children of white families from the United States. In New York City, the risk of high blood lead levels in children was five times higher predominantly for Haitian, Dominican, Pakistani, and Mexican immigrants. In the state of Michigan the majority of those concerned are Latin-American immigrants.[3] In both cases, these are low-income families living in old apartment units. These observations have not stopped some researchers from continuing to point to cultural causes or harmful behaviors. Still today, the Centers for Disease Control and Prevention even issue a list of idiosyncratic practices to be investigated, as well as other nonspecific ones such as the use of automobile batteries to generate electricity, or traditional ceramics for the preparation of food. Depending on the origin of immigrant or refugee families, clinicians are advised to inquire about the use of the following ingredients: *bo ying*, a Chinese medicinal herb; *daw tway*, a digestive tablet from Burma; *bint al zahab*, a powdered stone from Iran that is mixed with honey and butter to soothe colic; *tiro*, a Nigerian cosmetic used as eye shadow; *tamarind candies*, Mexican candies sold in ceramic pots; and many others.[4] Lead poisoning clearly continues to arouse a certain exoticizing tendency in public health circles.

The combination of these US epidemiological studies showing a high prevalence of lead poisoning both among Black children and, to a lesser degree, among Hispanic children, regardless of socioeconomic, environmental, and residential factors, and among children of immigrant families from the global South, regardless of alleged idiosyncratic practices, helps to explain a fact that also pertains in France. It is not immigration as such that fosters lead poisoning, but racial segregation. In France, childhood lead poisoning does not affect immigrants from Canada, Brazil, Iran, Poland, or Portugal. It is almost exclusively confined to children of people from sub-Saharan Africa. The housing precarity of these families, which often goes hand in hand with economic and legal precarity, is intrinsically linked to the color of their skin, and to a large extent to their past as colonized peoples. It is the racialization they are subject to that blocks their access to social housing, long after they have submitted their application, on the often-unspoken grounds of preserving (implicitly racial) diversity. The aim, though not officially acknowledged, is to avoid the proportion of tenants from minorities rising above a certain level, so as not to create "ghettoes" – this in cities with a predominantly working-class population, since wealthy cities do not tend to engage in the politics of social housing. In short, the relationship between immigration and health cannot be thought without taking into account the race issue, which is itself bound up with the colonial past.

Interest in the relationship between immigration and health is certainly nothing new. It is therefore surprising to note that in 2017 Patricia Frye Walker, president of the American Society of Tropical Medicine and Hygiene, chose to call her opening address to the society's annual meeting "Migration medicine: Notes on a young science."[5] In fact migration medicine was present throughout the nineteenth century and into the early twentieth century, principally in the form of border control. In 1832, the authorities in Canada, which had seen a steady rise in immigration during the preceding years, fearing that a cholera epidemic then raging in Europe might reach the banks of the St. Lawrence river, created an outpost at Grosse-Île, upstream of Quebec City. Immigrants were held there in quarantine, while the ships that had brought them were inspected and cleaned before being authorized to proceed to dock.[6] Conversely, in New York in 1847, the state governor appointed six commissioners to visit ships that docked and treat their sick passengers. These were indigent people, many of them from Ireland. Many were suffering from typhus and other infections. They were taken to hospitals with overcrowded wards, where they were treated before heading, if they survived, to the city's low-income neighborhoods.[7] Half a century later, health policy toward immigrants became more repressive, however, with the passing of the Immigration Act in 1891, which prohibited the entry of persons presenting contagious diseases described as "loathsome" or "dangerous." At ports, foreigners were subjected, aboard the ship, to medical examinations seeking out pathologies that, depending on the case, could lead to refoulement or to internment for prolonged treatment. First- and second-class passengers were seen quickly, while those in third class were subject to stricter selection. Over the years, the criteria gradually broadened, from the diagnosis of an infection to the identification of a generally poor state of health, but physicians were more tolerant toward Europeans than toward Asians. The US Public Health Service thus became a significant tool of immigration control, with more than two-thirds of rejections eventually being on medical grounds.[8] In 1897 the New Zealand parliament attempted to pass a law restricting entry of those carrying infections into this Commonwealth territory. The law focused particularly on people with tuberculosis, many of whom were coming from Great Britain because it was then thought that the southern hemisphere offered a more favorable climate. The law was not passed, but two years later, in a context of anti-Asian xenophobia, a clause restricting the

immigration of persons suffering from contagious diseases was slipped
into the Immigration Restriction Bill. Nevertheless, this clause did not
prevent the arrival in subsequent years of immigrants who managed
to conceal their disease and, remarkably, often gained the sympathy
of local physicians.[9] Finally, in Great Britain, the Aliens Order, a
1920 decree on foreigners that introduced major restrictions on entry
into British territory, also incorporated a medical element. At a time
of mass unemployment following World War I, the measure sought
to limit the number of workers arriving, establishing a link between
immigration policy and the labor market for the first time. But in
addition to being seen by an immigration officer, foreigners were also
subjected to a medical examination to determine whether their condition represented a health danger to the population, or whether there
was a risk that, because of the treatment required, they would become
a financial burden on society. In fact, however, detailed study of the
procedures and decisions at the ports of London and Liverpool shows
that the Ministry of Health played a much smaller role than the Home
Office, and medical bureaucracy remained secondary in the selection
process.[10] As these various examples show, public health has long been
associated with immigration control. Analysis of these cases prompts
two general observations.

First, border checks were informed by two distinct rationales, one
that attempted to screen for contagious pathologies, and the other
operating as a subsidiary function of the regulation of entries. With
regard to infectious diseases, it is obviously ironic that the Europeans
who settled in the lands they had colonized should seek to protect
themselves from anything coming from outside, when they themselves
had decimated entire populations through the germs they brought with
them, including smallpox, measles, diphtheria, syphilis, and tuberculosis. In terms of immigration control, the role of medicine was
essentially to back up and legitimize policies aimed at restricting the
entry of foreigners into national territory. Although the weight given
to either of these considerations varied depending on circumstances,
the first being reinforced during epidemics and the second taking precedence when there was tension in the labor market, over this period
there was a clear shift from the first to the second, from protection
against disease to reduction of immigration. This dual focus still persists. Australia, for example, has never had a case of cholera, thanks
to rigorous border control during times of epidemic. And international
students are required to fill out a medical questionnaire, to consult an
approved physician, and to undergo blood tests and X-rays before
being granted a visa.

Second, while public health is often instrumentalized in support of repressive policies, it can also be mobilized to implement benevolent initiatives. It is used to justify the refoulement of sick individuals at the border, or to stigmatize groups by associating them with pathologies. But it is also invoked to protect immigrants against pathologies or to provide them with medical care. This ambivalence also still persists. In the late 1980s, France instituted medical procedures at its consulates in African countries that included blood tests for AIDS, for the purpose of selecting individuals permitted to obtain a visa – in other words, to exclude those who tested positive. But from the beginning of the following decade, under pressure from humanitarian and human rights organizations, France began to grant foreigners with AIDS present in its territory, many of whom were African, temporary residence permits, and also allowed them to receive free care under the state medical assistance system.

But border control is not just a matter of the issues immigration presents for medicine and public health.[11] In fact the field that French specialists define as "migrant health" (which nongovernmental organizations prefer to term "exile health," to emphasize the fact that many of these migrations are impelled by war and persecution as much as by poverty and lack of prospects) has a complex genealogy, in which four main approaches can be distinguished. These can be described respectively as hygienist, tropicalist, differentialist, and epidemiological.[12] These four versions of "migrant health" roughly followed on from one another, starting at the beginning of the twentieth century. However, none of them has entirely disappeared. We might rather think of their succession as a process of sedimentation that, from time to time, when a health or immigration crisis arises, allows discourses and practices that seemed to have been superseded to resurface.

The public hygiene approach is a nineteenth-century legacy, with a conception of health in terms of populations, an experience of managing epidemics, a technical apparatus based on statistical processing, an ideology strongly informed by the principle of solidarity, and a practice that is essentially administrative in form. As Virginie De Luca Barrusse shows, public hygiene professionals were involved in immigration matters mainly in relation to recruitment of the foreign labor force that was increasingly necessary for economic growth, from the end of the nineteenth century but especially in the aftermath of World War I.[13] This labor force came both from neighboring countries and from the colonies. The high demand and insufficient resources meant that medical checks, usually conducted at the border, were perfunctory: immigrants were vaccinated against smallpox, those who might carry typhus were deloused, clothing was disinfected, people were made to take showers, and good physical condition was cursorily inspected. The same urgency and the same practices prevailed during World War I when soldiers were being recruited to reinforce the French contingents decimated at the front. During the 1920s, however, public hygiene professionals became stricter in their selection of immigrants (including Europeans) to ensure their fitness for work, and above all more insistent in their concern about potential contagious infections, particularly in people coming from the colonies.

In 1925 Léon Bernard, a professor at the Medical School (Faculté de médicine) in Paris, member of the Academy of Medicine, and an authority on social hygiene, published an article significantly entitled "The health problem of immigration." Noting that immigration was necessary for economic and demographic reasons, he argued, however, that it had risen to an "excessive level," posing a worrying problem as, he wrote, "a considerable number of sick people have been introduced into France through immigration," and "they are agents of transmission of infectious diseases, sources of unproductive and illegitimate yet unavoidable expense, and factors in the deterioration of the race."[14] As an example of good practice, he cites the restrictive policy of the United States, which, he explains, has introduced a set of medical criteria for rejecting immigrants in order to palliate this threefold negative consequence of contagion, economic cost, and racial degeneration. Drawing on this model, he proposes that, on the basis of a thorough medical examination, entry into France should be forbidden to individuals suffering from mental illness, epilepsy, blindness, deaf-mutism, drug addiction, alcoholism, or any active infection, and concludes his call for what amounts to health policing by asking whether France, like Italy, should not appoint "a general commissioner for immigration." Not long afterwards, Bernard's call was echoed by a declaration along the same lines from the Paris Society of Medicine (Société de médecine de Paris), and by the choice of the "problem of immigration" as the theme for the thirteenth Public Hygiene Congress. During these years when xenophobia was increasingly freely expressed in French society, public hygiene professionals imprinted the health grounds for rejection of foreigners in the public space, with the threefold warning that continues to inform certain political discourses to this day, although race science is now rarely expressed so explicitly. The pernicious image of being at once a vector of disease, a burden on the economy, and a threat to national identity still weighs on the immigrant.

The origins of the tropicalist approach are to be found in the history of the great colonial powers, particularly Great Britain, Spain,

Portugal, and France. In the French case, the Pasteur Institutes represented the golden age, with multiple branches spread over almost the
entire globe, from Madagascar to Montevideo, from Tehran to Dakar,
from Tunis to Hanoi. Thus, as Aro Velmet puts it, "at the dawn of the
twentieth century, bacteriology and imperialism came to symbolize
a new vision of the grandeur of France."[15] Both were involved in the
country's civilizing mission in Asia, Africa, and Latin America, with
bacteriologists conducting their research into plague, typhus, yellow
fever, sleeping sickness, and many other conditions. The first colonial
Pasteur Institute was opened in Saigon in 1890 by Albert Calmette, the
co-inventor of the BCG vaccine. Of this vaccine, Louis Pasteur Vallery-
Radot, in his apologia for his grandfather's work, stated emphatically
that all the overseas Pasteur Institutes, as they were called, should have
the statement that Calmette passed down to posterity inscribed over
their entrances: "Without Pasteur's discoveries, the development and
emancipation of indigenous peoples, the improvement of their lands,
the colonial expansion of France and other great civilized nations
would have been impossible."[16] In the colonies, however, physicians
found themselves faced not only with the bacterial and viral infections on which Pasteur and his disciples had worked, but also, and
above all, parasitic diseases. In the course of his research in Algeria,
Alphonse Laveran had identified in 1880 the hematozoa responsible
for malaria, a disease that until then had been ascribed to the noxious
air of marshes, and thus laid the foundations of what would become
"exotic pathology." A little earlier, Patrick Manson, a British physician working in China, had established in 1878 that a mosquito was
the vector for filariasis, earning him the title of the father of "tropical
medicine." Thus, Laveran set up the Société de pathologie exotique,
while Manson founded the renowned London School of Tropical
Medicine. The colonial world was thus the source of a new discipline,
known as either "exotic pathology" or "tropical medicine," depending
on which side of the English Channel one found oneself.

It might have been supposed that these disciplines would disappear
with independence, given their colonial past. Such was not the case,
however. On the contrary, immigration gave them a renewed lease on
life. In France alone, not only did the Pasteur Institutes continue their
research in exotic lands alongside the Office for Overseas Scientific and
Technical Research (Orstom, Office de la recherche scientifique et technique outre-mer), which later became the Institute for Development
Research (IRD, Institut de recherche pour le développement), but
specialists who had trained in the colonies retreated to dedicated
clinics, including in Paris those at the Claude-Bernard hospital, now

transferred to the Bichat hospital, and the Salpêtrière hospital. And it was to these so-called tropical disease departments that, almost as a matter of course, migrants from the African continent were most often referred, as if their origin determined the institution and the specialist department where they should be seen. A dogma known as "migrant health" became established in faculties of medicine. It instituted a nosography based on a triptych entirely conceived in relation to the chronology of migration: imported pathologies, usually parasitic, such as malaria, bilharzia, or filariasis; acquired pathologies, of which sexually transmitted diseases were supposedly the archetype; pathologies of adaptation, typified by depression due to isolation. The essentialization of migrants thus led to the naturalization of their pathology. Yet with the passing of time, this nosography made less and less sense – if, indeed, it ever had. The existence of tropical disease departments was increasingly less justified, since neither long-resident immigrants nor new arrivals, who were fewer in number and often came from cities, presented with these conditions any longer. Albeit marginalized, the discipline was nevertheless saved, if I dare say, by an opportune conversion related to the spread of the AIDS epidemic – both because infectiology was once more a global priority and because many patients happened to be African.

The differentialist approach has another way of particularizing migrants, on cultural rather than biological grounds. What is at play in this case is culturalism, which is a particular form of differentialism. As mentioned earlier, the characteristic features of culturalism are, first, a reification of culture, with the assumption that a given people or group corresponds to a specific culture, and, second, the desire to explain individuals' thinking and behavior in terms of their culture thus defined. Overall, it tends to radicalize alterity: the other is irreducibly different. It was in the domain of mental health that the differentialist approach was most explicitly applied; here again, the framework was developed in the colonial world. More specifically, the Algiers School (École d'Alger), under the leadership of Antoine Porot, developed a "Muslim psychiatry" during the 1920s, which made it, to quote Richard Keller, "the French empire's leading authority on the intersection of race and psychopathology."[17] During World War I, Porot, a neuropsychiatrist, had found himself chief medical officer of the Algiers military region, and encountered the Algerian recruits whom he described as "a shapeless mass of profoundly ignorant and largely credulous primitives." Although he recognized, from the experience of his medical practice, that "it is difficult to give even a rough outline of the psychology of the Muslim," he nevertheless presented a definitive picture that reveals not so much a fine clinical sense as a prosaic everyday racism. He writes of the Muslim native, as he calls him, that "his affective life is minimal and revolves in the restricted sphere of basic instincts," that his "passivity is the spontaneous manifestation of an often spiritless temperament," that his "mental childishness differs from that of children in the sense that there is no spirit of curiosity," that he has "no appetite for knowledge, no general ideas, and simple syllogisms, sometimes stupid in their conclusions," and finally that, faced with the experience of violence, his "rather unsophisticated and literal mind applies all its inert mass to the initial trauma," and that even if he did manifest symptoms, what was apparent was their "resemblance to our old Medieval hysteria." Having witnessed "legions of exaggerators and perseverators," Porot was therefore able to conclude: "The Muslim has therefore not been overly disturbed by the emotions of war."[18] This psychological portrait thus made it possible to ignore the kind of traumatic war neuroses observed among European soldiers at that time. Over the years, Porot would add to the portrait, not without some repetition, in various later articles on "the criminal impulse in the North African native," which emphasizes the constitutional nature of his "fundamental mental debility," and on "the primitivism of North African natives," which expounds an evolutionist theory about the "fragility of cortical integration" and the "predominance of diencephalic functions." The particularization of this "Muslim psychiatry" allowed the Algiers School to engage in the practice of aggressive treatment methods, ranging from electric shock therapy to lobotomy.[19] Some decades later, Frantz Fanon, a psychiatrist at the Blida hospital, was to put this race science, which was still prevalent on the eve of independence, on trial in his writings.[20] Pointing to the "number and depth of the injuries inflicted upon a native during a single day spent amidst the colonial regime," he contrasts it with a psychiatry that takes into account the mental disorders of both colonizers and colonized, deriving precisely from the colonial situation.

The Algiers School merits attention not just for the central place it occupied in the construction of colonial psychiatry,[21] but also for the imprint it left after independence on the definition of the mental health of migrants, particularly those from North Africa, at a time when Algeria, Morocco, and Tunisia were the main sources of non-European immigration to France. Although Porot's students practiced in mainland France, and some, such as Jean Sutter in Marseille and Yves Pélicier in Paris, occupied prestigious posts in teaching hospitals, this imprint was more evident in the authorized expression of a racialized clinical practice, often infused with racist stereotypes, in psychiatry but also in medicine. This is evident from two diagnoses that were frequently used to label patients originating from North Africa: "sinistrosis" and "Mediterranean syndrome." The first can be found in some psychiatry textbooks. The second was to be heard in hospital corridors and physicians' consulting rooms. The attribution of these diagnoses was influenced by gender, with sinistrosis being almost always a male disorder and Mediterranean syndrome most often diagnosed in women. Sinistrosis, a neurosis said to be related to a claim following an accident, was the name for a clinical picture in which the patient was alleged to suffer and complain of his suffering in order to obtain secondary benefits, such as extension of his sick leave and financial compensation for injury. Having been used to describe French workers during the first half of the twentieth century, in the latter half it was widely applied to North African workers injured on construction sites. As the name suggests, the negative image associated with the condition tended to invalidate the symptoms manifested and to obscure difficult working conditions that led to accidents. While sinistrosis thus has an official status, albeit no longer in use, Mediterranean syndrome belongs to a sort of clandestine medical language. It refers to a clinical picture characterized by diffuse pain that the physician is unable to interpret in his normal nosographic framework, and which he therefore ascribes to a geographically defined entity derived from a culturalist view of the disease. Here again the representation disparages the symptoms presented by the individual, which are deemed to have no organic cause, in other words no objective reality. Yet a diagnosis of Mediterranean syndrome might subsequently have to be corrected when cancer or another serious pathology was revealed to be the actual cause of the suffering the individual had complained of. Apart from the fact, then, that they point to the clinical shortcomings of psychiatry and medicine rather than their nosographic creativity, these two diagnoses manifestly bear a family resemblance to Porot's descriptions: they too incorporate the suspicion of malingering that he stigmatized, the difference being that elementary psychology underpinned by a simplistic evolutionism had been replaced by a psychoanalytic language in the case of sinistrosis, and a culturalist one in the case of Mediterranean syndrome. It is, however, hard to tell whether these representations have been transmitted through the scientific-sounding discourse of Algerian psychiatrists and propagated to distant followers, or, rather, whether a scientific-sounding discourse was legitimizing those same racial readings and racist prejudices, previously openly expressed in the colonies and now formulated in supposedly acceptable terms – in other words, whether this is a question of historical continuity or structural similarity.

But this offensive discourse has become outmoded, and is gradually disappearing. It is being replaced by another form of differentialism, more subtle and more complex: ethnopsychiatry. It could be said to have been founded by John Colin Carothers, as Jock McCulloch suggests.[22] This English physician, who was director of the Mathari hospital in Nairobi in the late 1930s, was self-taught in the discipline in which he subsequently distinguished himself, first in 1953, when he wrote the report *The African Mind in Health and Disease* for the World Health Organization, and then in 1954 when, as the British government's special commissioner, he wrote an account of the Kikuyu rebellion in Kenya, entitled *The Psychology of the Mau Mau*. In the WHO report, he explained Africans' intellectual inferiority in terms of a frontal-lobe laziness that made them resemble lobotomized Europeans. In his memoir, he ascribed the Mau Mau rebellion to a pathological deterioration in their forest mentality and their unhealthy obsession with the colonizers, eliding the political project of their nationalist and territorial demands. As the subtitle of his report for the WHO indicates, these are presented as works of ethnopsychiatry.

They are different, however, from contemporary ethnopsychiatry, which deals predominantly with "migrants." The origins of this variant are to be found in the psychopatholgy of Henri Collomb, at the Fann hospital in Dakar, and the ethnopsychoanalysis practiced by Georges Devereux at the EPHE (École pratique des hautes études) in Paris. In contrast to the colonial psychiatry practiced by Porot and Carothers, which claimed that the difference between North Africans and Africans, on the one hand, and Europeans, on the other, was anatomically based and often evolutionary, contemporary ethnopsychiatry ascribes this difference to the culture, which is supposedly characteristic of each people. There are two main versions of this French branch, which is without doubt the most widely known internationally.[23] One is a radical version, represented by psychologist Tobie Nathan, which holds that every individual belongs to an ethnic group and should be educated and treated in line with the principles of her or his ethnic group: the universalism of French republican schooling and clinical medicine is therefore fundamentally corrupting. The other, more open, version is represented by psychiatrist Marie-Rose Moro, who advocates both recognizing cultural differences and the practice of ethnic mixing, and collaborates with public institutions responsible for caring for children and adolescents from mainly African families. These distinct practices of ethnopsychiatry, which is sometimes renamed transcultural psychiatry, as it is known in Québec, are often based on collective therapeutic processes that ethnopsychiatrists claim are inspired by the traditional representations and practices of the societies from which patients originate. This approach therefore implies a specific treatment for patients who come from other worlds, or are imagined to do so because their parents emigrated, or because the color of the skin suggests they do, even if they are French and born in France. Moreover, paradoxically it is often schools and courts that turn to ethnopsychiatrists, as if specific solutions were required for these patients rather than ordinary law.

Finally, the epidemiological approach, which is the most recent, is distinguished from previous approaches by its focus on quantification as a means to objectively assess the health of immigrants. The discipline occupies a central position in the domain of public health, as the supreme technical system of knowledge production, whether that be characterizing groups, as in descriptive epidemiology, establishing causality, with analytical epidemiology, or measuring the efficacy of interventions, through evaluative epidemiology. For a long time, epidemiologists evinced little interest in the subject of immigration. There are many reasons for this indifference. In France these certainly included the fear of feeding xenophobia, as the public hygiene approach had done, the embarrassment around everything having to do with origins, and above all a predominant focus on explanation in terms of socioeconomic variables, inherited from the first studies of mortality inequality in the early nineteenth century. In the United States they included the fact that studies focused on ethnic and, particularly, racial categories made others less visible, since most studies differentiated between whites, Blacks and Hispanics but rarely considered immigrants as a category. In both contexts, it is also likely that the data were more difficult to obtain or construct, given the mobility of immigrants, the variety of their status, and the different lengths of time they had been in the country where they were living.[24] Conversely, the subsequent development of epidemiological studies on the subject was due partly to the growing prominence of the issue of immigration in often polemical public debate, and partly to the worrying increasing vulnerability of immigrants with regard to health and care, resulting from national and international policies concerning them. There was thus both a social demand and a social need for knowledge. But what epidemiological research showed was not exactly what might have been imagined.

First, there was what is known as the "healthy migrant effect," or more specifically for some authors, the "migrant mortality advantage": in general, people who migrate to a country are in better health than nationals, measured in terms of a series of indicators such as age- and sex-adjusted mortality, life expectancy, birth weight, and infant mortality. This result, which is surprising given that they come from poorer countries and settle in wealthier countries where they are often relegated to the lowest sector of society, recurs in studies of a range of groups, including Turks in Germany, southern Europeans in Sweden, and Latin Americans in the United States.[25] By way of example, in the latter country, the life expectancy of white immigrants is nearly a year longer than that of US-born whites, and when the comparison is extended to other groups, the gap increases to 3.8 years for Hispanic men and 8.1 years for Black men, depending on whether they were born in the United States or migrated there.[26] Incidentally, the initial advantage of people originating from Latin America is often described as the "Hispanic paradox," because the life expectancy at birth of Hispanic men is 79.1 years compared to 76.1 years for white men and 71.5 years for Black men, owing to the fact that Hispanic men make up a large proportion of immigrants. Remarkably, this advantage is greater for Hispanic individuals born abroad than for those born in the United States.[27] It has moreover been suggested that the term should be extended geographically, to identify a "Mediterranean paradox" in European countries.[28] These observations, which are surprising given that it is known that, in general, immigrants experience more adverse living conditions and find it harder to access healthcare than those born in the country, led to suspicions of a bias related to both the people entering and those leaving the countries in question. With regard to those entering, people who migrate are in fact on average more robust than those who remain: choices are made, prioritizing the "fittest," either by self-selection within families or through selection organized by consulates – at least as far as traditional emigration is concerned, for such choices do not operate in the case of departures impelled by conflict or persecution.[29] In the case of those leaving, it is assumed conversely that people in poor health return to their countries to die: this phenomenon is known as the "salmon bias," named for the salmon who at the end of their life return to the river where they were born. While this phenomenon does exist in the case of immigrants to the United States, its effect is modest, except for Mexicans, probably for reasons of geographical proximity.[30] However, these biases are not sufficient to explain the better health outcomes of immigrants, at least in many studies.[31] It is thought that a healthier way of life, particularly as regards alcohol consumption and smoking, food, and exercise, plays an important role, helping to explain the paradox of migrants' good health. But the extent of the paradox varies in relation to country of origin and host country, and even depending on cohort, with more recent migrants having poorer health than those who arrived earlier.

However, the advantage observed on arrival does not last. The terms "unhealthy assimilation" and "health convergence" describe the gradual reduction in the initial advantage. A European study of 100,000 older individuals in nineteen countries showed that, in terms of a number of indicators, the health of immigrants, which was initially better, dropped to the level of nationals after they had been in the country for a certain length of time. Reaching this point of convergence took twenty years for self-reported health, twenty-seven years for excess weight, thirty years for chronic disease, and fifty-two years for restrictions on everyday activities. This accelerated deterioration is more marked among immigrants from poor countries.[32] Similar observations have been made elsewhere with regard to other indicators such as complications in pregnancy and premature birth. In France, a study of a nationwide sample of 1 percent of the population confirmed, first, the initial health advantage of immigrants, interpreted as the result of healthier practices in the country of origin and selection of the most robust for migration, and, second, the unhealthy acculturation, owing to the adoption of harmful behaviors in terms of alcohol and tobacco consumption, diet, and activity, but also to multiple disadvantages in living and working conditions.[33] In the United States, the observations initially made solely with regard to Hispanic populations have been generalized, and analyses have been refined in relation to regions of origin, showing, on the one hand, that Black immigrants also had an advantage over Black people born in the country, and, on the other, that those from the Caribbean gradually lost it, while those from Africa retained it: these facts confirm the effect of selection, and differentiate the process of deterioration.[34] Thus, over the course of a few decades, the epidemiology of immigration established solid facts, demonstrated in relation to a variety of indicators and in diverse contexts: first, despite the difference in standard of living between the country they leave and the country where they settle, immigrants are in better health than those born in the country when they arrive; second, with time, they lose their advantage and their health deteriorates. Thus, unlike the other three approaches, the epidemiological approach makes space for the social dimension of the migration experience, by taking into account differences in the poverty of the country of origin, or living conditions in the host country. Yet this aspect of the experience still receives little attention. It is in the fine detail of the figures that the effect of the social is to be sought. These statistics are precious, but they are still discussed primarily in technical terms.

The four approaches I have outlined here – public hygiene, tropical-ism, differentialism, epidemiology – succeeded one another over time, but none of them disappeared completely. The public hygiene approach resurfaces in times of epidemics, with the resurgent temptation to close borders and control immigration. Tropicalism is reinvented with so-called emergent infectious diseases that have little to do with the old exotic pathologies. Differentialism has freed itself from the original evolutionist, organicist, and offensive tendencies of colonial psychia-try, re-emerging as ethnopsychiatry. Epidemiology itself changes by taking on new questions. A remarkable feature of these changes is the way the expression of xenophobia and racism, so open during a large part of the twentieth century, is fading out. Except within far-right ide-ology, it is no longer acceptable to talk of racial degeneration caused by immigration, or Muslims' mental fragility. Culture often replaces race in the explanation of behaviors or the justification of treatment. Conversely, the French so-called republican ethos rejects any distinc-tion based on origin, skin color, or religious affiliation in surveys and services. It is as if the colonial legacy of xenophobia and racism had been forgotten, suppressed, as if the reality of racial discrimination linked to immigration had become transparent, impossible to articu-late. Hence the silence around the selective exposure of children of African families to the risk of lead poisoning, and the embarrassment around accounting for it once it had become difficult to deny.

Despite the sedimentation of these four approaches over time, they did not merge. But whatever distinguishes them from one another, two elements unite them: they particularize the migrant population, and they ascribe to it its health conditions one way or another. For public hygiene professionals, migrants are potential vectors of infec-tion. For tropicalists, they suffer the effects of the physical environ-ment in which they live. For differentialists, they inherit physical or cultural traits that explain deviant behaviors and mental disorders. For epidemiologists, they benefit from favorable health practices in their country of origin but lose the advantage when they assimilate into their new country. Each of these ways of viewing immigrants has its own logic and its specific relevance. Prevention of the spread of epidemics can justify certain border controls. Knowledge of parasite cycles is essential to the treatment of parasitic infections. Attention to immigrants' self-representation and their ways of treating disease can be helpful in caring for them. The counterintuitive evidence of a better state of health on arrival and subsequent deterioration is important in understanding the consequences of migration. But it is clear that particularizing migrants and focusing on their characteristics leads to considering them as separate from the rest of the population, as if they had enough in common among themselves to justify distinguishing them from others, even though they may have very different life journeys and situations. Whether these approaches stigmatize migrants, as in the case of the interwar public hygiene professionals or the colonial psychiatrists, or aspire to benevolence, as contemporary tropicalists or ethnopsychiatrists do, or even whether they attempt to neutralize their topic through quantification, as in the case of epidemiology – in other words, whether they adopt one or other moral position – is not the point. For the problem is not a moral one. It is doubly political, from the point of view of science and from the point of view of society. Here again, if children of African families make up almost all of those affected by childhood lead poisoning when most of them are French nationals born in France, it is the result of policies that researchers and physicians must acknowledge and integrate into their analyses, simply because these children are no longer immigrants.

The question then becomes whether it is possible both to cease singularizing immigrants and to stop ascribing health conditions to them. Continuing to talk about "migrant health," as is still the case in most public health textbooks and teachings that devote a chapter to the subject thus defined, often means unconsciously applying the same exceptional treatment to exiles as immigration policies have long imposed on them. And continuing to think of "migrant health" as if it were an entity that can be described using a language (vectors, risks, syndromes, transmission, acculturation) and variables (self-reported health, life expectancy, country of origin, length of residence, age on arrival) to characterize this population means depriving ourselves of tools that could help us to reflect on the simultaneously objective and subjective reality of what the World Health Organization calls the physical, mental, and social well-being of these exiles who, often by force of circumstance, move from one country to another to try to build a better life. I shall consider two examples.

The first example concerns occupational health. Various studies show that migrants are much more often employed than nationals in jobs that present a higher risk of workplace accidents and work-related diseases, particularly in agriculture, cleaning, construction, and public works.[35] A survey of 30,000 people in thirty-one European countries showed that they are significantly more exposed to onerous working conditions known to have repercussions on health.[36] Among men, nonmanual workers more often suffer psychological pressure linked to shiftwork, with variable hours and a fast pace of work, and unfavorable working arrangements, including Sunday presence and enforced changes to working hours. Manual workers are more frequently exposed to high temperatures, high noise levels, uncomfortable body positions, intense machine vibrations, and repetitive hand movements. Among women, there are also adverse differences, including the length of time spent standing during the day. In parallel, an analysis in the United States compared mortality from workplace accidents among foreigners, who represent 16.5 percent of the labor force, and nationals.[37] Out of 39,000 deaths recorded over eight years, the risk of dying, after adjustment for age, sex, and profession, was 15 percent higher for foreigners, and even 30 percent higher for Mexicans. It was particularly high in security, construction, cleaning, and catering. It should be added that these official data do not take account of workers without residence permits, who are employed clandestinely and are known generally to accept particularly punishing working conditions. However that may be, in the light of these studies, can the data collected be said to reflect "migrant health," that is, the health condition of migrants as related to their migration? Or is it rather that they reveal the way migrant labor is treated in the various areas of work, the way immigrants are exploited in the name of flexible production, the fact that they are exposed more than nationals to a variety of harms, not as well protected against dangers, given less time to train in risk prevention? If this is the case, we need to speak not of migrant health, but of occupational health, and to link their health condition not to their migration as such, but to the practices of corporations that penalize them because of their social vulnerability.

The second example relates to humanitarian medicine, as practiced in the various more or less informal spaces where people, mostly undocumented foreigners or asylum seekers, gather.[38] In Calais, in the waste terrain generally known as "the Jungle," where the French government permitted several thousand people to set up camp in 2015, and where nongovernmental organizations have opened clinics, a number of surveys have been carried out among a population consisting primarily of young men who at that time came mainly from Sudan, Eritrea, Ethiopia, Afghanistan, Iraq, Iran, and Syria.[39] These studies noted in particular the high frequency of respiratory infections, in a quarter of patients, and of scabies and other skin conditions, in a fifth of patients. Most significantly, they showed that two-thirds of exiles reported having suffered violence, a quarter of them in Calais at the hands of the police; they complained of beatings, tear gas inhalation, and being held at the precinct. The Syrian students I met in "the Jungle" all wanted to show me their scars from nightstick blows and dog bites. A report by Human Rights Watch, written following the French government's destruction of the camp, showed that repression of the migrant and refugee families who subsequently set up precarious camps on the beaches and in public spaces has become still harsher, with the police using pepper spray at night to disperse them, confiscating their sleeping bags and clothing, and preventing humanitarian organizations from distributing food.[40] At a more global level, a number of studies have been carried out in various countries on the effects of detention on the mental health of asylum seekers. A meta-analysis assembled data from twenty-six studies relating to 2,099 individuals, including twelve studies in centers in Australia and five in the United States.[41] The frequency of mental disorders was high: two Australian studies, for example, showed that between 95 and 100 percent of children were suffering from severe depression, 80 percent were self-harming, and 50 percent of adolescents presented with enuresis. Among adults, in two US studies, 86 percent were suffering from depression, 77 percent from anxiety, and 76 percent from post-traumatic stress. Although some of these psychiatric and psychological disorders may stem from violence suffered in the country of origin, the higher levels of psychic distress among individuals detained than among those not detained indicate that detention conditions play a part, often duplicating earlier suffering. Reading Kurdish journalist Behrouz Boochani's memoir *No Friend but the Mountains*, about his five-year imprisonment on the island of Manus off Australia, where he had gone to seek asylum, gives an insight into the degree of dehumanization to which refugees can be reduced and to which, at the same time, a nation can stoop.[42] Such situations might be imagined to be isolated cases, but the United Nations High Commissioner for Refugees states that, in a number of countries, "putting people in detention has become a routine – rather than exceptional – response to the irregular entry or stay of asylum-seekers and migrants." It should be borne in mind that in Australia, the United States, and many other countries, there is generally no provision for filing a request for asylum, and therefore any applicant for refugee status is by definition irregular and detained.[43] Once again, are we to analyze these pathologies and sufferings in terms of "migrant health," as if migration in and of itself characterized or determined the health of exiles? Or should their respiratory infections and skin conditions be seen as the result of winters spent confined without heating in the insalubrious, overcrowded shacks and tents set up in more or less tolerated encampments, and the mental disorders developed by adults and more so by children as the consequence of fear, waiting, and uncertainty, and of the bullying, harassment, violence, and destruction of their shelters and their meager belongings perpetrated by the police?

In this interpretation, in humanitarian situations too we must speak not of migrant health, but perhaps invert the viewpoint to consider instead the health of the society that treats those who have come to seek refuge in this way.

These two illustrations of occupational health and health in the camps relate to the conditions encountered by recent and more long-term immigrants in so-called host countries. However, we need to heed Abdelmalek Sayad's warning: "Any study of migratory phenomena that overlooks the emigrants' conditions of origin is bound only to give a view that is at once partial and ethnocentric. On the one hand, it is only the immigrant – and not the emigrant – who is taken into consideration, rather as though his life began the moment he came to France. On the other hand, the problematic, both explicit and implicit is always that of adaptation to the "host" society."[44] To some extent, it could be said that taking an interest in "emigrants' origin" is what the public hygiene, tropicalist, differentialist, and even the epidemiological approaches each do in their own way, by highlighting respectively the risk of infection, unhealthy environment, cultural particularism, and good health practices. But leaving aside the taint of racialism, and indeed racism, in some of these approaches, at least in the past, none of them really attempts to grasp the social, historical, and political dimensions of emigration. Yet the sons of rural Malian families who came to work in French factories in the 1960s have sociologically very little in common with Congolese asylum seekers fleeing persecution in their country in the 1990s. Even for emigration from one specific region, for example Syria, there are major differences between the generation of political dissidents who came as refugees in the 1980s and the generation of students and executives attempting to escape the civil war during the 2010s. In this regard, Sayad himself describes what he calls the "three ages of emigration," corresponding to three generations, each of which develops a particular form of the "double absence" – absence from the country of origin, to which emigrants return less and less, and absence in the host country, where they do not find their place.

In the contemporary world, however, we need a broader understanding of "emigration," encompassing not only the origin, nor even the departure, but also the journey. The journey has become an increasingly significant part of the migration adventure, as Western countries close their borders to people from poor countries, which may also be countries in the grip of war, countries where minorities are persecuted, countries where people suffer from destitution or simply the lack of a future – countries which, for diverse, sometimes tragic, reasons, people

have had to leave. While a few decades ago all they needed to do was
take a plane or a boat, when they could afford it, to get to the country
to which they were emigrating, those from poor countries now have
to make the clandestine, grueling, interminable journey by road. And
"road" is to be understood in broad terms, for it is often a matter of
fording turbulent rivers, venturing along unmarked paths, hiding in
suffocating containers. This is the paradox of the present. While technological advances, especially in aeronautics, combined with tourist and
business economics, have put the most remote destinations less than a
twenty-four-hour flight away, itineraries have never been so long or so
dangerous for those who travel not for pleasure or work, but to survive
or simply to make their life more livable. In the study Anne-Claire
Defossez and I have been conducting in the Alps among exiles who
had crossed the Montgenèvre pass from Italy into France, the men and
women who arrived had left their country between two and five years
earlier. From West Africa, Ivorians traveled through Burkina Faso
and Niger, the Senegalese through Mali and Algeria. Crossing the
Sahara was fraught with danger owing to violent extortion from armed
gangs in zones partly controlled by terrorist organizations. In Libya,
through which it was virtually impossible to avoid traveling, these
exiles were imprisoned, in some cases several times, and liberated only
upon payment of a ransom. If they were unable to pay, a local employer
could settle the sum in exchange for a month of forced labor. Finally
there was the perilous crossing of the Mediterranean, during which
many had seen their traveling companions drown. From the Middle
East, the journey was longer, though perhaps a little less dangerous.
Afghans, often helped across borders by Kurdish smugglers, traveled
through Iran and Turkey, where they sometimes stayed for several
months to save the money needed for the perilous passage through
the Greek islands; they then continued through Greece, Albania or
Bulgaria, Montenegro or Serbia, Bosnia, and Croatia, where they were
severely beaten and stripped of their goods, before reaching Slovenia.
Whether they came from West Africa or the Middle East, once they
were in Italy, some exiles received the minimum welfare assistance
from the government and local support organizations, until the day
when the policy changed, their meager subsidies were cut, hostels were
closed, and temporary residence permits were not renewed. They then
had to set out on the road again. Once they had crossed the Alps,
sometimes taking serious risks in the cold and snow, avoiding roads
and paths and venturing into the mountains so as not to be seen by
the border police, they took the train, in the best cases to join a family
member or friend who would put them up, and otherwise to gather in

makeshift shelters around Paris or Calais, with no water supply or sanitation, dependent on food aid from support organizations and subject to brutal expulsion by the police. Thus, today, given how long it takes and the risks to which it exposes people, migration as such is taking on a new meaning: it is a life stage, indeterminate, unpredictable, with a beginning but rarely an end. Exiles, always at risk of being rejected and deported, at least until they have obtained a residence permit, never know what tomorrow will bring. Even when they are allowed to apply for asylum, their request no longer protects them from deportation if they have been forced to provide their fingerprints in the first country they passed through. A product of contemporary anti-immigration policies, their form of life is undefined and ungrounded.[45] This is not without its consequences for their health.

A final paradox, then. Having wished to departicularize "migrant health" by questioning the association of migrants with infection risk, a physical environment, cultural traits, and behavioral characteristics, I have finally to reintroduce a particularity of the exile's condition by showing how it affects the physical, mental, and social well-being of those who experience it. This is a paradox, but not a contradiction. Here, mine is a radically different perspective, one that focuses not on the qualities of individuals, but on the form of life imposed on them by state authorities, one that takes into account historical developments and their effects on this form of life. Just as working and living conditions explain the deterioration in a state of health that on arrival was on average better than that of nationals, so restrictive and repressive immigration policies, with the concomitant lack of cooperation between European countries in taking responsibility for refugees and the externalization of border controls to Turkey, Libya, and Morocco, make migrants' journeys dangerous and sometimes fatal. The implications of this observation are clear.

A meta-analysis of nineteen studies over three continents shows that unfavorable policies with regard to entry into the country, access to rights, social protection, and integration have deleterious consequences for the general health, particularly the mental health, and the mortality of immigrants.[46] This result is of course unsurprising. However, it reminds us that in a time when these restrictive and repressive policies are becoming normalized, when ethnic and racial discrimination is becoming routine in many spheres, it is on the basis of the consideration, treatment, and dignity accorded to exiles that the ethics of the host society are to be judged.

Carceral Ordeals
9 June 2021

A peculiar source of criminal career. – The parallel history of the internment of lunatics and criminals. – The general hospital, a place of indiscriminate internment for undesirables. – The time of the reformers. – The birth of the asylum and the prison. – The aborted humanization of places of internment. – Psychiatric and penitentiary establishments of the Jacksonian era. – The penalization of the lower classes. – Contrasting the evolution of asylum and prison populations. – Fewer crimes, but more prisoners. – Omnipresence of mental disorders and lack of specialist care in prisons. – Penal practices and carceral condition as sources of excess suicide. – Physical death, social death. – Punishing in lieu of caring.

The most unexpected result of epidemiological studies of childhood lead poisoning, as presented earlier, was the establishment of a presumed causal link between lead poisoning in childhood and the perpetration of delinquent and criminal acts in adolescence or adulthood. It is indeed, to say the least, surprising that the presence of lead in old paint, water pipes, or air polluted by vehicle emissions could account at least in part for delinquency and criminality in poor neighborhoods. The first suspicions of a link between the two phenomena date back to a study from the 1960s of children in Philadelphia, who were followed over a period of twenty years from birth, but it was not until the 1990s that research on this subject began to proliferate in the United States. Most of this research was based on one or the other of two different methodological protocols. The first method consisted in following a cohort of children presenting with varying levels of lead contamination over a given period, and recording the occurrence of a range of disorders such as attention deficit, hyperactivity, aggressiveness, and impulsivity, and the subsequent incidence of criminal acts, and then calculating whether there was a statistical association between blood lead level during childhood and these various so-called antisocial behaviors late in life. The second method worked not on an individual but on a territorial scale, comparing rates of delinquency and criminality in counties or cities with different levels of lead in the air, or in the water supply systems.[1] The first approach is known as prospective, the second as ecological. The frame of reference in the former is temporal, and in the latter spatial. Whatever the method employed, the statistical association between presence of lead and the perpetration of criminal acts was almost always demonstrated, though the strength of the relation varied. Subjects presenting with lead contamination were more likely than average to show attention-deficit hyperactivity disorder in childhood and criminal behavior in adolescence and adulthood. Researchers estimated that, in the United States, lead poisoning at an early age was responsible for one-fifth of crimes committed, and that the reduction of lead contamination explained half of the dramatic fall in violent crime in the late twentieth century.[2] But was there not a bias in the establishment of this association between the two phenomena, given that other variables, particularly socioeconomic factors, could also contribute to the incidence of these issues. The interpretation of the data therefore poses problems that are not only technical, but also moral and political.

Sociobiological explanations – biological explanations of social facts – are not new, and they have been widely criticized in the past. But here the alignment between studies based on different methods, either following children to adulthood or analyzing at the level of regions or groups, backed up by both anatomopathological and epidemiological evidence of the toxicity of lead for the brain, throws strong suspicion on the role of lead in the onset not only of cognitive deficits but also of mental disorders and even criminal practices. Are children living in dilapidated buildings, contaminated by tap water, or exposed to vehicle emissions more at risk of becoming delinquent adolescents? The difficulty, of course, lies in the existence of what are known as confounding factors. Two phenomena may be statistically associated owing to the influence of a third that affects both simultaneously. In this case, the proportion of dilapidated housing and rates of juvenile delinquency are particularly high in low-income neighborhoods and among racial minorities, and these social variables – poverty and minority status – are associated both with high levels of lead poisoning and with the frequency of criminal acts. We might therefore wonder whether it is because those most at risk of lead poisoning belong to these marginalized and disadvantaged groups that they are also more often involved than others in crime. Aware of this problem, most authors strive to control statistically for these variables in order to provide results formulated in terms of "all things being equal," as the time-honored phrase has it.

Thus, in one study carried out in Pennsylvania, a high bone lead level was detected four times more frequently in adolescents convicted of various offenses than in others of the same age and from the same city who had no criminal record, even after adjustment for racial category, parents' level of education and profession, household composition, and neighborhood crime rates. But in another study conducted in New Zealand, after adjustment for sex, blood lead levels measured at age 11 were only weakly associated with the frequency of criminal convictions in adulthood, and paradoxically appeared to be more predictive of nonviolent than of violent offenses, and of a first offense than of repeat offending. However, it is difficult to compare these two conclusions, given the difference in methodologies, since the Pennsylvania research was a cross-section study using a measure of bone lead level, while that in New Zealand was a thirty-year longitudinal study based on an initial measurement of blood lead level. Furthermore, over and above the national differences, the composition of the groups (Black minorities in Pennsylvania versus white-majority subjects in New Zealand) and the type of exposure (in one case from paint, with widely varying distribution, and in the other from vehicle emissions, with no social differentiation) probably explain these divergent results.[3] Notwithstanding these apparent contradictions, in light of research carried out on at least three continents, it can be asserted that there is a statistical association between childhood lead poisoning and the perpetration of offenses.[4] This association usually persists when adverse socioeconomic conditions are taken into account. All the same, James Feigenbaum and Christopher Muller conclude their historical study establishing a relationship between lead poisoning and violent crime: "If lead exposure increases crime, then the solution is to invest in lead removal ... Even if lead removal will not reduce crime, it will remove a dangerous toxin from the environment."[5] Without overstating their significance, these studies are useful in that they remind us that material conditions, such as the state of the housing in which people live, the water they drink, and the air they breathe, have a major impact not only on the physical health of children, but also on their mental health and, as a result, on their way of being in the world – which in its turn influences their social outcomes. In this case the perpetration of offenses, even minor, or even simply the adoption of behaviors considered asocial, draws them into the police–justice–prison cycle from which, as interactionist theories show, it is extremely difficult to escape. In increasingly punitive societies, a criminal career is inextricably bound to a penal and, ulti-

mately, a prison career.[6] At least this is the case for those from poor
backgrounds and racial minorities, for in most countries the police and
justice system is probably the most inegalitarian arm of the state, the
one that penalizes the disadvantaged classes most inequitably. This is
what I showed in the case of France through the research I conducted,
over a twelve-year period, into the police, immediate arraignment, and
the world of prison.[7] This disparity in the distribution of sanctions, and
hence in the acknowledgment of offenses, is a further factor that invites
a degree of caution in establishing a causal relationship between childhood lead poisoning and criminal careers, since the epidemiological
studies conducted in various countries count convictions rather than
crimes actually committed. It would therefore be more correct to speak
of a statistical association between lead poisoning and penal sanctions.

This interpretation of an association between cognitive and behavioral disorders assumed to be caused by lead, and the perpetration of
offenses presumed to result from them, can be seen as a new avatar in
the long history of the relationship between the treatment of psychic
disorders and the treatment of social disorder. The genealogy of this
relationship is illuminating. It is remarkable that the management
of "madness" and "illegalities," to adopt the terms used by Michel
Foucault, its most percipient analyst, was conceived in identical form
in the last years of the eighteenth century, with an internment specific
to each, in the asylum or the prison respectively.[8] In both cases, this
modernization was seen as a humanization, liberating the insane from
their chains and softening the sanctions on criminals. The asylum and
the prison were imagined as moral progress. Admittedly, given what
each became during the nineteenth and twentieth centuries, this might
seem hard to believe. And yet. We must remember the conditions to
which both the mentally ill and offenders were subjected during the
seventeenth and eighteenth centuries, that is, before the creation and
development of both asylums and prisons.

Many treatments for mental patients had been dreamed up over
time, from sedatives to stimulants, from hellebore to bleeding, from
the dancing processions of the Middle Ages to the post chaise vibra-
tor of the Enlightenment.[9] Internment was reserved for those of the
mad whose behavior created disturbance in public space or family
life. There were two types of institutions. A minority were cared for in
hotels-Dieu, or medical hospitals, the largest of which was located in the
center of Paris: although the care was rudimentary, these insane people
were seen as sick and were treated by physicians. But the majority
ended up in a *hôpital general*, or confinement house, such as Salpêtrière
or Bicêtre, where the mad found themselves among the destitute, the

old, the invalids, the criminals, and (in the women's quarters) the prostitutes: medical care was only given when they fell sick from another cause. Some were also placed in poorhouses or houses of correction, in other words among the indigent or prisoners. All these mental patients, who thus found themselves in nonmedical institutions amongst the outcasts of society, and were treated as causes of public disorder rather than sufferers from a mental pathology, were subjected to a desperately painful experience of internment. In a report written in 1818, the psychiatrist Esquirol described the misfortune of mental patients in most of the establishments where they were locked up: "To how many insults, abuses and privations are these lunatics not exposed on the part of villains who make a joke of their condition? What humiliation for the sick man, if he has a few moments of lucidity, to find himself mixed in with criminals!"[10] The material conditions were particularly grueling. "Almost everywhere the indigent mental patients, and often those who pay for board and lodging, are naked or clothed in rags ... Many of them have barely any straw to protect them from the damp floor and the cold air." And the methods of restraint for those called "raving mad," and more generally those who appeared agitated, only aggravated their torment and increased their distress: "The abuse of chains is revolting. Iron collars, iron belts, shackles and manacles are used." Furthermore, paradoxically, although the policy of exclusion of the insane was designed to remove them from the public gaze, they reappeared in public displays of their condition, presented to onlookers, sometimes for payment. As Foucault notes, "until the beginning of the nineteenth century ... madmen remained monsters – that is, etymologically, beings or things to be shown."[11] In short, the treatment of the insane consisted of undifferentiated internment, dissociated from any therapeutic intention, deaf to their psychic suffering. A mixture of rejection and cruelty that the invention of the asylum would not eliminate, even if it took other forms.

By contrast, until the end of the eighteenth century, internment occupied only a marginal place among the arsenal of sanctions for perpetrators of crime.[12] Punishments varied widely, from fines to banishment, from flogging to mutilation, from exposure in the pillory to being sentenced to the galleys, from wearing a garment bearing the sign of moral degradation to indelible marking of the skin. Executions were rare but, being held in public, were spectacles for the crowd, from burning at the stake to hanging, to being tortured on the wheel. Internment was for a long time reserved for people charged and awaiting trial, held in buildings with a few miserable cells, or in the case of prisoners held on the king's orders, incarcerated in state fortresses that were generally more comfortable.[13] It was therefore not punitive, but either preventative or political. However, it gradually became more extensively used during the second half of the seventeenth century, with the creation of confinement houses. But the people housed there, apart from the mentally ill, were beggars, vagrants, and prostitutes, as well as children and women whose fathers or husbands paid for them to be interned there for "correction." In most cases, decisions to intern people were not made by the courts. They were not sentences, but a way of getting rid of individuals whose very presence disturbed public order, or even a way of administering private order through the policing of families. In the same spirit, poorhouses began to be created in convents and abbeys during the eighteenth century, and correction quarters in the confinement houses. Petty offenders and sometimes felons began to be interned there, in addition to the beggars and vagrants. The Conciergerie and the Grand Châtelet were the two largest prisons in Paris. The report on these establishments produced by Lavoisier, a member of the Royal Academy, for Necker in 1780, paints "a distressing picture for humanity."[14] They consisted of "very small and low rooms, housing too considerable a number of prisoners, rooms so distributed that air and light reach them only with difficulty, the air being already foul and contaminated when passing from one space to the other," with "pallets on which prisoners are rather piled up than lying," on "straw that is often rotten," "the floor and the tiles almost everywhere flooded with water that is stagnant, because often it cannot drain away," and "everywhere filth, vermin and degradation." During the years preceding the Revolution, true prisons were also being constructed, varying widely in levels of comfort depending on the social status of those housed in them, but also with differentiations between institutions depending on the crimes committed. In Paris, the Grande Force was designed for those awaiting trial or serving short sentences, generally from good families, the Madelonnettes being the equivalent for women, while prostitutes were interned in the Petite Force, and those serving medium-length sentences, along with debtors, in Sainte-Pélagie. But the most degrading conditions were reserved for those sentenced to long terms or forced labor while awaiting their transportation, who were interned at Bicêtre; the equivalent for women was Saint-Lazare.[15] As Foucault notes, "the penal system begins to be conceived as a mechanism intended to administer illegalities differentially."[16] Although confinement houses such as Bicêtre and Salpêtrière continued to mix criminals with the poor and insane, it was gradually recognized that murderers could not be housed alongside the unfortunate.

To sum up: until the late eighteenth century, the "great confinement" was applied almost indiscriminately to all undesirables. By and large, its function was neither to treat madness nor to correct illegalities. With the exception of those who found a place in the general hospitals, the insane did not receive any medical treatment. They were left at the mercy of other detainees and the discretion of staff, and if they behaved in an unseemly or aggressive manner they would be put in chains. Until the eve of the Revolution, the device of internment in confinement houses, houses of correction and poorhouses was applied principally to the needy, vagrants and prostitutes – in other words, those whose presence in the public space disturbed a particular moral order and who were locked up without any judicial process. Only a few prisons specifically incarcerated individuals who had been convicted or were awaiting judgment, their number increasing during the revolutionary period. In these diverse institutions, all of these rejects from society were locked up for an indeterminate length of time in insanitary, deprived, and abject conditions, and were often subject to untenable violence.

What I have described here in relation to France had parallels throughout Europe, with some substantial variations. In England, for example, the insane began to be separated out earlier, for example in the Bethlem Royal Hospital, where they were housed from the fourteenth century on.[17] Later on, treatments based on cold baths, purgatives, emetics, and bleeding were introduced; these were so punishing that the patients likely to be able to withstand them had to be specifically selected. At the same time, the exhibition of the mad to curious spectators represented a lucrative attraction for the hospital. The terrible conditions imposed on the patients contributed to the sinister reputation of Bedlam, as it became popularly known. It was in part as an alternative to these practices that St. Luke's Hospital for Lunatics was founded in 1750. As for prisons, in the eighteenth century there were more than 300 in England, most of them consisting only of a guardroom or a single cell, but the largest, Newgate, housing up to 300 prisoners.[18] Those incarcerated there usually stayed only a short time, awaiting the arrival of a judge for their trial or payment of their debts, with impecunious debtors representing over half the prisoners. The rooms were filthy, the air foul, water unavailable, the odor pestilential, the noise unbearable. Food was minimal and of poor quality, and inmates were dependent on their personal resources and the goodwill of their jailers. Some prisoners who were acquitted were not allowed to leave until they had paid the jailers what they owed. Men and women were rarely separated during the day. The mentally ill and deficient mingled with the other inmates. In short, while it was earlier and more

extensively differentiated in England than in France, the internment of
madness and illegalities still remained a degrading exclusion.

It was precisely this exclusion, and its conditions that were seen
as inhumane at a time when the idea of humanity itself was taking
shape, that sparked the indignation of reformers at the very end of
the eighteenth century. Philippe Pinel in France and William Tuke in
England embarked on a campaign for better treatment for the insane.
Pinel, a psychiatrist, was appointed to Bicêtre in 1793, and followed
the example of a warder, Jean-Baptiste Pussin, who removed patients'
chains and thus calmed their agitation. Transferred to Salpêtrière two
years later, Pinel in his turn freed mental patients, in what became an
iconic gesture, and wrote an influential treatise in which he described
them as subjects of their illness. Tuke, a Quaker philanthropist, discovered how patients were being treated after a woman suffering from
melancholia died in York Lunatic Hospital, and in 1796 decided to
create a more welcoming place for them, the Retreat, also in York.
The methods used to treat patients were less aggressive, the diet more
balanced, and physical exercise was prioritized. Remarkably, Pinel
and Tuke described their vision of care for mental patients in the
same terms: "moral treatment."[19] At the same time, a movement for
reform of penal law and penitentiary institutions was emerging. With
regard to penal law, the treatise *Dei delitti e delle penne* [*On Crime and
Punishments*], published by Cesare Beccaria in 1764, found immediate
success throughout Europe. In it, the Italian 26-year-old legal scholar
and philosopher defined the foundations of the right to punish and
posited the limits on it, rejected torture and the death penalty, proposed that the severity of the punishment should be proportional to
the seriousness of the crime, asserted the presumption of innocence
and the non-retroactivity of the law, and prioritized prevention of
crime over repression. His treatise inspired reformers in several countries, including France, and exerted a lasting influence on penal law
throughout the world. With regard to penitentiary institutions, the
Calvinist philanthropist John Howard visited hundreds of prisons
in England and Wales, but also in continental Europe, and returned
from his tour with a report, *The State of Prisons*, published in 1777,
which excoriated English and Welsh penitentiary institutions, and his
country's backwardness in comparison particularly with the Dutch
model. He contrasted the insanitary, dirty, disordered, and irrational
British prisons with the hygiene, cleanliness, order, and rationality of
correction facilities in the Netherlands. His position as High Sheriff of
Bedfordshire, the Crown's representative in administrative and judicial affairs, lent his analyses and recommendations an incontestable

legitimacy. Interestingly, though troublingly, Beccaria and Howard, through their respective interventions into penal law and penitentiary institutions, both contributed to placing the prison at the center of the punitive apparatus, whereas previously it had been used unspecifically, and often as a subsidiary measure. In Beccaria's view, it avoided the cruelty of corporal punishments and made it possible to fit the punishment to the crime. For his part, Howard worked to make it more functional and more efficacious, better fitted to its mission of rehabilitation and better governed by its administrators.[20] The hitherto marginal and repugnant prison, thus revised – at least as these humanist reformers saw it – could take its place at the heart of the new architecture of punishment. It was to remain there for more than two centuries.

That the promises of the psychiatric asylum and the carceral institution were not kept, and that the ideal of those who tried to promote them was not realized, is evident simply from a reading of the plethora of reports on one or the other produced throughout the nineteenth century. The humanization of the mad through moral treatment did not take place. The softening of punishments with proportional imprisonment did not occur. Such is Foucault's diagnosis in *Madness and Civilization*, and later in *Discipline and Punish*. His thinking is surely subject to some amendment, and indeed he himself was not so categorical in his analysis. In the asylum and in the prison, a different kind of coercion was exercised. Mental patients were no longer chained up, but they were subdued by authority. Criminals were no longer tortured, but they were subjugated by discipline. A new kind of intervention on minds and bodies was being put in place. And this intervention gained ground, because both types of establishment, reputed to be less violent and assumed to be more effective, made it possible to intern many more people by doing so for shorter periods. However, in the case of France two factors suggest that both the reform of treatment of madness and the reform of treatment of crime were much less real on the ground than in the minds of those who conceived either of them. First, descriptions and testimonies from asylums and prisons show that overcrowding, lack of hygiene, the arbitrariness of sanctions, brutality on the part of warders, and absence of medical or moral rehabilitation persisted. Second, the separation of mental patients and criminals, the sick and the poor, was very partial, and the shortage of places for the insane meant that they continued to be detained in poorhouses and even in penitentiary establishments.

During the first half of the nineteenth century, the country that most fascinated visitors seeking solutions for the mad and the criminal, especially visitors from France, was the United States. As David

Rothman notes, from the 1820s onwards a dual process unfolded, with the construction of asylums and prisons in most states.[21] What historians call the Jacksonian era, which extended up to the Civil War, was marked by a degree of extension of the democratic space, from which women, Blacks, and Native Americans nevertheless remained excluded. Regarding people with mental illnesses, on the one hand, the proliferation of asylums was driven by the enthusiasm of psychiatrists who believed that madness could be cured. The dominant explanation of madness, strongly tainted by conservatism, was that it was caused by civilization, a poorly defined term. Specifically, social mobility, religious freedom, civic participation, and the political openness that characterized the period were seen as prejudicial, producing mental disorders in some people. Constructed some distance away from the overstimulation of cities, asylums therefore offered an environment, a disciplinary regime, and a work routine that were supposed to return the insane to sanity. But in fact the predominant features for these patients were isolation, since they were cut off from their families, and rigidity, for the doctrine was strictly applied. With time, victims of their own success in some sense, asylums became overcrowded and, during the second half of the nineteenth century, maintaining order began to take precedence over care. Not all patients were to be found in these asylums. Some of them were interned in almshouses, workhouses, and local jails. For petty offenders and felons, on the other hand, a network of prisons developed, based on two well-known models that worked in different ways toward moral rehabilitation of inmates without the use of physical force. The first, "congregate" system, inspired by Auburn Prison in New York State, was based on collective labor in absolute silence during the day, and solitary confinement at night. The second, "separate" system, implemented in the Eastern State Penitentiary in Philadelphia, involved solitary confinement day and night, where the only contact possible was with the prison staff. Apart from the obvious differences between them, one integrating the economic benefits of free labor, the other focusing on the moral reform of isolated prisoners, the principle in both cases was to remove them from an external environment deemed corrupting, to the extent that neither visits nor mail were permitted. Gradually, however, in a number of prisons the rule became blunted, leading to violent repression of recalcitrant inmates by guards, contrary to the claimed values of these penitentiaries. There is thus a remarkable parallel between the philosophies of mental health and corrections institutions of the Jacksonian era: madmen and criminals should be removed from their harmful social environment; the asylum and the prison can put them back on the right path; but this is more a matter of order than of medicine, in the first case, and of constraint rather than rehabilitation in the second. Soon enough it was a question of coercion pure and simple.

Visitors seem to have been drawn more to the carceral than the psychiatric facilities. Well-known figures were eager to discover the new models of internment. Having been entrusted by the July Monarchy – the constitutional monarchy that started with the revolution of 1830 and lasted until 1848 – with a mission of inquiry, in 1831 Alexis de Tocqueville and Gustave de Beaumont toured US penitentiaries, and returned with a report for the French parliament in which they described the Philadelphia prison as a "magnificent establishment," rhapsodized about the "admirable order" that prevailed in prisons such as Auburn, and found the discipline in these penitentiaries "both moral and just."[22] To be sure, "solitude is a severe punishment, but such a punishment is merited by the guilty," they write. Moreover, "separation, which prevents the wicked from injuring others, is also favourable to himself. Thrown into solitude, he reflects. Placed alone, in view of his crime, he learns to hate it." Furthermore, "labor is introduced into the prison. Far from being an aggravation of the punishment, it is a real benefit to the prisoner." Yet their enthusiasm contrasts with the remarks of Charles Dickens, who visited the same places just eleven years later, in 1842, but presented a very different picture of them. Having spoken with a number of inmates in the Philadelphia prison sentenced to several years' imprisonment for a mere theft or possession of stolen goods, he describes them as "buried alive; to be dug out in the slow round of years; and in the meantime dead to everything but torturing anxieties and horrible despair." At the end of his account he concludes, with regard to this form of punishment: "My firm conviction is that independent of the mental anguish it occasions ... it wears the mind into a morbid state, which renders it unfit for the rough contact and busy action of the world. It is my fixed opinion that those who have undergone this punishment, must pass into society again morally unhealthy and diseased."[23] Indeed, while the "separate" model was rarely reproduced in the United States, unlike its rival "congregate" model, which was much less costly and more profitable, and was widely taken up, it nevertheless left a deep mark in the genealogy of prisons, creating a system that later became generalized and normalized in all US prisons, and well beyond: solitary confinement. It is the most radical practice and the most damaging experience of contemporary imprisonment, now known to foster the development of psychotic manifestations and the risk of suicidal impulses. While this system might have been morally justified in the minds of its designers, it quickly became apparent, in the form it was then given, for what it in fact was from the outset: an extreme punishment designed to destroy the person rather than rehabilitate him.

Thus, from the Ancien Régime to the post-revolutionary period, from France and England to the United States, the treatment of madness and the treatment of crime remained closely linked over centuries and across continents. They were bound together in various ways: either mental patients and criminals were locked up together, or they were interned separately but drawing on the same repressive or moralizing principles, with asylums adopting methods of coercion and repression similar to those of prisons, and symmetrically, with prisons developing methods liable to cause psychological harm to prisoners. There were of course substantial temporal and geographical variations: the Salpêtrière of the early nineteenth century was not that of the mid-eighteenth century; Bicêtre was not Philadelphia. But the internment of the mentally ill can never be thought in isolation from the imprisonment of offenders, or the imprisonment of criminals separately from the internment of mental patients. However, there was a third factor uniting them: social status. If the insane were interned in poorhouses, and vagrants in houses of correction, it was because poverty, at least when it was displayed by beggars or nomads, became, like madness and crime, a disturbance of public order, and ultimately the response was the same – removal of the individual. Mental disorder and criminal acts on the part of poor people were not subject to the same laws as mental disorder and criminal acts on the part of rich people. Internment was reserved for the lower classes.

Given that responses to madness and criminality were closely associated, both in terms of the ideologies on which they were based and the technologies they used, it is interesting to observe their evolution over time, through the institutional statistics available. A surprising discrepancy can be observed in the case of France.[24] On the one hand, there was a progressive increase in the number of patients hospitalized in psychiatric establishments from the early nineteenth century up to the eve of World War II in both absolute and relative terms: 11,500 in 1835; 43,000 in 1875; 71,500 in 1905; 108,800 in 1939 – an almost tenfold rise in the asylum population over 100 years. But the evolution of the carceral population over this period is intriguing, with first a slow rise, then a gradual decrease interrupted by a spike after the Commune in 1871, and marked by a drop during World War I: from 34,400 in 1831 the number of prisoners rose to 51,300 in 1852, then fell to 28,000 at the end of the century, to reach its lowest level in 1939, with 12,300 prisoners. The prison population had fallen to less than a quarter of what it was in the mid-nineteenth century.

Remarkably, the two graphs thus show opposite trends. On one side, the growing institutionalization of mental illness means that the lunatic asylum became the dominant mode of managing madness. On the other, the spectacular fall in the carceral population in a little less than a century seems to indicate a contrary pattern. But this development is deceptive, and reflects contradictory processes. In 1885, the French parliament passed both the law on banishment of repeat offenders, who on their fourth conviction would be transported to the overseas territories of French Guyana and New Caledonia, and the law introducing parole, which allowed prisoners to be released halfway through their sentence, on certain conditions. Although these two laws moved in opposite directions in terms of their intention, one being harsher and the other more lenient, combined, they helped to empty prisons in mainland France. Furthermore, there were 48,000 people sentenced to hard labor, who were not included in the prison statistics, between 1874 and 1938, the year when transportation for forced labor was abolished. Finally World War I, with its 1.7 million dead and 4.3 million wounded, decimated the young male population, which in normal times makes up a large proportion of the prison population. All these elements thus suggest that the fall in the French prison population should not be taken at face value. By contrast, analysis of how the asylum and prison populations changed in the United States during this period is simpler, with both showing a similar rise.[25] The construction of psychiatric hospitals accelerated through the nineteenth century, but the number of patients continued to exceed their capacity: in 1830, the average size of the nine asylums then existing was 80 beds; in 1875, one-third of the seventy-one asylums had more than 500 beds; by the early twentieth century, some establishments housed more than 3,000 patients. At the same time, the number of prisoners was also increasing, although somewhat less rapidly, from 6,700 in 1850 to 165,000 in 1940, representing a rise from 29 to 125 per 100,000 of the population – in other words more than quadrupling. However, unlike France, the United States did not have overseas colonies to which it could send its hardened criminals and repeat offenders. Moreover, in proportion to its population, its losses during World War I were one-thirtieth those of France. To sum up, as soon as asylums and prisons became autonomous in the early nineteenth century, they saw major expansion, more rapid in the case of asylums than of prisons, with national variations in the prison population owing to specific penal policies and particular historical circumstances.

But in the mid-twentieth century, a radical change occurred, and this time the trends in the two countries aligned, with a fall in the asylum population and an increase in the prison population.[26] In France, during World War II, the mentally ill were abandoned, and this was reflected in tragic mortality rates, estimated at 48,500 excess deaths. Following liberation, the number of patients rose again over two decades, and then began a rapid decrease: the rate of patients hospitalized fell from 236 to 73 per 100,000 between 1969 and 1998, reducing in-patient numbers by more than two-thirds in three decades. This shift arose out of the move to deinstitutionalize psychiatry and the creation of a plethora of alternative treatment regimes, out of the development of a range of psychotropic drugs, but also out of budget concerns. More broadly, society became more tolerant of mental illness and handicaps: their image changed, they were better integrated, and anti-discrimination laws were introduced. Conversely, the prison population, which had been very high just after World War II, with many people incarcerated for collaborating with the Nazi regime, fell to its lowest point in the mid-1950s, but since then has risen inexorably: there were 20,000 people in prison in 1955; 43,000 in 1985; 66,000 in 2015; and 72,000 in 2020. Even taking into account the growth of the overall population, this represents a tripling in sixty-five years. This increase bears no relation to trends in serious offenses, and rather reflects the criminalization of minor offenses and the increase in length of prison sentences, both resulting from lower tolerance of crimes committed by certain groups, and a penal populism promoted across almost the entire political spectrum.

In the United States, the evolution of the asylum and prison populations also shows the two curves moving in opposite directions, the first falling and the second rising from the mid-1970s, as shown by Bernard Harcourt. Rather than seeing this evolution as a phenomenon of communicating vessels, with inmates moving from asylums into prisons, as many believe, Harcourt argues that there is a sort of mirror image demography in the two institutions: whereas previously poor white women populated the asylum, now poor Black men fill prisons. The same is true in France, where, formerly, older white women comprised a large proportion of the population of psychiatric hospitals, but today the majority of the prison population consists of young men of color from low-income backgrounds.[27] The question therefore is no longer whether the deinstitutionalization of mental health is filling prisons, which may be true in a certain number of cases, but rather, to what extent the psychological fragility or indeed psychiatric vulnerability of some sections of the disadvantaged classes influence life journeys that culminate in prison sentences.

Epidemiological studies in France give an unequivocal answer to this question: a large proportion of those who enter prison present more or less serious mental disorders. A study conducted in five prisons in the Picardy region showed that a quarter of the 1,780 newly arrived prisoners, 95 percent of them men, had previously received psychiatric care, a fifth were currently under psychiatric treatment, and one in fifteen had been in an in-patient psychiatric facility within the past year. In addition, one in six presented excessive alcohol consumption, the same proportion were receiving opioid substitute treatment, and one in four regularly used drugs, a quarter of those being addicted to heroin. Another study conducted in prisons in the Nord and Pas-de-Calais regions, of the 653 new arrivals, 96 percent of them male, refined the analysis using an internationally validated psychiatric question-naire that identified one or more mental disorders in seven out of ten individuals. Out of the cohort of new prisoners, 27 percent had experienced a depressive episode in the previous two years, 26 percent had experienced generalized anxiety in the previous six months, and 15 percent showed a moderate or high risk of suicide. In addition, 7 percent presented psychotic-type symptoms, 7 percent described past episodes of mania, and 5 percent showed post-traumatic stress. The authors of the study compared these figures with those observed in the general population, after adjustment for sex, age, marital status, and employment situation, using the same questionnaire. They found that depression, anxiety, and psychosis were almost twice as frequent, the risk of suicide and previous episodes of mania were three times as frequent, and post-traumatic stress ten times as frequent. Furthermore, 23 percent of those arriving in prison were dependent on alcohol and 26 percent addicted to drugs, a frequency four times higher than in the general population.[28] It is clear that people sentenced to imprisonment – and it is well known that prison sentences are socially differentiated – are often disproportionately likely to suffer from psychic disorders and psychiatric pathologies, some serious, often coupled with dependencies, compared to the rest of the French population. Thus, while we cannot be certain that those who are imprisoned today would in the past have been interned as mental patients, it is nevertheless clear that many of them have need of psychological or psychiatric care at least as much as of a carceral institution, the sad reality of which is that it can only make them worse and does not have the resources to care for them.

The rigorous study conducted by Bruno Falissard and his team gives a measure of this situation. It concerned 800 male inmates selected at random in twenty prisons, who were assessed separately by a junior clinician using a questionnaire, and a senior clinician conducting an unstructured interview, with the two diagnoses subsequently being compared and discussed. Taking into account only those cases where there was consensus on the diagnosis, it showed that only 13 percent of prisoners were judged to have no psychiatric disorder; 51 percent presented slight or moderate disorders, 23 percent presented manifest ones, and 13 percent serious ones, with 2 percent showing very serious disorders. The pathologies thus identified were as follows: 6 percent of respondents were suffering from schizophrenia, 24 percent from severe depression, 18 percent from generalized anxiety, 14 percent from trauma neurosis, 11 percent from social anxiety, and 10 percent from agoraphobia. Moreover, 12 percent were dependent on alcohol, and 15 percent on drugs.[29] These figures reveal the scale of the problem of mental illness in prisons, where only one prisoner in eight presents no symptoms, and one in eight is suffering from a serious or very serious mental disorder. In the absence of similar studies from the past, it is impossible to affirm with certainty that the situation has deteriorated, but two explanatory factors that arose in the late twentieth century suggest this is the case. First, outside the prison, publicly funded psychiatric care for young working-class adults presenting psychic disorders is increasingly difficult to organize, owing to the lack of professionals in their locality, although it is among this age group that acting out is most frequent. Second, in court, diminished responsibility is less frequently cited by psychiatric expert witnesses, and less accepted by judges, and, under new legal provisions, mentally ill individuals are increasingly often convicted of their offenses, being deemed dangerous by the "new criminology."[30] Consequently, in the crime–insanity alternative, the scales of justice have moved strongly toward crime. In the eyes of both legislators and judges, a mentally ill criminal is first and foremost a criminal. Should prison then become the place where he is treated? Surely not: it is above all the place where he is incarcerated. Official administrative data leave little doubt as to this.

While there are many of them in prisons, inmates presenting mental disorders, in some cases serious, receive limited care. In France the 26 Regional Medical-Psychological Services (SMPR, Services médico-psychologiques régionaux), or, where this specialist body does not exist, the 129 general psychiatry departments that stand in for them, offer consultations in prisons.[31] The fact that consultation rates are three times higher in the SMPRs than in the general psychiatry services clearly suggests that a substantial proportion of the demand for care goes unmet in the majority of prisons. Moreover, while waiting times for consultations are often short in emergency situations, such as suicide risk, psychotic decompensation, or drug withdrawal (provided that the emergency is recognized by the prison officer communicating the request), consultations in less serious cases may be postponed for weeks, and psychological consultations are never offered before six months. In the prison where I conducted my ethnographic study, those serving short sentences, often vulnerable, since many of them were in prison for the first time, therefore had to go without any care. The others who stayed there longer were kept waiting, like the anxious, insomniac man who had asked to see a psychologist eight months earlier and still had not had a consultation. It is easy to imagine the ordeal represented by the gulf between suffering a panic attack or a depressive syndrome, in this prison world that generates anxiety, and the experience of such a long wait, or indeed the lack of any support.

In many respects, the situation is still worse in the United States, for at least three reasons: the forced closure of psychiatric hospitals has ejected many patients without care, because they lack health insurance; the outsize prison system, with its enormous facilities, generates a high level of violence on the part of both staff and inmates; and the delegation of some prison operations to private companies, more interested in the profits they can make than in the services they are supposed to provide, has led to a drop in the standard of care in these institutions. A US study of 1,256,000 prisoners revealed a prevalence of mental disorders of 45 percent in federal prisons, 56 percent in state prisons, and 64 percent in local jails.[32] In local jails, which generally contain those unable to make bail who are awaiting their sentence, as well as those sentenced to short terms, 54 percent of prisoners reported symptoms of mania, 30 percent signs of depression, and 24 percent manifestations that suggested psychotic pathology – in other words, serious mental illnesses. Compared to the general population, they had twenty-five times more symptoms of mania, four times more signs of depression, and eight times more psychotic manifestations. Interestingly, three prisoners in ten in federal and state prisons, and four out of ten in local jails, presented mental disorders but had no history of psychiatric problems, whereas the proportion of those who had a clinical history but no symptoms was twice as high in state prisons as in local jails. Two important findings thus emerge from this study. First, the prevalence of psychiatric pathologies in prisons is quite high compared to the rest of the population, and a significant proportion of these pathologies results from the condition of incarceration itself, since they did not exist before. Second, the higher rates of mental illness in local jails show that those awaiting sentence and those who have committed minor offenses are more psychologically vulnerable than those who have committed serious crimes and receive long sentences.

The observations made in France and the United States are repeated in many other locations. A meta-analysis of sixty-two studies carried out in twelve countries, relating to 22,790 prisoners, found an average prevalence of 4 percent for psychoses, 10 percent for serious depression, and 65 percent for personality disorders, including 47 percent described as antisocial behavior (a problematic description on both the psychiatric and the sociological levels, but explicit nevertheless).[33] These rates were two to four times higher than in the general population for psychosis and serious depression, and ten times higher for so-called antisocial behavior. However, the authors highlighted a disturbing scientific issue: while prisons in Western countries house one-third of the world's prisoners, 99 percent of studies on mental health relate to these institutions. In other words, the situation in other countries, particularly those of the global South, remains virtually unknown.

In short, even though nosographies vary from one country to another, and methods are somewhat heterogeneous, what emerge from this set of studies are solid facts: the frequency of serious mental disorders, including psychoses; the role of incarceration in producing these disorders, since a proportion of prisoners had no psychiatric history; the aggravation of these disorders during the prison sentence, indicated by the panic attacks, social anxiety, and agoraphobia; and the massive failure of care by inadequate specialist services. Particularly because of behaviors sometimes described as antisocial, people suffering from mental disorders are more likely to commit acts that will lead them to prison, and, once incarcerated, are more likely to commit acts that will lead to punishment – usually solitary confinement, extensions of their sentence, sometimes with tragic complications.

Shortly after I finished my four-year study in a prison, a young man of African origin who presented psychic disorders was incarcerated there after receiving a short prison sentence for a minor offense. A few weeks later he argued with another prisoner, and, notwithstanding his vehement protests, was placed in solitary confinement. Rebelling against this decision and distressed by the isolation, that same evening he set fire to his mattress in a gesture of despair, but his clothes quickly caught fire. Alerted by his shouts, prisoners in neighboring cells called for help. The night shift officer ran up, but not having the key to the security door, could not open the gate to the cell: at night only the duty officer had the key. When the two guards returned a few minutes later and managed to put out the fire, the man was lying unconscious in the smoke, amidst an acrid smell of burned flesh. Transferred to the hospital with second- and third-degree burns over 80 percent of his body, he died several weeks later in a resuscitation unit. In the interim, a judge, to whom his case had been referred, had ordered that he be released so that symbolically he could die free – or perhaps more cynically so that his death would not be counted as a prison suicide. However that may be, the very psychic vulnerability that had given rise to the minor offense and led him to prison had contributed to his altercation and, once he was in solitary confinement, to his desperate reaction.

In this respect, suicide is the most tragically inarguable indicator of psychological fragility, whether it is linked to an underlying pathology, particularly depression or psychosis, or to the torment of incarceration. In 1960 there were four suicides for every 10,000 prisoners in France. In 1996, the rate was twenty-four per 10,000: it had increased sixfold in thirty-six years. In 2018, following the introduction of a prevention plan, the rate had fallen back to eighteen per 10,000, still four times that of a little over half a century earlier. This is around twice the rate observed in England, Germany, Italy, or Denmark, and four times higher than in Spain, Ireland, and the Czech Republic. France is the European country where the most people take their lives in prison.[34] It is sometimes pointed out that the suicide rate in the general population is high, suggesting that French people have some kind of proclivity for ending their lives, but this comes down to overlooking the fact that the rate is ten times higher in prison than outside, whereas in the mid-twentieth century fewer prisoners committed suicide than people who were free. International comparisons are hardly flattering in this respect. Some countries, such as the United Kingdom, have a low suicide rate among the general population, but a marked excess of suicides in prison, while others, such as Germany, have a high suicide rate among the general population but only a small excess of suicides in prison. France has high levels for both indicators: hence its rating in the classification.

Why is it that what demographers call "carceral excess suicidality" is so high in France? Attributing it to the state of prisons, as people tend to do, is too simple. In fact, two factors combine: on the one hand, the penal process, at the end of which lies prison; on the other, the carceral condition, which refers to the reality of life in prison. A first series of statistics reveals the importance of what is played out in the penal process. First, the more the prison population increases, the higher the suicide rate rises, not because of the over-occupation of cells, but because of the severity and perceived injustice of sentences. The growth in the number of prisoners is due in large part to sentences for offenses which, a few decades earlier, would not have received such a punishment. Second, the rate of suicide in prison is three times higher among those awaiting trial, and therefore presumed innocent until their case is judged, than among those convicted: these prisoners awaiting trial represent almost half of those in short-stay correctional facilities. Finally, the rate is twice as high among people who receive a prison sentence and are incarcerated than among those who receive a prison sentence but remain on probation, usually with electronic monitoring: the decision is made to incarcerate in 85 percent of cases. These three factors show that, in the punitive moment that reigns in contemporary France, penal policy and judicial practices that prioritize imprisonment over other possible measures, including for those awaiting trial, contribute to the high number of suicides.[35] But the carceral condition itself also plays a decisive role. More than one suicide in ten takes place during the first week after admission, and a quarter in the first two months; this shows how lethal what judges call "incarceration shock," a condition that they believe serves as a beneficial lesson for those who commit crimes, can be. For shock there is, under the accumulated weight of all the deprivations the prisoner experiences from one day to the next: deprivation of freedom, of course, but also of movement during twenty-two hours of confinement in a cell, of privacy in a single cell compulsorily shared with two or three people; deprivation of sports or intellectual activity, work, or training, at least during the first few months; deprivation of autonomy to make the most mundane decisions such as taking a shower; deprivation of affective and sexual life, of psychological care; and even deprivation of expression of permanent frustrations, for fear of being taken before the disciplinary committee. This committee, which issues in-sentence sentences, almost always punishes transgressions with solitary confinement, which is particularly feared by the most vulnerable. The risk of suicide in solitary confinement is ten times higher than in regular cells, and half of these tragedies occur on the day of, or the day after, the issue of a punishment whose harmful effects on the psyche are well known. It should be emphasized, moreover, that a third of those who commit suicide had a history of psychiatric illness, that half had received psychiatric treatment, and that half had already attempted suicide.[36] To sum up, many people commit suicide in France because of both sentencing and incarceration practices.

Comparison with the situation in the United States is once again instructive. On the one hand, surprisingly given the length of sentences and the harshness of life in prison, in the United States the suicide rate is an eleventh of that in France in state prisons, with 1.6 per 10,000 prisoners, and just over one-quarter in local jails, with 4.7 per 10,000 prisoners. On the other hand, the same link can be observed between punishments of solitary confinement, which are especially frequent in local jails, and rates of suicide and self-harm, which are eight times higher when prisoners are moved to punishment cells.[37]

But with 2.2 million prisoners, the orders of magnitude are different: there are around 500 prison suicides each year in the United States, but it is estimated that every day there are 80,000 prisoners in solitary confinement. The discrepancy between the relatively low number of suicides and the extremely high number of people in solitary confinement calls for deeper reflection on what Lisa Guenther calls "social death." For as Lorna Rhodes's ethnography in maximum security prisons in the United States shows, many of those incarcerated in these establishments, and still more in special units within them, suffer from severe mental illness, or develop manifestations of psychosis secondary to solitary confinement.[38] Solitary confinement may last years: three members of the Black Panthers were sentenced to this punishment for four decades in the notorious Louisiana prison known as the Angola Penitentiary.

This difference between an excess of physical deaths in France, the country with the highest suicide rate in the West, and an excess of social deaths in the United States, the country with the largest population in solitary confinement but the lowest suicide rate, is indeed troubling.[39] It suggests that psychic suffering, whether it leads to suicide or results from isolation, is an integral part of the violence of the carceral condition. Nevertheless, there is clearly a difference between taking one's life and having death imposed on oneself. In the first case, it is an act of desperation expressing the individual's desire to react to an intolerable situation from which he wishes to escape, or to an unjust one that he rejects; it is, then, at the very least, a gesture of resistance. In the second case, there is extreme coercion whereby, sometimes through the use of physical force, the institution subjects the individual by depriving him almost entirely of autonomy, including the possibility of suicide: this is an almost absolute form of subjection.

Having reached this point, it is useful to trace the journey in this parallel between the treatment of mental illness and the treatment of criminal acts. Until the late eighteenth century, little distinction was drawn between the mentally ill and the criminal, and both usually found themselves in the same places, confinement houses, houses of correction or poorhouses, alongside beggars and vagrants. The twofold revolution that removed the chains from the insane, interning them in an asylum, and replaced corporal punishment with internment of criminals in a prison, appeared to introduce a radical separation between pathology and deviance. But very quickly in the second half of the nineteenth and the first decades of the twentieth centuries, for many the asylum became a prison from which it was difficult to escape, and the prison often served to house the massive overflow from asylums. However, from the 1970s this trend altered radically, and the two graphs moved in opposite directions, with, on the one hand, the deinstitutionalization of mental illness, leading to the decline of psychiatric hospitals, and, on the other, the increasing recourse to imprisonment for more and more minor offenses, leading to an inflation of the prison population – a trend that was particularly marked in the United States.

Fewer asylums, more prisons, then, but within this institutional movement a sociodemographic shift took place: those who were locked up came predominantly from low-income backgrounds, now supplemented by ethnic and racial minorities. With a greater tolerance of mental disorders in society came a growing intolerance of minor offenses, particularly where these groups were concerned. But in this swing of the moral pendulum, the confusion between the sick person and the criminal reappears: the perpetrator of an offense often presents psychological fragility or a psychiatric condition, and the subject suffering from psychotic symptoms, manic disorders, or substance addiction more easily tends to commit deviant acts. At this interface between vulnerability and criminality, which is surely not new, a choice has to be made between medical care and penal sanction. And judges and psychiatrists seem increasingly inclined, respectively, to punish and to justify the punishment, simultaneously following what are often seen as the contradictory philosophies of Kantian retributivism (every crime deserves to be punished) and Benthamite utilitarianism (the danger of the criminal must be reduced for the good of society), rather than being able to imagine another way of dealing with the problem. Thus, in the world of prison, there are prisoners with serious pathologies as well as prisoners with less serious vulnerabilities, but in both cases these generate deviant behavior on the outside that leads them to the courts where they are sentenced to imprisonment, and inappropriate conduct inside that brings them before disciplinary committees where destructive isolation is the usual punishment.

The situation, then, is less different than might have been imagined from that which prevailed three centuries ago. In this respect, it is interesting to note that in France, the independent authority set up in 2008 to ensure respect of the fundamental rights of incarcerated individuals, the General Inspector of Places of Detention (CGLPL, Contrôleur général des lieux de privation de liberté), is tasked with inspecting not only correctional facilities but also psychiatric institutions. This link derives from the fact that mentally ill individuals or fragile personalities, as soon as they disturb public order, are defined as delinquents or even criminals, to be punished rather than cared for, or at least for whom punishment takes precedence over psychiatric or psychological

care. And if, in addition, they behave badly, there is solitary confinement, today in a disciplinary cell that replaces the dungeon of the past.
It might be tempting to compare solitary confinement with the "separate system" of the nineteenth-century Philadelphia prison. But while
the latter had an – albeit problematic – concern with moral reform, the
former is only interested in repression. As to the social composition
of these places of internment, while the confinement house brought
together the mad, the criminal, and the poor in the same space, current
correctional facilities, especially short-stay prisons in France and local
jails in the United States, gather the same people, since a significant
proportion of prisoners present mental disorders and belong to disadvantaged groups. Today, as in earlier times, they are undesirable. It
is therefore clear how important it is to consider the management of
mental illness and offenses and of psychiatric and judicial institutions
– in short, the asylum and the prison – together, since they all involve
moral values and political choices that define the most neglected and
most unknown area of public health.

Readings of the Pandemic
16 June 2021

Thinking events as they take place. – A unity of time, place, and action. – The course of events. – From outright denial to martial rhetoric. – Unpreparedness and incompetence. – Restrictions and delocalizations. – The ordeal of uncertainty. – Hypotheses about the origin of the virus. – Absorption of the attention economy. – Enemies, heroes, and victims. – Divergent forecasts. – Controversy around a medication. – Global conspiracy. – Tragic choices. – Exiles between detention and exclusion. – Reason of health and reason of security. – Protecting lives at all costs. – Critiques of biolegitimacy. – Lives lost, lives ruined.

With the Covid pandemic, public health found itself in the spotlight. It was of course not an entirely unknown concept, but for the majority it occupied a minor space on the fringes of medicine. People were perhaps aware of its role in sanitation, vaccination, and disease prevention. They knew vaguely that it was called on during flu epidemics, or to control emerging diseases from Asian countries, or enlisted in the fight against endemic pathologies in Africa. But it was a somewhat impenetrable domain of technicians and administrators, programs and numbers, far removed from the glamor of great biomedical advances. And all of a sudden, it was in the name of public health that billions of people found themselves confined to their homes, under threat of sanctions if they ventured out without duly formulated authorization, that schoolchildren no longer attended their schools or students their universities, that many men and women stopped going to their places of work. It was in the name of public health that most of the world's economies were partially put on hold, that in some places a hitherto unchallenged dogma of budget austerity was abandoned, that governments decided voluntarily to go into recession. It was in the name of public health that restrictions on civil liberties, suspensions of fundamental rights, police surveillance, and digital tracing were imposed. All aspects of life, from the most trivial to the most essential, were decided on the basis of what public health experts said. Life moved to the tune of statistics of new cases, hospitalizations, deaths. People learned to read tables, graphs, and forecasts. They awaited the prophecies of the oracles of mathematical modeling. They hoped for announcements from the seers that might herald the return of freedom. They compared the political responses of their countries, and their effects on the development of the epidemic. They speculated about the success of some and criticized the inability of others, seeking to draw some lessons from this experience. Fundamentally, they now interpreted the world purely in terms of public health.

The health crisis did more than just make public health visible. It became a total social fact. There was therefore no question of ignoring it. But there was equally no question of refocusing my entire project around it. The social sciences have a duty to resist the absorption of the entire attention economy by a current issue, however important and dramatic, whether it be a terrorist attack, a presidential election, or an unprecedented pandemic. A solution to this dilemma emerged when I realized that each of the themes I had chosen as the focus of my first seven lectures could shed light on one facet of the health crisis, thus offering a richer, more complete, and occasionally more unexpected interpretation of it. Rather than being beside the point, the themes of the birth of public health, the truth in numbers, epistemic boundaries, conspiracy theories, ethical crises, precarious exiles, and carceral ordeals that formed the core of each of these lectures became strikingly topical in the pandemic context, proving their pertinence as keys to reading public health. In the midst of what was presented as an unprecedented event, the already shaped pieces of what might have seemed an unlikely jigsaw puzzle gradually fitted together to create a credible picture of the scene that was being played out. Not the only conceivable picture, but one of several possible ones.

In a short text written in 1973, a year when his lectures focused on the punitive society and he was politically engaged in many issues, from prisoners to immigrants, Michel Foucault stated: "I see myself as a journalist, insofar as what interests me is current affairs, what is going on around us, what we are, what is happening in the world." In doing so, he explicitly aligned himself with Nietzsche: before Nietzsche, philosophy's "raison d'être was eternity;" after Nietzsche everything changed, for he was "obsessed with the present."[1] This twofold assertion, about himself and about the thinker who was probably his greatest influence, may seem surprising. On the one hand, it is a sort of provocation. In what we might call his serious works – and we know that the word "works" held a particular significance for him, to the extent that he made it the title of the Seuil series he edited with Paul Veyne and François Wahl – he hardly ever considered the present, although of course the subjects he chose to address from a genealogical perspective, from madness to prison, from security to neoliberalism, resonated strongly with the contemporary moment.[2] However, Foucault did address the present in interviews, talks, panel discussions, and of course at demonstrations, press conferences, and indeed traveling to the places where events were unfolding, from Attica in 1972, where prison riots had been violently repressed a year earlier, to Tehran in 1978, where he reported for the Italian press on the eve of the Iranian revolution. This was where he practiced the "radical journalism" he claims to uphold – not in his books or his lectures at the Collège de France. On the other hand, it may seem paradoxical to consider Nietzsche a philosopher of the present, given that he is known for the four essays gathered together under the title *Untimely Meditations*.[3] But this is a problem particularly of the translation of the word *unzeitgemäss*, which means "untimely," but also "inopportune" and "obsolete," literally "against time." It is because Nietzsche is, as he puts it, "a pupil of earlier times, especially the Hellenic," that he thinks "counter to the time" in which he lives, and "for the benefit of a time to come." In other words, he considers his present with a critical gaze.

This brief digression via Foucault and Nietzsche is by way of proposing the idea of an unsettling approach to the contemporary moment. Here, what I mean by unsettling is an analysis of the contemporary moment that uses different keys to interpretation than those habitually used for this purpose. These are the keys proposed in the seven preceding lectures, which, as I have shown, can offer a new understanding of a range of controversies, arguments, dissidences, divergences – in short, critical situations – precisely the sum of ordeals testing contemporary societies under the pandemic. This approach "against time," since I propose my analyses without the passage of time as the events go on, makes it possible to take some risks, to explore unmarked paths, as commentators, researchers and laypeople, decision-makers and dreamers have done. Perhaps, with time, some of my analyses will be confirmed, and others invalidated. Perhaps what appeared innovative at a given point will become commonplace, or conversely, erroneous. But the benefit of this approach to the present is that it opens a field of possibilities, of what could have happened and what might have been thought. A field of possibilities that is at risk of being shut down by the course of events and the consolidation of narratives.

At the outset, I should establish unity of time, of place and of action. I began to write this text in April 2020, during the first lockdown, and completed it in March 2021, at the point when, after much hesitation, the third lockdown was announced in France. It therefore covers the first year of the pandemic. At the point when I began to revise it, the milestone of 3 million people reported to be infected with corona-virus worldwide had just been passed. Of these, 200,000 had died. Internationally, France ranked fourth, with 130,000 cases and 24,000 deaths, while the United States, the epicenter of the pandemic, was in first place with 1 million cases and 60,000 deaths. This was a time when people were hoping for a vaccine, without really believing it would come. When I completed the revision, it was estimated that 122 million people had been infected, 2.7 million of whom had died; the United States was still the country worst affected, with 30 million cases and 540,000 deaths. France was in fifth place in the world and second in Europe, with more than 4 million cases and 92,000 deaths; there were now several vaccines available, and the proportion of the population who had received at least one dose was 30 percent in the United States, but only 12 percent in France. However, people were beginning to wonder whether the long-awaited vaccine would really mark the end of the crisis, or whether, given the doubts as to the duration of immunity and the spread of new variants of the virus, they needed to prepare themselves for living with the pandemic indefinitely.

Before embarking on my analysis, however, I need to retrace the course of events, because it is in the nature of the present that it dissipates as new events occur and, however insignificant, replace the previous ones, just as footprints left in the sand fade with each new wave that rises upon the beach. The following account is based primarily on two countries, the comparison of which is illuminating for both their similarities and their differences. These countries are the United States and France, though I will occasionally venture beyond them.

On 31 December 2019, the Chinese authorities reported several dozen cases of pneumonia of unknown cause to the World Health Organization; a physician had attempted to draw attention to these earlier, provoking the wrath of his government.[4] In the days that followed, researchers identified a new coronavirus and sequenced its genome, which they made available to scientists throughout the world, enabling them to produce diagnostic tests almost immediately. Although for a short while Chinese physicians believed that there was no person-to-person transmission, they soon acknowledged this mode of contagion. Faced with the proliferation of cases and also with deaths, the authorities decided to place a strict cordon sanitaire around Wuhan, and then to cancel all celebrations of Chinese New Year, a period when millions of people travel around the country. On 30 January 2020, the World Health Organization declared a global health emergency: nearly 10,000 cases had already been reported in twenty-one countries, including the United States, where a man returning from Wuhan was diagnosed on 21 January, and France, where three cases, also imported from Wuhan, two of them in Chinese tourists, were reported on 24 January. Twenty-four hours after this announcement, the United States government banned the entry of persons coming from China, except for US citizens and permanent residents. On the same day, the first two cases were diagnosed in Italy, a Chinese couple from Wuhan, and the first case in Spain, a German tourist. These two countries were to become the global epicenter of the pandemic for several weeks, with a particularly high death rate. On 1 March, Italy had 1,700 cases and 34 deaths; one month later it had 120,000 cases and 15,000 deaths, with Bergamo and its surrounding region being the most affected. In Spain there were 85 cases and 1 death on 1 March; by the beginning of the following month the figures had already reached 126,000 cases and 12,000 deaths. These data are in fact underestimates of both the number of cases, owing to the limited availability of tests, and the number of deaths, because those occurring at home were not registered.

In the United States, the development of the epidemic was a little slower. A few cases were reported in February, with only twenty-four by 29 February, but the main reason for this low figure was that there were no diagnostic tests available. At the highest level of government, the risks were being minimized. On 30 January, Donald Trump stated that the infection was "very well under control." On 10 February, he asserted that "when it gets a little warmer, [the virus] miraculously goes away." On 28 February, he described the concerns expressed by Democrats about the epidemic as "one more false alarm." On 2 March, he affirmed that the epidemic had "a much smaller range" of deaths than the flu. On 10 March, when the number of cases had reached 936, doubling every forty-eight hours, the president declared: "We are prepared, and we're doing good work. It will go away. Just stay calm." Yet during the month of March, when no lockdown guidelines had been issued at the national level, the number of cases rose from 42 to 186,000, and the number of deaths from 2 to 3,800. This did not prevent the president from stating, on 24 March, regarding Easter Sunday, which was two weeks away": "Wouldn't it be great to have all the churches full all over our country?" At this point, not only were there still not enough diagnostic tests just to confirm infections, but medical personnel did not have masks, gloves, or scrubs, and were sometimes forced to reuse disposable equipment and to dress in cut-up garbage bags. The situation became particularly acute in New York, which went from 1 to 63,000 cases in thirty days, with more than 2,000 deaths. Intensive care services were overwhelmed and respirators were in short supply. A hospital ship with 1,000 beds was sent to the port of Manhattan, and a conference center was converted into a 4,000-bed hospital in the heart of the city, but as, strangely, both refused to take people infected with the virus, they received only a few dozen patients. On 20 March, the governor of New York state issued the order for lockdown. Other governors had preceded him, including in California, which was less affected. But without federal coordination, which the president was refusing, each state had its own policy, with some imposing lockdown and others opposing it, and all in fierce competition in the market for the scarce disposable equipment of masks, gloves, scrubs, and respirators. Each evening, during this presidential campaign period that had been brutally interrupted for the other candidates, the president, surrounded by his advisers, engaged in an hour-long question-and-answer session with the media, which he used mainly to boast about how he had managed the crisis from the start. On 11 March, he announced the ban on foreigners from Europe entering the country, with the exception of residents. On 13 March, he declared a national emergency, allowing the release of emergency funds to combat the epidemic. On 23 March, he stated: "We are at war with an invisible enemy." On 27 March, he signed the law passed by Congress introducing a 2 trillion-dollar relief program to support economic activity and provide financial assistance to the population. However, most of this sum was earmarked for large corporations, with a quarter of the total even being left to the president's discretion, with no oversight from Congress. At that time, a 34 percent recession was being predicted for the second quarter, and the aim was to avoid both the closure of businesses and the dismissal of their workers. The employment situation was already critical, with 5 million additional people unemployed each week, in a country where unemployment benefits are limited. On 14 April, the president announced that he was going to stop funding the World Health Organization, claiming that it was responsible for the United States' delay in responding to the epidemic. On 17 April, when the death toll was the highest since the start of the epidemic, he declared his support for angry Republican demonstrators who were noisily protesting lockdown in Virginia, Minnesota, and especially Michigan. In the latter state, they had gathered on the steps of the Capitol in Lansing, armed with automatic weapons, in a threatening demonstration that prefigured the invasion of the Capitol in Washington on 6 January 2021. But the president demanded that the governors of these states "free" their population. The same day, he announced a plan for a rapid return to normal, still without any real policy for testing.

In France, the epidemic developed along an almost identical trajectory, and the response was equally inadequate, except for two things: the government almost immediately appointed a scientific council, whose recommendations it followed, at least during the earlier months, and the country's centralized administration allowed for nationwide coordination, managing shortages thanks to measures of solidarity between regions. Apart from this, the two countries had much in common. Despite the appearance of clusters of infection in the Oise and Bas-Rhin departments, the epidemiological situation evolved fairly slowly during February: at the end of the month there were 100 cases and 2 deaths. The virus began to spread more quickly in early March, reaching 52,000 cases and 3,500 deaths by the end of that month. On 7 March, when there were already 949 cases and the figure was doubling each day, President Emmanuel Macron publicly attended a theater performance, and seeking to reassure people, even encouraged his fellow citizens not to change their habits: "Life goes on. There is no reason, with the exception of those who are vulnerable, to stop going out." The next day his culture minister tested positive for coronavirus. In the days that followed, progressively stricter measures were introduced: a ban on gatherings of more than 1,000 people on 9 March, then of more than 100 people on 23 March; closure of daycare centers and all educational establishments on 12 March; suspension of all non-essential activity in public spaces on 14 March. But on 15 March, when there were already more than 5,000 cases, fifty times more than two weeks earlier, and 127 deaths, the first round of municipal elections was held as normal, after the scientific council appointed four days previously gave approval for them to go ahead. Forty-eight hours later, in a radical change of tune, the president declared, in an address to the nation, that "the country is at war," and announced a general lockdown with sanctions for failure to comply. The Greater East region was the most affected at this point, following an evangelical celebration attended by several thousand people in Mulhouse in mid-February, and demand for intensive care beds surpassed capacity at the end of March, with patients having to be transferred to other regions or even neighboring countries: Germany, Switzerland, and Austria offered their help. Then it was the Île-de-France region's turn to see its hospitals overflowing, particularly in

Seine-Saint-Denis, the poorest department in the country. In addition
to the shortage of beds for seriously ill patients, there was a lack of
masks, gloves, and protective clothing, including for medical personnel. Owing to the shortage of diagnostic tests, these too were soon
reserved for hospitalized patients, the seriously ill, those at risk, and
medical personnel. Nursing homes were excluded from statistics, and
the many cases and deaths there were not counted during the initial
weeks. At the same time, the economic situation worsened, with the
stock market losing two-thirds of its value. In order to stem the fall in
gross domestic product, then estimated at 9 percent for the year 2020,
the threat of bankruptcies, and the rise in temporary layoffs, the government implemented a 110-billion-euro emergency plan, and agreed
to guarantee loans up to a total of 300 billion euro. Significantly, most
of this aid was given to the largest corporations, with no obligation
of repayment, thus enabling them to use money provided by the state
to pay dividends to their shareholders, while continuing to lay off
employees. On 13 April, the president announced that the lockdown
would be gradually lifted beginning 11 May.

The events of these first three months of the pandemic reveal that,
despite their presidents' differences in style, and beyond the shared
martial rhetoric that followed the initial denial, the United States and
France had two factors in common: neither country was prepared for
the emergence of a pandemic, and their governments did not have the
capacity to respond. As Richard Horton phrased it, this was a dual
failure leading to a "catastrophe."[5] The two factors are distinct, and
each merits attention.

The lack of preparation is certainly not unique to coronavirus.
In a book significantly titled *Unprepared*, Andrew Lakoff analyzes
twenty years of epidemics, from bird flu to swine flu, from Ebola to
Zika, which tested "the fragile and still uncertain machinery of global
health security."[6] If, as one United States health official elegantly put
it, "preparedness is a journey, not a destination," the Covid pandemic
exposed a brutal interruption of that journey. Unpreparedness was
manifested in the fact that pandemic response plans had not been
updated, that hospitals were not equipped to react to the need for
intensive care, that stocks of medication were not sufficient to meet
demand, and essential personal protective equipment was unavailable,
even for those on the front line caring for patients, or whose jobs made
it impossible for them to stay at home, for example in the food and
transport industries. In the United States, a number of reports had
alerted successive governments to gaps in the system for responding
to a potential future pandemic; the most recent, from 2019, had noted

inadequate funding and coordination following a preparation exercise called Crimson Contagion, which had, in almost premonitory fashion, imagined an infection causing nearly 8 million hospitalizations and 600,000 deaths.[7] The epidemics caused by the H1N1 virus in 2009 and then Ebola in 2014 had been full-scale tests, and it was thought that lessons had been learned from them. In the White House, a directorate with special responsibility for this preparation had been created within the National Security Council, and in the handover between the Obama and Trump administrations in January 2017 an exercise had been organized for members of government responsible for these issues, including the secretary of state and the Homeland Security secretary. Two years later, the main participants in this exercise had been dismissed by the president, and the special directorate disbanded. In February 2020, as the first cases were being reported, the government was proposing, in its budget for the following year, a reduction of 700 million dollars in the funding for the Centers for Disease Control and Prevention, representing 9 percent of their budget. In France, the emblematic example of the shortage of masks reveals an equally edifying history of unpreparedness.[8] As early as 2005, a parliamentary report emphasized the importance of masks in the case of major epidemics. The following year the General Secretariat for Defense and National Security (SGDSN, Secrétariat générale de la défense et de la sécurité nationale), drew up a plan for the stocking and distribution of masks to combat a potential flu epidemic. It was put into operation in 2009 during the H1N1 pandemic. But that virus proved less serious than had been predicted. A new, much more economical plan was then drawn up, and the Ministry of Health now delegated the responsibility for buying masks for their agents and employees to healthcare establishments and to companies. Within ten years, 1 billion surgical masks destined for patients and, possibly, the public, was divided by nine, while the number of FFP2 filtering masks reserved for medical personnel and some in exposed professions fell from 700 million to zero. At the same time the Health Emergency Preparation and Response Unit (ÉPRUS, Établissement de préparation et de réponse aux urgences sanitaires), saw its funding from the state and state medical insurance scheme being reduced from 281 million euro in 2007, when it was first set up, to 26 million euro eight years later, although this sum was augmented by funds rolled over from previous years. Thus, in both the United States and France, unpreparedness was due to the difficulty of taking seriously the probability of a rare event involving substantial resources. As Michel Callon and Pierre Lascoumes note, the 1990s culture of precaution gradually disappeared.[9] Of course, it is difficult to prepare for the worst when the worst is an exceptional situation, but that is precisely what preparation means, whether for a terrorist attack, a natural disaster, or a pandemic.

But even once the pandemic had been declared, the governments' response did not allow them to change course. Of course, much like the villagers hearing the boy cry "wolf" in Aesop's fable, their fingers had been burned in the earlier epidemic of the H1N1 virus, better known as swine flu, which had given rise to what Carlo Caduff, in *The Pandemic Perhaps*, calls "prophetic discourses" announcing catastrophic developments and justifying mass vaccination campaigns against an infection that ultimately proved less serious than seasonal flu.[10] With the Covid pandemic, the response of the authorities thus revealed an inability to grasp the seriousness of the situation. Following the belated recognition of the urgency involved, healthcare systems struggled to put effective preventive measures into operation. The management of diagnostic tests is telling. These tests were essential in order to confirm cases of the disease, but still more in order to identify healthy carriers who transmitted the virus all the more easily because they had no symptoms, and in both cases to isolate them. In the United States, the tests produced by the Centers for Disease Control and Prevention, which had the monopoly on their manufacture, proved ineffective because they were contaminated, but the authorities refused those offered by the World Health Organization and set up regulatory obstacles to tests developed by research laboratories at the universities of Stanford, Washington, and Nebraska.[11] Several weeks were thus lost in the identification of cases. As of 1 March, fewer than 500 people had been tested in the entire country, representing 2,000 times less than was the case in South Korea, where testing combined with contact tracing and isolation of patients allowed the epidemic to be rapidly contained. In France, other bureaucratic hurdles slowed down the production of tests, as private clinics and veterinary laboratories, which had offered their services, were not called upon to help a struggling public system.[12] During the month of March 2020, a little over 200,000 tests were conducted, whereas in Germany 500,000 tests were conducted each week – that is, around ten times more. Moreover, owing to the shortage of tests, their use was limited to serious cases only, resulting in no patient isolation or contact tracing.

Clearly, prevention was deficient in both the United States and France, although the specific reasons differed somewhat in the two countries. But the same failures were observed in healthcare. The seriousness of the crisis was due not only to failures of preparation and response. It also resulted from the difficulties healthcare services had in meeting the influx of patients, despite the extraordinary efforts of medical personnel. The origin of these difficulties lay in two choices made long before, and particularly marked in the French case: the reduction in public spending on healthcare, which explained the shortage of resources in hospitals, and the delocalization of the production of medical goods, which accounted for the problems in the supply of medication and protective equipment. First, the public healthcare system had been subject to major budget cuts.[13] The shortage of intensive care beds was thus set in a more general context of the reduction of the number of hospital beds, which had fallen by 15 percent over fifteen years while, at the same time, the population had risen by 10 percent, and the proportion of people aged 65 and older had increased by 35 percent. In 2018 alone, French hospitals lost nearly 4,200 beds. This situation created a chronic difficulty for the emergency services in finding hospital beds for the patients who needed them. This problem, which was regularly heightened during flu epidemics, became insurmountable during the Covid pandemic. With regard to intensive care in particular, in 2020 France had only 5,000 beds, compared to Germany's 25,000. With regard to physicians, while the rate per 1,000 of the population was above the OECD average in 2000, it had fallen below since that time, having remained at the same level, whereas in Germany it had increased by a third to meet new needs. Finally, in terms of nurse salaries, France was in twenty-ninth place out of thirty-three countries. It was the program of public spending cuts that explained the shortage of material and human resources, the latter being exacerbated as healthcare teams themselves became infected. In the year prior to the start of the epidemic, French medical personnel had continuously protested this shortage, going so far as to strike, to no avail. The pandemic showed how justified their diagnosis was, and how legitimate their demand. But the processes described above were not limited to France, and in the United States, where the public contribution to healthcare remains modest, there was strong pressure to reduce it still further, particularly through cuts in the Medicaid system for people on low incomes. Second, shortages of medication and protective equipment revealed the consequences of the delocalization of production, particularly of healthcare products.[14] As the epidemic spread and the need for certain products increased, tensions arose around the supply of medicines, particularly curare- and morphine-based drugs used in intensive care, as well as antibiotics and steroids, and a shortfall arose in the supply of masks. It proved impossible to meet the increased demand, owing to the fact that most of these products were manufactured in China, which suddenly found itself subject to global demand from highly competitive countries. But this situation, which threatened France's sovereignty in the domain of health, illustrates a more general phenomenon of economic dependency generated by the constant drive for lower labor costs and higher profits. Trade with China represented 90 percent of France's total trade deficit in 2018. The United States' dependence was even greater, and had even grown under Donald Trump's presidency, exceeding 400 billion dollars in 2019.[15] Thus, in varying ways, depending on the country, the combination of a neoliberalism concerned with reducing public spending at all costs and a capitalism keen to minimize its production costs, thwarted prevention and treatment of the disease, aggravating its spread.

The pandemic is often presented as an inevitability. Yet the differences observed show that this is not the case. The countries that were best prepared and most reactive generally suffered less than others. At the end of the first peak, in June 2020, the death rate from coronavirus per million inhabitants was four times higher in France than in Germany, and sixty times higher in the United States than in South Korea. With an efficient healthcare and hospital system, Germany was quicker than France to develop tests, and therefore able to screen, isolate, and trace, and it had many more intensive care beds, enabling it to reduce the disease's case fatality rate. Learning from the experience of previous epidemics, South Korea, in contrast with the United States, also put a testing system in place immediately, accompanied by quarantine for those infected and contact tracing, at the same time reinforcing its hospital provisions by setting up temporary facilities and recruiting short-term staff. Remarkably, neither of these countries resorted to lockdown, whereas France and forty-two of the fifty states in the United States had to take extremely restrictive, harshly enforced measures. Of course, the account of these differences observed during the first six months of the pandemic cannot encompass the diversity of situations, or their evolution over the first year: while in early 2021 the epidemic was still under control in South Korea, it was rising in Germany, although the death rate from Covid remained much lower than in France, where the vaccination campaign took a long time to be rolled out, unlike the United States, where mass immunization of the population led to a slowdown in the epidemic.[16] The level of preparation, the quality of the response, the competence of the authorities, and their honesty in public statements have all been essential to interpreting the differences in epidemiological and economic performance between countries.

Although all too brief, this summary of the events offers an Ariadne's thread, allowing us to retrace our steps, returning to the themes of the various lectures in this course and the multiple stakes identified in each of them. In this way, it becomes possible to put forward a novel reading of the pandemic, while remaining aware that, at the time when this lecture is written, there are still many unknowns – from the origin of the virus and the medium-term efficacy of vaccines, to the consequences of measures taken to combat infection in poor countries, and the conditions of a return to what is too hastily being called "normality." The first year of the pandemic is definitely marked by the ordeal of uncertainty.

Let us begin then, by returning to the distinction established earlier between social production and social construction. The concept of social production refers to what gave rise to the pandemic, what unleashed it, what explains it. Here the question is: what caused it to arise? By contrast, the notion of social construction relates to the way various agents contributed to the representation of the pandemic, and how that representation in its turn was involved in the way it was experienced in different places and communities. Here the question is: how was it seen, and how, therefore, have people lived through it? In the social production the objective aspect of the phenomenon is emphasized. In the social construction, it is the subjective aspect. Both are partially connected.

Analysis of social production involves asking, first, how the disease emerged and, second, how it spread, hence distinguishing the virus from the pandemic, although the former is obviously necessary to the latter. The origin of the virus is the subject of various conjectures. In light of studies on the epidemiology of what are assumed to be the first cases, the virology of flu syndromes that occurred prior to the official start of the epidemic in China, the comparison of genomes of the virus in humans and those of coronaviruses present in animals, and the visit of a group of researchers under the aegis of the World Health Organization in early 2021, the most likely hypothesis points to contact between humans and animals, probably bats, in Hubei province, with an intermediate host – although the possibility of an accident at the laboratory in Wuhan has not been entirely ruled out.[17] But specific conditions were necessary in order for this infection to become a pandemic. The increased international circulation of people, initially through Chinese tourism across the world and economic cooperation with China, seems to have been a decisive factor, but subsequently all travel was involved. Passenger air travel has doubled in a decade, with the most rapid growth in the Asia-Pacific region, where it rose by almost 10 percent every year.[18] It is indeed ironic that the countries of the global North, which prohibit entry of migrants and refugees from the global South into their territory on grounds of the infectious risk they present, were themselves the purveyors of the epidemic to those countries. On 17 March 2020, the French president called for the closure of the borders of the Schengen Area, at a point when the European continent had become the global epicenter of the pandemic. Yet, the first cases in Mali, Senegal, and Burkina Faso, among others, involved citizens of those countries returning from France. The president of the United States announced the closure of his country's southern border on 19 March, a time when the United States had 73 times more cases and 175 times more deaths than neighboring Mexico. In fact, the first Mexican cases concerned men returning from Italy. In any case, the globalization of both tourism and trade was a major factor in the spread of the infection.

But if we wish to understand the many different reactions to the pandemic, not only at the political level but also within the population, it is essential to grasp its social construction. The most obvious fact in this respect was the way in which, during the first months, it almost entirely absorbed media attention. From mid-February onwards, Western media began to devote an increasing proportion of their output to it.[19] The most dramatic rise occurred in Italy: beginning on 23 February, the day when 100 cases were first recorded, the coronavirus infection took up more than half the daily news bulletins. By mid-March, in the United States, France, Spain, the United Kingdom, and of course in Italy, this proportion had reached, and even gone above, 70 percent. Lockdowns intensified this phenomenon, both because journalists had difficulty traveling to carry out their usual work of reporting, and especially because of the fascination the pandemic exerted on an audience now confined to their homes. Rolling news channels were dedicated almost exclusively to the subject, and the other media reorganized their schedules to better respond to the public expectation they imagined and helped to create. The daily report of statistics on cases and deaths, the evening press conferences by the French Director General of Health and the president of the United States, the testimonies from healthcare workers and relatives of people who had died, the opinions of scientists questioned about the potential evolution of the pandemic, how long it would take to produce vaccines, the psychological consequences of isolation, and practical ways of emerging out of lockdown – all charted a dramaturgy that, opinion polls showed, initially generated a high level of anxiety, and then became more reassuring as a degree of knowledge was disseminated, making every citizen an expert. It was remarkable how, in the United States, the Democratic primaries, initially a focus of interest and strong feelings, disappeared almost entirely from television screens and the press, while in France the pension reform that had led to so many debates and protests seemed no more than a distant memory, the proposed changes no longer discussed in the media.

The shift of attention to the pandemic accentuated two pre-existing phenomena in both the United States and France, as well as in many other countries: the news produced focuses on national situations, and the audience feels its own involvement through the expression of each individual's experience. This self-focus, at both national and individual level, fostered a consensus around a shared destiny, and the recognition of subjectivities affected. The government called for all to unite in this common cause. Citizens celebrated the work of introspection that lockdown made possible. This attitude was bound up in a degree of retreat from politics as conflictual but also as collective endeavor. It also went along with the quiet concealment of the fate reserved for certain groups who were implicitly seen as less legitimate members of the national community, and whose individual experience was not explored. The voices of residents in disadvantaged neighborhoods were barely heard, despite the fact that they were the most affected by the epidemic. Few people wondered what life was like for inmates in the overcrowded prisons, where social distancing was a fiction. Few spared a thought for the undocumented foreigners interned in detention centers. As for the rest of the world, it seemed to disappear: the hundreds of migrants dying in the Mediterranean, the thousands of refugees crowding into camps in Greece, the hundreds of thousands of Syrians stuck without shelter at the Turkish border, the millions of Yemenis facing famine under bombs supplied by Western countries – in short, everything that until February 2020 was called a "humanitarian crisis" – had all vanished. The world only existed insofar as it was exposed to the pandemic. Except that this was a very limited world, essentially restricted to Western countries, with China and, to a lesser degree, Russia as useful negative images.

Within this restricted context, the pandemic was constructed in a twofold relationship of alterity, to the viral other and to the human other, both in antagonistic mode. The virus was described as an "invisible enemy," in a martial rhetoric championed by Donald Trump and Emmanuel Macron, with Trump describing himself as a "wartime president," and Macron repeating at every opportunity "we are at war."[20] This language had a dual function: to raise the status of the person who used it and posed as the defender of the nation, attempting to rise to the stature of a Roosevelt or a de Gaulle; and to call for the people to fall in line behind the leader, silencing criticism at the moment when the state's weaknesses had become most visible. The enemy was often located geopolitically: some spoke of the "Chinese virus," a phrase that was used by journalists in the United States and France, and insistently by the US president. There was a swift move from hostility toward the virus to animosity toward human beings.[21] In the United States, France, and elsewhere, Chinese people, or nationals of those countries who were of Chinese origin, or even by approximation people from other East Asian countries, were subjected to racist abuse and even attacks. Conversely, in Guangzhou in the south of China, it was Nigerians who were suspected of being infected and driven out of one neighborhood. The identification of scapegoats at times of epidemic is a common phenomenon. But it rarely comes out of nowhere. Almost always, this is a reactivation of an older hostility or mistrust, for which the disease offers new justification.

However, positive images need to be constructed to offset these negative effects. During the first lockdown, a strong heroicizing dynamic developed in relation to healthcare workers. The gratitude shown to them by the thousands of people who applauded them at 8 p.m. each evening in many places was reinforced in the media, where journalists praised their courage and thanked them for their commitment. Those in government joined their voices to this unanimity of gratitude. But in this exercise, President Trump proved less fortunate than President Macron. While the US president made public statements about suspected theft of equipment by medical personnel, prompting indignation at his lack of sensitivity, his French counterpart managed to redirect his elitist discourse about the merits of "front runners" toward a humanist discourse about the honor of the "front line" formed by those who were saving lives, thus striving to erase the memory of the police repression of their protests against their working conditions just weeks earlier. But if there were heroes, there were also victims, the seriously ill and those who died; the media, unable to display their suffering, exhibited the grief of those who had lost a loved one, and sometimes even the tears of the journalists interviewing them. But this desire to create empathy focused on people with whom a majority of the public could identify. A moral economy therefore emerged, promoting a selective coming-together, in the admiration of heroes and compassion for victims that offset the sad passions mobilized toward those who were held responsible.

At the boundary between production and construction of the epidemic, quantitative data saturated the media, raising once again the question of the "truth in numbers." Never before had the statistics of a disease so taken over the public space. The numbers of cases, of deaths, of recoveries, of hospitalizations, of intensive care patients, of tests carried out, of positive tests. And also: the basic reproduction number, doubling time, case fatality and mortality rates, the proportion of the population that had received one vaccine, and the proportion fully immunized. For many, submerged in this sea of data that scrolled across the bottom of television or computer screens, the experience of the pandemic proved a real education in epidemiology. Not that people became experts, but they became familiar with these data that seemed to determine how both the near and the more distant future would unfold. Day after day the figures were churned out, worrying in their progression, but reassuring in the knowledge they appeared to accumulate, and even the transparency they seemed to be demonstrating. Rather than the discourse of experts and images of the sick, what brought the epidemic into existence as a fact, aroused fears, awoke consciences, and fed conversations, were the figures. Yet what is the power of veridiction of numbers, I asked at the start of this course? China was suspected of not transmitting trustworthy data. Authoritarian regimes such as Turkey and Iran were accused of not communicating their data honestly. But observers often lacked this critical eye when they looked at statistics from Western countries, quoting them and commenting on them as if they represented the reality of the epidemic. However, there could be serious distortion. In both the United States and France, for example, the low number of diagnostic tests carried out for a long time led to serious underestimates of the number of cases, while the failure to take into account deaths outside hospitals, whether in private homes or nursing homes, considerably understated the number of deaths. Yet experts would discuss case fatality rates calculated by the division of an incorrect number of deaths by a still less correct number of cases identified. In the United States in mid-April 2020, for example, this produced a probability of 4.5 percent that someone with the virus would die – a quite excessive value given what was beginning to be understood from the more reliable data in countries where population-wide testing was being carried out. People expressed surprise that Germany had 20 percent more cases of the virus than France, but only 20 percent of the number of deaths, forgetting that, in addition to the much higher availability of intensive care beds, Germany was carrying out five times more diagnostic tests and was therefore producing data much more faithful to reality.[22] As sociologist Emmanuel Didier notes, these data were glossed over without any serious discussion as to the quality of the quantities that were alternately feeding the public's fears and hopes, grievance and pride.[23] Given these considerable margins of error, which are as certain as they are impossible to evaluate, it is remarkable that figures were able to impose their truth to the point

that these doubtful, not to say improbable, values were used to formu-
late forecasts, on the basis of which experts advised rulers and rulers
made decisions that committed their respective countries to onerous
and costly policies. The forecast industry, indeed, boomed, with a proliferation of research centers producing data that diverged wildly: at
the end of April 2020, estimates from the ten main institutions producing these forecasts for the situation only three weeks ahead predicted
death rates that differed by a factor of as much as four, depending
on the simulations used and the hypotheses adopted. Governments
therefore had the choice of which figure to base their initiatives on.
The White House, determined to minimize the seriousness of the situation, prioritized the forecasts from the Institute for Health Metrics and
Evaluation, funded by the Bill and Melinda Gates Foundation, despite
the fact that 70 percent of its optimistic predictions were invalidated
the day after. By contrast, the French government, concerned about
an evolution that the health authorities were clearly unable to manage,
followed the pessimistic analyses of Imperial College London, which
predicted a potentially massive death toll of up to 500,000 deaths in
France, in the unlikely case that absolutely no preventive measure was
taken.[24] Consequently no restrictive measures were implemented at the
federal level in the United States, while strict lockdown was imposed
in France. To paraphrase Pascal's famous maxim: truth in numbers on
this side of the Atlantic, error on the other side.

While the statistics were thus discussed and argued over, the same
was not true of "epistemic boundaries" as far as the virus was concerned. In late December 2019 the strange pneumonia was described.
Two weeks later its genome had been sequenced by Chinese researchers. A month after that, the name of the virus, SARS-CoV-2, and
the official name of the disease, Covid-19, had been determined by
the International Committee on Taxonomy of Viruses and the World
Health Organization, respectively. Thus, within a very brief time the
nosology was established, and very shortly afterwards its polymorphous clinical presentation. Even the prolonged form, in which debili-
tating fatigue is accompanied by drowsiness, disorders of memory,
concentration and mood, chest tightness or palpitations, headaches,
muscle pain, skin eruptions, and digestive symptoms – in other words
a picture very similar to chronic fatigue, especially in that the large
majority of sufferers are young or middle-aged women – was almost
immediately taken seriously by physicians, with no one venturing to
challenge it as they had Gulf War syndrome or chronic Lyme disease.
"Long Covid," as it was named, was thus entered into a provisional
nosography, neither official nor contested. In fact, it was around the

issue of treatment that epistemic boundaries were most powerfully challenged, testing both the medical community itself and its relations with the public and the authorities. The most high-profile case, in France, centered around the drug hydroxychloroquine. Initially, a clinical study was conducted by a team in Marseilles on forty-two patients with a mild form of the disease, of whom twenty-six were treated with hydroxychloroquine and sixteen formed a control group who received conventional treatment.[25] On the sixth day, fourteen of the twenty treated no longer showed any trace of the virus, compared to two out of sixteen in the control group, leading the authors to claim that their treatment was effective. However, many infectiologists had reservations about the study. To begin with, the two groups had not been selected at random and presented differences at the outset, making it difficult to assert that the effects observed were solely due to the treatment. Second, the conclusions omitted the troubling fact that six of the patients taking hydroxychloroquine – nearly a quarter – had disappeared from the analyses because they had not completed their treatment: three had been transferred to intensive care and one had died, raising concerns about a product whose cardiac toxicity was well known. Two camps then formed. The orthodox held that it was necessary to await the results of a properly conducted randomized controlled clinical trial, in order to be sure of both the efficacy and the safety of the treatment. The heterodox, on the other side, convinced that hydroxychloroquine saved lives, felt that the drug should be widely put to use immediately. The former argued for science and precaution, and the latter for pragmatism and urgency. This dispute was also played out in the political arena, with the health minister forbidding physicians in private practices to prescribe the medication for this purpose, while one of his predecessors launched a petition, signed by several hundred thousand people, for its authorization. Although disavowed by the majority of the scientific world, the heterodox won the battle for public opinion. A poll conducted in early April 2020 showed that 59 percent of respondents thought that hydroxychloroquine was effective against coronavirus, compared to only 20 percent who were not of this view.[26] In a classic example of displacement of the source of legitimization, the science heretics, deprived of rational legitimacy, sought recognition in popular legitimacy. It was probably in order to absorb some of this legitimacy that President Macron, in a gesture that many saw as populist, paid a surprise visit to the physician responsible for the Marseilles trials. Yet this fringe controversy would have remained a minor French story, had the president of the United States not himself become involved, publicly promoting the drug on several occasions, declaring that there was strong evidence of its efficacy, and going so far as to release 25 million doses from the national stocks to be distributed throughout the country.[27] On 16 April, when a scientific journal published a retrospective study of 368 patients infected with coronavirus, showing that the death rate among those who had received hydroxychloroquine was 2.6 times higher than among those who had not received it, President Trump changed his tune. However, the controversy did not end with this article, which was challenged in its turn as not being a randomized controlled trial.[28] Thus, whether they relate to diseases, as in the cases studied in my previous lectures, or treatments, as with the pandemic, epistemic boundaries form where there is uncertainty, or, more often, contested certainties. Then an orthodoxy that lays claim to scientific norms – in this case double-blind clinical trials – comes up against a heterodoxy that challenges them, winning an alternative legitimacy outside the scientific world, particularly among patients seeking answers that medicine has not given them.

This is undoubtedly fertile soil for "conspiracy theories." The hydroxychloroquine affair fed them on social media. Presenting himself as a victim of the medical establishment, the dissident physician laid the ground for allegations about truths the health authorities were suspected of trying to hide. More generally, in March 2020 half of those interviewed in France thought it likely that the government had withheld information about the epidemic from them.[29] It may reasonably be assumed that they began to doubt the honesty of ministers after they had heard them repeat for weeks, when there was a shortage of masks, that masks were "pointless" for the general public, even too "complicated" to use, and potentially "counterproductive," only to start encouraging people to wear them a month later, and subsequently making them compulsory. They were told similar untruths about tests for the virus, which one day were of no use and the next became essential. It is hard to imagine that such fallacious assertions from the French government contributed nothing to the development of conspiracy theories, which in these cases might indeed appear to be lucid assessments of official discourse. The authorities, moreover, occasionally fanned or even stirred up these theories. The most internationally widespread conspiracy theory related to the origin of the virus. The city of Wuhan, where the epidemic started, is home to one of China's two P4 laboratories, which house the most dangerous infectious agents, the ones with a high mortality for which there is neither treatment nor vaccine. Without citing its sources, but hinting that the information came from within the intelligence services, the

conservative 24-hour news channel, Fox News, asserted on 15 April
that sources believed "with increasing confidence" that the epidemic
originated in this laboratory, owing to the Chinese government's desire
to challenge the United States by demonstrating its country's superior
capabilities in the fight against viruses, and that the World Health
Organization, aware of the facts, strove to cover them up.[30] While not
confirming these maneuvers, several members of the US government,
including the president himself, also disseminated this suggestion in
interviews with journalists. Despite the fact that most scientists considered this hypothesis the least probable, media and politicians close
to President Trump continued to proffer their insinuations, fanning
an anti-Chinese sentiment that mingled open accusations with latent
resentment. Chinese social media networks, for their part, encouraged
by the authorities, teemed with messages pointing to the United States
as the true source of the virus, in an inversion of the blame. Like all epidemics, that due to the coronavirus thus generated conspiracy theories
in which coincidences became proof, popular imaginaries coalesced
with political strategies, and the most incoherent fantasies mixed with
the most disturbing facts. Two films released within a few months
of one another in 2020, on each side of the Atlantic, encouraged the
spread of these theories: *Plandemic* and *Hold-Up*, produced, respectively, in the United States and France.[31] Both drew in researchers,
some of them already discredited for their earlier work and views. They
accused the authorities of having withheld the facts, particularly the
efficacy of hydroxychloroquine and the danger of masks. They asserted
that the virus originated from manipulations in a laboratory, with
Wuhan as the favored candidate, with Fort Detrick and the Institut
Pasteur also being mentioned. They accused Bill Gates of having disseminated the virus in order to profit from vaccine revenues, and even
of taking control of those immunized by injecting them with nano-
particles. More broadly, linking back to the classic trope of alleged
plots by Jews or freemasons, they expounded the theory of a world
conspiracy of the powerful who sought to dominate humanity, and
even eliminate the poor. The remarkable popularity of these two films
suggests more than mere curiosity: it indicates a particular receptivity
to the language of conspiracy.

But the language of the pandemic is also one of "crisis." While
some of those in government drew on a martial metaphor, the most
commonly used expression was that of health crisis. The rhetoric of
crisis is performative, in two ways: it brings the crisis into being, by
dramatizing the situation – in this case through discourse, images,
and, above all, figures; but it also, through the crisis, brings into being

a set of facts. First, it enables the event and the response applied to it to escape the normal order of things: literally extraordinary decisions can be taken, set in the context of a state of exception. Second, it shakes up the temporality of political action: there is a need to act urgently, removing decisions from democratic scrutiny and leaving aside analysis of structural causes, which in theory will be taken into account at a later date. Finally, it suspends critique: unity in adversity must prevail, and objections are condemned on the grounds that they sow division. These three sets of circumstances – escape from the normal order, disruption of temporality, and suspension of critique – can together be categorized as a state of shock. It is both the cause and the consequence of the collective fear, in the face of which governments find themselves caught in a dialectical relationship, needing it in order to encourage citizens to acquiesce to a state of exception, but at the same time needing to calm it in order to avoid uncontrollable panic. Among the various aspects of health crises, one is particularly important to consider – the ethical dimension. Given that what led to the health crisis was, in practice, the fear of seeing hospitals and, above all, intensive care units overwhelmed because there were not sufficient beds, decisions had to be made as to who could be hospitalized, or indeed transferred to intensive care. Such decisions are what sociologists call tragic choices – choices that have life-or-death consequences in a context of scarce resources.[32] In this case, deciding who was to be hospitalized or transferred to intensive care effectively meant deciding between those who were to be given a chance to live and those who were to be exposed to the risk of dying. This kind of "triage" occurs daily but invisibly in medicine, especially when the question is whether an elderly person in fragile health should receive intensive care that might pointlessly, and sometimes against their wishes, prolong their suffering without significantly increasing their life expectancy. During the pandemic, these tragic choices were often spoken of in the context of the Bergamo province, where more than 3,000 people died in March and April 2020.[33] There was much less discussion of decisions made in many places in the United States and France not to hospitalize elderly patients, whether they lived at home or in an institution, so as to save hospital beds for younger patients.[34] But focusing merely on tragic choices obscures other elements of the ethical crisis of the pandemic, which arose in terms of social justice. Think, for example, of the obligation for people in high-exposure jobs to continue their work without protection, or the stigmatization of residents of low-income neighborhoods held responsible for the high numbers of cases and deaths, due in fact to their living conditions and accommodation.

These inequalities had a particularly harsh impact on "exiles." The legal precarity that goes hand in hand with socioeconomic precarity for migrants, refugees, and asylum seekers increased during the 2010s in most countries. By 2021, the majority of exiles were not like those of the preceding generation, in whom a "healthy migrant effect" had been discovered. Because they came from countries riven by conflict or poverty, because their journey had been long, grueling, and dangerous, and because the conditions to which they were relegated in the country where they sought refuge were often degrading – forced out onto the streets, into train stations, constantly at risk of arrest and maltreatment – their physical and mental health deteriorated, making them vulnerable to the pandemic. Some no longer had a residence permit, some had never had one; their lack of official status often led them to risk their health in dangerous jobs without protection that they could not refuse, and if they fell sick they were faced with the dilemma of risking being reported to the authorities or going without care.[35] They were extremely vulnerable to two dangers: detention and exclusion. The first was a matter of punishment, and the second stemmed from indifference. On the one hand, locking exiles up in detention centers is effectively an imprisonment that punishes individuals who have committed no offense, since they are accused merely of lacking a residence permit. In France, around 50,000 foreigners, just over half of them in the mainland, pass through these centers, which have a little over 1,800 places, each year. With the pandemic, when the first cases arose in these centers, detainees became anxious: some went on hunger strikes while others self-harmed in order to draw the authorities' attention to their situation, which was both dangerous and absurd, since, given the suspension of international flights, deportations could not take place. Notwithstanding these desperate gestures, and despite the intervention of the Observatory on the Detention of Foreigners (OEE, Observatoire de l'enfermement des étrangers) and the Defender of Rights (DDD, Défenseur des droits) calling for the closure of the centers, and judges' decisions to free detainees given the circumstances, there were still 150 exiles confined at the end of March 2020, and their number began to rise again as soon as the first lockdown ended.[36] However, the conditions in which tens of thousands of undocumented foreigners were detained in the United States were even more troubling, in view not only of the risks of contagion but also simply of the abject treatment of these men, women, and children herded into vast hangars. On the other hand, exclusion was most obviously manifested in the presence of exiles camped in public spaces and empty lots. In France, they crowded under bridges and on waste ground on the outskirts of Paris, in public parks and on the beaches around Calais, and in many other cities, sometimes in tents donated by humanitarian organizations. Because there was not enough space in hostels for all the asylum seekers, some of them, even if they had an accommodation voucher, were in the same situation. The police regularly drove away these undesirables, sometimes tearing down their makeshift shelters, destroying their belongings, and spoiling their food. During lockdown some were provided with temporary accommodation in emergency hostels, in hotel rooms where they found themselves isolated, or in gyms where social distancing was impossible.[37] Beyond France, what was happening at the borders of Europe could be seen as a combination of detention and exclusion. In the Moria camp on the island of Lesbos at the end of April, there were 19,000 migrants and refugees forcibly confined in a precarious space designed for 3,000.[38] An appeal by Human Rights Watch, Amnesty International, and Médecins du monde to reduce the population of the camp, in order to avoid an epidemic as soon as the first case arose, received no response from either the Greek government or the European Union.

But it was in the "carceral" world that enforced confinement created the conditions most conducive to the spread of the epidemic. Prisoners cohabiting may be due to overcrowding, as in France, where in early 2020 the average density per cell was 1.38 percent in short-stay prisons: more than 14,000 prisoners were living in overcrowded cells, with more than 1,600 sleeping on mattresses on the floor, indicating that the same number of cells designed for one prisoner were occupied by three. It may also be due to the organization of the correctional facility itself, as in the United States, where the local jails that house prisoners awaiting trial or serving short sentences sometimes have dormitories with several dozen bunk beds. In many countries, the first reaction of the authorities was to attempt to reduce prisoners' contact with the outside world, or with one another, by banning visits from lawyers, chaplains, and family members, as well as sports, cultural, and educational activities. The effect was immediate, with a rise in tensions, incidents, and, in some cases, deadly mutinies, particularly in Italy, Mexico, Venezuela, and especially in Colombia. The reduction in prisoner numbers was often belated, but sometimes spectacular, as in Iran, where 54,000 prisoners were released.[39] In France, the CGLPL, the DDD, and judges' and lawyers' unions and human rights organizations alerted the public authorities early on, and demanded that incarceration in individual cells, as prescribed by the law, be respected. Within three months, the prison population fell by 19 percent, from 72,000 to 58,000, thanks to the combined effect of a lower number of convictions since courts had reduced their activity, and measures decided in favor of early release for prisoners nearing the end of their sentence. However, as soon as the first lockdown ended, the number of prisoners began to rise again, by 1,000 each month, thus increasing by 10 percent in only eight months.[40] In the United States, public health experts, advocacy organizations, elected representatives, and judges appealed to federal and state authorities to approve early release of nonviolent offenders, and older, disabled, and sick prisoners, but with only limited results, as governors feared losing some of their support on the eve of national elections. In mid-April, out of 50,000 prisoners in New York, 1,100 had been released; in California 3,500 out of 130,000. When the state of Ohio undertook the effort to test all prisoners during the same period, in one of the largest correctional facilities, 1,828 prisoners, 73 percent of the total, tested positive.[41] Thus, while confinement of the general population, though applied with varying degrees of rigor depending on the country, helped to protect healthy people from circulation of the virus, confinement in prison operated, on the contrary, as forced exposure to the risk of infection, with no way of avoiding it. The authorities, then, had a choice between health rationale and security rationale. In France, the former seems to have prevailed, at least during the first lockdown, but this choice meant imposing still harsher conditions of incarceration. In the United States, the latter was the rule, with tragic consequences for inmates. By early June there had been one death from Covid in French prisons, and 510 in US prisons. In proportion to the carceral population in each country, the death rate was twenty times higher in US than in French prisons.

Thus, the various themes identified over the course of the previous lectures – social production and social construction, the truth in numbers, epistemic boundaries, conspiracy theories, ethical crises, precarious exiles, carceral ordeals – help to redefine the boundaries of the Covid pandemic, offering fresh perspectives on it and retrospectively validating the choice to use them as keys to interpret public health. But one crucial dimension of the pandemic remains that cannot be explored in terms of these themes, and which was the subject of my inaugural lecture:[42] the question of life and the unequal treatment of it.

What makes the event unique is not the global diffusion of the virus, for flu often evolves in the same way, nor the seriousness of the infection, for more people have died of AIDS. It is the reaction it provoked – which in the majority of countries was the confinement of the population and the suspension of most activities, imposed with varying degrees of rigor and for varying lengths of time. The confinement was of course not total, since some workers were considered indispensable to the smooth functioning of society, and certain sectors such as health and social care, transportation of people and goods, security on the streets and in prisons, were therefore exempted, but confinement at home with limited possibilities for going out, and the interruption of work with the exception of those working from home, were the rule. The response to the pandemic was therefore achieved at the cost of a double sacrifice to what can be called health police. First, civil liberties and, more broadly, democratic life, were temporarily impacted.[43] Moving around, or simply being outside one's home, or in the company of others, was deemed an offense punishable by a deterrent fine. Assessment of the certificate that was supposed to authorize going out was left to the discretion of the police, who in some cases abused this power, especially in low-income neighborhoods. Even the right to privacy was threatened by the introduction of invasive surveillance technologies that traced those infected and their contacts. In many countries the state of emergency also gave the government decision-making powers with virtually no parliamentary oversight, since this was restricted by the impossibility of gathering together. Second, the interruption of economic activity meant that recession, unemployment, and the impoverishment of large sections of the population loomed.[44] In 2020, gross domestic product in the United States saw its largest fall since 1946, namely 3.5 percent, with the loss of 9 million jobs, while the reduction in the GDP in France was 8.3 percent and unemployment rose by 7.5 percent. According to International Monetary Fund estimates, sub-Saharan Africa saw negative growth for the first time in a quarter century, with an increase in poverty and multiple food shortages. However, it would be wrong to imagine that these shocks on both the political and the socioeconomic levels were entirely due to the pandemic. The rollback of democracy had already begun in many countries. To take just Europe into consideration, this was certainly the case in Viktor Orbán's Hungary and Andrzej Duda's Poland, but many other countries had also embarked on this road, including France, where in 2017 the president only ended the two-year state of emergency following the 13 November 2015 terrorist attacks after a law was passed that actually integrated the main emergency measures into the ordinary legislation. In 2018, philosopher Michaël Foessel drew a troubling parallel with the French situation eighty years earlier, on the eve of World War II.[45] The socioeconomic regression, too, was already under way. For some companies, the arrival of coronavirus was a godsend that allowed them to put through redundancy packages and restructuring programs that had been planned before the health crisis.[46] Others often needed only to not renew contracts, to ask for voluntary redundancies, to stop recruiting temporary staff, and to put employees on temporary layoff – in other words to use all the provisions for precarization and flexibilization of employment that had been introduced over the previous years.

As a catalyst for pre-existing tendencies, which it accelerated, the pandemic thus demanded a considerable double sacrifice from people, often the most disadvantaged. There was only one justification for this sacrifice – saving lives that were at risk of infection. It should be remembered that during the early months some experts were predicting as many as 100 million deaths to come.[47] But rather than the potential number of victims, which was both abstract and uncertain, it was the dramatization of deaths through the daily statistics, images of mortuary bags piling up, accounts of overwhelmed intensive care units, and testimonies of relatives of those who had died that imprinted in people's minds the necessity of doing everything possible to reduce mortality due to the pandemic. Lockdown, despite its encroachments on democracy and its economic and social consequences, seemed to all – or almost all – the only possible response. A consensus formed, which few politicians or intellectuals dared to challenge.

This sudden consecration of life as sacrosanct calls for appraisal. It may seem to go without saying. Yet, it is a relatively recent phenomenon. One need only think of the 20 million dead, half of them civilians, that were accepted as the price of victory during World War I, barely a century before the beginning of the Covid epidemic.[48] Moreover, even today, when those dead are on the enemy side, they certainly do not have the same value, as evidenced by Madeleine Albright, then US Ambassador to the United Nations, cynically asserting that the more than 500,000 children who died as a result of US sanctions against Iraq were the price to pay for the fall of Saddam Hussein's regime.[49] Even when the dead are simply foreigners, and not foes, they hardly count. Think of the more than 20,000 men, women, and children who have been left to drown in the Mediterranean between 2014 and 2021: not only were they not helped, but humanitarian activists were prevented from helping them.[50] It is, then, when it is a matter of "our own," or at least those we can consider as belonging to our moral community, that life deserves to be protected. Hence the substantial sacrifices people consented to in order to limit mortality due to the pandemic.

But the life for which these sacrifices are consented to is the physical life. The efforts to preserve it did not extend to social life – life exposed not to a virus, but to degradation and injustice, the lives of African families whose children suffer from lead poisoning, the lives of exiles in internment camps, the lives of prison inmates. This disconnection between two forms of life – physical and social – and the promotion of the former over the latter, characterize what can be termed bio-legitimacy, the recognition of physical life as a supreme good, which is a signature of Western modernity, and perhaps increasingly of modernity itself.[51] Of course, one can retort that there is a glaring paradox in the way governments in certain countries – China, which makes its dissidents disappear, Saudi Arabia, which executes them in public, the United States, which continues to practice the death penalty – made the choice of more or less generalized lockdown, partial suspension of civil liberties, and temporary interruption of economic activity, all to protect human life.

Yet, the consensus was not total. The critique of biolegitimacy, albeit marginal, arose out of two distinct perspectives, economic and political. In the arena of the economy, the most prominent dissident was Dan Patrick, Lieutenant Governor of Texas, who pleaded "Don't sacrifice the country," asking that older people be allowed to take care of themselves. He added that if he was asked: "Are you willing to take a chance on your survival in exchange for keeping the America that all America loves for your children and grandchildren?" he would not hesitate to agree to it, in order to save the economy.[52] This remark, which resonated with the discourse of heads of state like Donald Trump and Jair Bolsonaro in Brazil, shocked people because it prioritized the situation of the economy over the life of older people: "wealth over health," as the saying goes. But there was little discussion of the bad faith of this declaration, given that, thanks to the privilege of his office, his material circumstances, and his working conditions, the risk this public figure said he was willing to take was much lower than that run by workers in construction, transport, and food production, most of whom belonged to the lower classes and to ethnic and racial minorities. In the political arena, the intellectual who expressed himself most vehemently in Europe was Giorgio Agamben, who, after denying the existence of a pandemic and accusing the Italian government of using the situation as an excuse to impose a state of exception, presented a more acceptable version of his critique, stating during the first lockdown that "just as, faced with terrorism, it was claimed that freedom had to be suppressed in order to defend it, similarly we are now told that life has to be suspended in order to protect it."[53] The problem in his view was that his fellow citizens were "prepared to sacrifice virtually everything, their normal conditions of life, social relationships, work, and even friendships, political and religious affects and beliefs, to the danger of infection," adding that "even the dead no longer have a right to a funeral." Thus, the meaning of life was at stake, between what he calls bare life and qualified life, or, to put it another way, between simply being alive and fully being in the world. These are therefore two very different contestations of the restrictive and sometimes repressive measures taken by governments: in Patrick's version, the protest is in the name of a life at the service of the economy (living means contributing to the wealth of the nation); in Agamben's version, it is based on a conception of life as a human and a citizen (living means participating in the construction of the city). Which life do we want? This is the question that, according to those who resist confinement, we are asked to give up thinking about.

However, I would like to pose a different question, to ask not whether the right choice was made, but whether it was rightly implemented in light of the principle it claims to be based on. I want to shift scrutiny of the policy of confinement from the normative (was it right to make this decision?) to the descriptive (what happened in practice?), thus moving toward a different form of critique. Lockdown was presented as a universal measure, but in reality it excluded not only the workers required to meet the essential needs of healthcare, food supply, and transport, but also, and often in a hidden manner, workers who were simply useful to the smooth running of certain sectors of the capitalist economy, insofar as their precarious status or their lack of resources made them likely to accept dangerous conditions – and it became clear how spikes of infection could arise in some of these places, from abattoirs to construction sites. The modalities of enforcement of lockdown varied widely between areas, with a higher police presence in low-income neighborhoods, where punishment of breaches of the rules was more strict and abuse of power more frequent, despite the fact that living conditions in these neighborhoods made it more difficult to comply with the measures. Finally, in some cases, enforced confinement was not protection against the disease but, on the contrary, exposure to the risk of contracting it, as we have seen in the case of foreigners locked up in detention centers, inmates incarcerated in short-stay prisons, and migrants gathered up into gyms. In short, what was presented as a measure that applied to everyone in fact set up deep divisions, effectively indicating the inequality of the value of lives. In the United States, a study at the level of counties showed that an increase of 1 percent in socioeconomic inequalities translated into a 2 percent rise in the incidence of infection, and a 3 percent rise in mortality; an increase of 1 percent in racial disparities was associated with a 4 percent rise in the incidence of infection and a 7 percent rise in mortality. These discrepancies resulted in a fall in life expectancy of 2.7 years for Black people, compared to 0.8 for whites in 2020, representing a difference of almost six years between Blacks and whites, the widest gap observed since 1998.[54] In France, the Seine-Saint-Denis department, the poorest in the country, has a population density sixty-four times that of the country as a whole, a proportion of immigrants three times above the national average, and only a quarter of the hospital provisions of Paris. In March and April 2020, the excess mortality there compared to the previous year was 134 percent, much higher than in other departments, and was even as high as 169 percent in its most disadvantaged district.[55] Thus, at the very moment when those in government were seeking to generate consensus, epidemiological reality made it clear that, in the face of the pandemic, not all lives were equal. Biolegitimacy is an unfairly distributed principle.

But the question of the value of lives needs to be extended beyond the pandemic, to ask about the predictable consequences of the suspension and then slowdown in economic and social activity during the high point of the health crisis. There is a risk of these consequences remaining largely invisible. Resulting from job losses, business closures, evictions from housing, the rise in poverty, the weakening of social links, and the perception of the lack of a future, their delayed translation will have little echo in the public sphere. They will manifest all the more violently when social protection is reduced, solidarity weaker, and the idea of justice more contested. As is already the case, they will hit vulnerable groups and discriminated minorities hardest. They will impact the young and adults of working age, unlike the pandemic which affected the oldest most. They will take two main forms.

First, there will be the lives lost: excess deaths that only recorded death statistics will be revealed several years afterwards, for these deaths will usually be from nonspecific causes such as cardiovascular disease, but also in some cases have a more characteristic etiology, such as suicide, overdose, and complications from alcoholism. This is the phenomenon Anne Case and Angus Deaton have called "deaths of despair."[56] In the United States, it reflects a deepening of inequality since the 1980s, which intensified following the 2008 financial crash, reversing the hitherto positive graph of life expectancy.[57] In France it is manifested in a death rate among the unemployed that is three times higher for men and twice as high for women than among those of the same age who are employed.[58] Unlike deaths due to the epidemic, the numbers of which were the subject of a daily public announcement that dramatized them, these premature deaths, which will inevitably be unequally distributed, will go unnoticed. They will disappear in the annual death statistics only discussed in the academic circles of demography and epidemiology.

And then, there will be the lives ruined, as they already have been, by this deterioration in economic and social conditions. These lives will not even be counted, because the damage to them is not measured by statistical tools, and perhaps above all because, being no longer productive, they no longer count. They suffer the ordeal of "moral injuries" that Axel Honneth describes as violations of the three elements essential to self-realization as a social being: self-confidence, self-respect, and self-worth.[59] For the victims of the emerging crisis, the loss of value experienced through their relationships with others, whether family members, potential employers, or assistance providers, feeds a state of suffering that affects individuals much more deeply than the disease.[60] It is crucial to recognize this collective affliction, for both moral and theoretical reasons, because to do so is to refuse to limit life to what Walter Benjamin called "mere life."[61] This is one final lesson for public health from the pandemic: the life it has to protect cannot be reduced to physical life; it must also, and above all, be a politically and ethically dignified and full life.

Notes

Introduction

1 Among the various ways of referring to the disease caused by the coronavirus designated SARS-CoV-2, I have chosen to simply use the term "Covid."
2 The title of Foucault's 1979–80 course at the Collège de France is somewhat deceptive, since the series actually focuses on the government of the self and subjectivation through submission to pastoral power.
3 Ulrich is the protagonist of Musil's book (1996 [1955], vol. 1, p. xx), who in the first drafts of the work was tellingly and ironically named Anders ("the Other") and is thus gifted with "a sense of the possible." As Jean-François Vallée notes (2004, pp. 28–29), Musil's writing is entirely geared toward producing an "effect of strangeness, or at the very least, 'defamiliarization'" in the reader.
4 The allusions here are respectively to the work of Edward Evans-Pritchard (1940), Claude Lévi-Strauss (2011 [1955]), Jeanne Favret-Saada (2015 [1977]), and Margaret Lock (2013).
5 Making a distinction between alterity and difference, Bazin argues (2008, p. 48): "However strange, and sometimes absurd, human actions appear to us initially, there must be a point of view from which, once they are better known, they prove to be merely different from our own: it is this that renders the description of them anthropological."
6 See Rey (2001), Gaffiot (1934) and Brown (1993).
7 This choice to narrate is partly justified by what Laurent Demanze (2019, p. 113) calls "the democratic power of storytelling," which I use in a slightly different sense, since my aim is, through narrative, to meet with a broader audience and thus facilitate their access to the research.
8 These worlds are distinct from the "social worlds" that interactionists such as Anselm Strauss (1978) have theorized, which are constituted around activities that involve technologies and evolve within organizations.
9 See, for example, George Rosen's classic history (1958).
10 See, of course, *The History of Sexuality*, vol. 1 (1978 [1976]).
11 Readers who followed the lectures online will note some differences between the spoken and written versions. This is because the written lectures were a little too long for the Collège de France's one-hour format. In addition, some parts of the preface were included in the spoken version of the first lecture,

since the point of them was to introduce the course. The final lecture has been substantially augmented in the book, in order to construct a partial history of the pandemic that a reading more distant in time might have obscured. In other respects, the two versions are very similar.

The Birth of Public Health

1 Winslow's definition (1920, p. 30) is in his article in the journal *Science*, the published text of a speech given to the American Association for the Advancement of Science.

2 Porter adds (1999, p. 1) that this history "conjures up an image of investigating toilets, drains and political statutes through the ages," owing largely to the way mid-twentieth-century historians approached the subject, in a spirit that "reflected the ideals of nineteenth-century public health reform."

3 It is in Foucault's lecture of 31 January 1979 that he describes this imaginary conversation (2008 [2004], pp. 76–77). In the "Course summary," he writes that his lectures "ended up being devoted entirely to what should have been only its introduction," liberalism and neoliberalism.

4 In *L'Espace politique de la santé* [*The Political Space of Public Health*], in contrast to Foucault (1978 [1976]), who talks of a "biopower" deployed in the Western world from the eighteenth century, I have proposed the concept of "government of life" (1996, p. 199), attempting to identify early forms of it in first-century Rome, and in the Inca empire in the fifteenth century, and later in precolonial African societies, linking these forms to the constitution of a sovereign state that bases its legitimacy on the protection of its subjects not only against external and internal enemies, by means of the army and the police, but also against disease and death.

5 This research, carried out with the invaluable collaboration of Anne-Jeanne Naudé, then a doctoral candidate in social sciences, was funded by the Ministry of Research (Naudé and Fassin 2004).

6 Clear-sightedly, but leaving open the possibility of a happier outlook, Fee (1990, p. 572) adds: "The history of lead paint poisoning as a public health problem is not yet a success story."

7 See Régis Cohen (1987). This article, like others published in pediatric journals at the time, reports blood lead levels in μg/deciliter, but in order to facilitate reading and comparisons over time I have converted these into μg/liter in line with current practices in epidemiology. I have discussed Cohen's article elsewhere (2003), comparing it with another published in the same journal two years later.

8 See Expertise Collective (1999), particularly the chapters "Effets sur les fonctions cognitives de l'enfant" ["Effects on children's cognitive functions"], "Diagnostic et traitement de l'intoxication" ["Diagnosis and treatment of poisoning"], "Imprégnation des populations et strategies" ["Population absorption and strategies"] and "Synthèse et recommandations" ["Summary and recommendations"], as well as the memorandum "Plomb dans l'habitat urbain" ["Lead in urban housing"]. For a clearer grasp of the financial sums at stake, I have converted French francs into euros (the amount would be slightly superior in dollars). I discussed the report in an earlier text (2008), parts of which are incorporated here.

9 Although childhood lead poisoning had become a national priority, the limited response from the authorities can be judged from the fact that three years after the Inserm expert report was published, the budget dedicated to this disease by the Ministries of Housing and Health represented 0.5% of the estimated sum required to address high-risk buildings, and 7% of that required to take care of the children at risk (Tratner 2003).

10 These two surveys were conducted by a doctor at the mother and child clinic and a biologist from the City of Paris Health Laboratory (Laboratoire d'hygiène de la Ville de Paris), Marcelle Delour and Fabien Squinazi (1989a and 1989b).

11 The first study was by Herbert Needleman et al. (1979). It prompted dozens of further studies, some transversal, carried out at a given point in time, and others longitudinal, following a cohort over a certain period (Expertise Collective 1999). While not all showed the same results, a consensus formed around the link between lead poisoning and cognitive disorders (Canfield et al. 2003).

12 Herbert Needleman, the great expert in childhood lead poisoning, was the first to raise this statistical link (1990), even suggesting that it was "possible that 20% of crime is associated with lead poisoning." Although various studies appeared to confirm this association, either through clinical studies based on following children for long periods (Denno 2008) or through ecological studies based on spatial data on the presence of lead in the air (Stretesky and Lynch 2004), these results should still be interpreted with caution given the many confounding factors between the two variables.

13 See, for example, the article by Michel Duc et al. (1986) on water-derived lead poisoning, which was published during this period of uncertainty.

14 Although the first clinical publications on childhood lead poisoning that pointed to lead-based paint as the cause date back to the early twentieth century in the United States, the first studies suggesting the extent of the problem and its link to dilapidated housing date from the 1950s, with R. K. Byers' influential literature review (1959). Research establishing the toxicity of low levels of saturnine impregnation for cognition and behavior proliferated from the 1980s, stimulated by the work of Herbert Needleman and David Bellinger (1991).

15 In his preface to the mission report by François Bourdillon et al. (1990), the director of the Department of Public Health at Bichat hospital joked that "the gang of four" had returned from the USA to "tell of the conquest of the West."

16 The book begins: "This book is about space, about language, and about death; it is about the act of seeing, the gaze" (Foucault 1987 [1963], p. ix).

17 As Naudé and I have shown (Fassin and Naudé 2004), the French had to travel the same path, strewn with hesitations, errors, and obstacles, as the United States a few decades earlier.

18 The history of Baltimore's pioneering program is recounted by Elizabeth Fee (1990). The slow change in gaze and hence in practices is analyzed by Barbara Berney (1993).

19 In their history of childhood lead poisoning, Gerald Markowitz and David Rosner (2013 [2002], p. 300), write: "These industries responded to potent evidence of the danger of their products by hiding information, controlling research, continuing to market their products as safe when they were known to be dangerous, enlisting industrywide groups to participate in denying that there was a problem, and attempting to influence the political process in order to avoid regulation."

20 Remarking on their research, Alain Fontaine and his collaborators (1992) note this proportion without appearing to devote more attention to it than to the data on other variables, such as the number of children in the family or the mother's job, except for saying that these high numbers reflect the fact that screening was rarely carried out among children "originating from Europe or Asia."

21 As Éric Fassin and I have shown (2006), race long remained an unspoken issue that was eventually exposed by a series of events, including the uprisings of fall 2005.

22 As Olivier Monso and Thibaut de Saint Pol have shown (2006), the history of the many versions of the census since 1851 reveal the ambiguity of French society, which, on the one hand, constantly reasserts the principle of no differentiation between citizens, and, on the other, continually produces new forms of distinction on the basis of origin. I have described and analyzed (2002) the belated beginnings of public recognition of racial discrimination in France, and the long history of the disavowal of any statistical measurement of it.

23 The debate on what are called ethnic statistics, but should rightly be termed ethno-racial statistics, has been analyzed by Patrick Simon, one its most active proponents (2014). For a discussion of the debates around the word "race" in France, see Sarah Mazouz (2020).

24 Practical culturalism is to be distinguished from theoretical culturalism, an anthropological concept developed in the United States during the 1920s under the aegis of the Culture and Personality movement, whose leading lights were Margaret Mead and Ruth Benedict. Drawing on case studies of maternal mortality in Ecuador and AIDS in France, I have made (2001) a critique of "practical culturalism in public health."

25 While they acknowledge the role of housing conditions in substandard apartments, Nadia Rezkallah and Alain Epelboin (1997, p. 190) highlight, in addition to mothers' tolerance for their children consuming paint flakes, a series of cultural factors such as eating with the hand and then licking the fingers, and even being familiar with the sight of crumbling clay walls.

26 In the concluding paragraphs of their epidemiological study of the distribution of childhood lead poisoning in Chicago, Robert Sampson and Alix Winter (2016, p. 261) describe lead toxicity as an "environmental pathway through which racial segregation has contributed to the legacy of racial inequality in the United States."

27 For a discussion of the concept of moral economy and a redefinition distinct from the apparently irreconcilable versions of E. P. Thompson (1971) and Lorraine Daston (1995), see my article (2009).

28 These case studies, analyzed in my *Life: A Critical User's Manual* (2018a), focus on the tension between treatment and social justice in the prevention of AIDS transmission from mother to child in South Africa, and the contrast between the fall in acceptance of asylum requests and the rise in the awarding of resident status to undocumented migrants on medical grounds in France. More recently, I have shown how the Covid pandemic seemed to push this logic to its extreme (Fassin 2022a).

The Truth in Numbers

1 Organized by the General Directorate of Health in collaboration with Inserm and the National Institute for Health Monitoring (INVS), this conference brought together around thirty institutions and forty experts from the worlds of health, urban planning, housing, and research. See the 2008 interim expert assessment report, *Saturnisme: Quelles stratégies de dépistage chez l'enfant?* (available at Publi.Inserm.fr; quotation from p. 280).

2 As Rainhorn shows (2019, p. 169), in that period when "epidemiological statistics [was] still in its infancy," quantified data on *"cérusiers"* (painters who used lead-based paint) became a major issue because, by underestimating lead contamination, they contributed to the "grammars of opacity."

3 Though the question of truth is present throughout his work, it was only later that Foucault (2001, vol. 2, pp. 841 and 1451) began to use the term "regimes of veridiction," which he associated with "regimes of jurisdiction," in an effort to defend and justify his historical method, which had been criticized by historians. "Analyzing 'regimes of practice'," he writes, "means analyzing ways of programming behavior that have effects that are both prescriptive in relation to what is to be done ('jurisdiction' effects) and codifying in relation to what is to be known ('veridiction' effects)." What interests him, he explains, is "the history of 'veridictions' understood as forms according to which discourses that can be said to be true or false are articulated in a domain of things."

4 In Hacking's view (1990, pp. 4–5), the revolution of probabilities – their success story – is manifested in four great fields of thinking: metaphysics, epistemology, logic, and ethics: "Probability is ... *the* philosophical success story of the first half of the twentieth century."

5 Paradoxically, as Desrosières notes (1993, pp. 9 and 26–27), the tools of what we now call "statistics" were inherited not, despite its name, from German statistics but from English political arithmetic. German statistics was more of a descriptive accumulation designed to provide an exhaustive representation of the state (the word statistics coming from *Stadt*, or town), while political arithmetic produced methods of calculation that made it possible to measure mortality, life expectancy, and total population on the basis of a sample.

6 A paradox that Hacking points out (1990, pp. 5 and 145): "Nothing better typified a positive science than a statistical one – an irony, for Comte himself despised merely statistical enquiries."

7 Himself a mathematician and author of several texts on mathematics, Russell (1950, p. 3) believed that philosophy rests on logic. He distanced himself from the Vienna circle of logical positivism, whose doctrine was nevertheless partly inspired by his work.

8 In an edited book on "positivism and its epistemological others," Steinmetz (2005) discusses and criticizes what he describes as the "positivist hegemony" that has come to prevail in all the social sciences in North America, first in economics, then in sociology and political science.

9 According to King (2014, p. 165), "quantitative social science ... had a part in remaking most Fortune 500 companies; establishing new industries; hugely increasing the expressive capacity of human beings; and reinventing medicine, friendship networks, political campaigns, public health, legal analysis, policing, economics, sports, public policy, commerce, and program evaluation, among many other areas."

10 The 192 volumes of *Annales d'hygiène publique et de médecine légale* [*Annals of Public Hygiene and Forensic Medicine*], published between 1829 and 1922 (BIUSanté.ParisDescartes.fr), constitute a precious archive of the beginnings of public health, revealing the diversity of its themes and the role of numbers.

11 For evidence of the gap between the old and new epidemiologies, the reader need only compare the "Que sais-je?" volume of *L'Épidémiologie* by Hervé Harant and Alix Delage (1984), which is in fact a revised edition of a 1953 book in the same series, entitled *Les Épidémies*, with Arnaud Fontanet's inaugural lecture at the Collège de France in 2019, *L'Épidémiologie ou la science de l'estimation du risque en santé publique*.

12 On the history of community health in Canada, see the article by Michel O'Neill (1983); on the history of primary health care in what is known as the Global South, see Marcos Cueto (2004).

13 There is substantial literature on evidence-based medicine. One frequently cited summary is that by David Sackett et al. (1996), published in the *British Medical Journal*, which has systematically promoted evidence-based medicine in its pages. For an application to public health, see the summary by Ross Brownson et al. (2009).

14 A presentation of the techniques used to measure the global burden of disease can be found in the World Health Organization report "Global Burden of Disease (GBD) 2002 estimates," at WHO.int. Vincanne Adams (2016) offers a critical analysis of the QALY and DALY measures used in decision-making in public health.

15 This study is often cited as an illustration of the method of the "randomists," of whom Abhijit Banerjee and Esther Duflo (2011) are the most illustrious representatives. According to Séan Mfundza Muller et al. (2019), in sixteen years of its existence, their research center, the Abdul Latif Jameel Poverty Action Lab, or J-PAL, conducted 876 trials aiming to decide policy in eighty countries, and received 300 million dollars in subsidies. Their influential model led the World Bank to increase the share of this technique in its project evaluations in the Third World from zero in 2000 to two-thirds of them in 2019.

16 Banerjee and Duflo's approach to economics (2011) is presented in a general-audience book that gives numerous examples of randomized trials and concludes with a section titled, significantly, "Against political economy." The Sveriges Riksbank Prize in Economics in Memory of Alfred Nobel originated from the desire of this central bank's governor to create an award to commemorate the bank's tercentenary. It was set up in negotiation with the Nobel Foundation and the Swedish Royal Academy of Sciences, so that it could be associated with the actual Nobel prizes.

17 The influential article by Julia Walsh and Kenneth Warren (1979) cites numerous examples. It is noteworthy that economists who use randomized trials rarely acknowledge their scientific debt.

18 There is a discipline of biostatistics that concerns the application of statistics in biology and medicine; this discipline has its own courses, conferences, textbooks, and journals. Here I use the term biostatistics more broadly, in the same way that Michel Foucault talks of biopower and biopolitics.

19 For an analysis of the growing influence of randomized trials in economics, notwithstanding the scientific and political problems posed by this method, see the article by Florent Bédécarrats et al. (2020).

20 Edward Miguel and Michael Kremer published a very long article in the journal *Econometrica* (2004). An analysis of the controversy and its significance for RCTs was put forward by Nassima Abdelghafour (2017). The key sources on this story can be found on the World Bank website, under the heading "Worm wars: The anthology."

21 Evidence Action's Deworm the World Initiative is presented by GiveWell as one of its top charities. The organization's name is interesting, in that it combines the ambitious aim of "deworming the world" with a reference to "evidence-based action." The answer given to the question "What do I get for a dollar?" is that the cost of a treatment is 0.66 dollars. The precise answer is therefore one and a half treatments ("Evidence Action's Deworm the World Initiative," GiveWell.org).

22 The "reanalysis" of the original study, carried out by Alexander Aiken et al. (2015), found, after verification, that only 3.9% of the increase in school attendance was actually due to the program, a result that was not significant. The same team proposed a different method of analyzing the data, and found an improvement in school attendance but with substantial biases owing to missing data (Davey et al. 2015).

23 See David Taylor-Robinson et al., "Deworming drugs for soil-transmitted intestinal worms in children: Effects on nutritional indicators, haemoglobin and school performance" (CochraneLibrary.com, 23 July 2015); "New deworming reanalyses and Cochrane review" (GiveWell.org, 24 July 2015).

24 On this point, Marion Fourcade et al. (2015) reveal, in their article on "the superiority of economists," both their dominant position in the domain of science and their influence on the circles of power, two factors that distinguish them from social scientists.

25 On this theme, the idea of "opening the black boxes" of science, as Trevor Pinch puts it (1992), has made a substantial contribution to social studies of science, but has rarely been applied to the work of economists.

26 In this report Deaton and Cartwright (2016) criticize the partisans of RCTs for a form of arrogance that consists in thinking they can ignore previous studies and reject all theoretical analysis.

27 Against these reductionist approaches, Biehl and Petryna (2013, p. 8) propose to examine public health problems from the perspective of those who are affected by them.

28 See the 2017 Instituto Nacional de Estadísticas y Censos report on maternal mortality: *Estimación de la Razón de Mortalidad Materna en el Ecuador*, June 2017, available at EcuadorEnCifras.gob.ec.

29 Oni-Orisan's chapter (2016, pp. 82–85) opens with the case of a young pregnant woman, Blessing, who dies in the hospital, but who is reported to have died before she arrived, so that, for "political" reasons, as the doctor who received her explains, she is not counted in the maternal mortality data.

30 Vincanne Adams (2016, pp. 48–49) herself titles the final section of the collection of case studies she edited "Storied metrics." The combination of the power of stories and the "power of numbers" was the subject of a literature review by Pierre Pluye and Quan Nha Hong (2014).

31 A study by Jean-Marie Robine et al. (2007) revealed two peaks of excess mortality in June and July 2003 that affected several countries but were not identified as such and did not give rise to any alarm.

32 Brard's paper (2004) focuses on the media treatment of the 2003 heatwave.

33 This chronology is based on a reading of all the articles published by leading daily newspaper *Le Monde* on the subject during this period. The Inserm report was written by Denis Hémon and Éric Jougla (2003).

34 The most interesting account is that by Lucien Abenhaïm (2003), who was forced to resign in the middle of the crisis, a scapegoat, as most commentators noted, for the troubles of the Ministry of Health. The most complete analysis is that by Richard Keller (2015).

35 Analyzing the management of the 2003 heatwave crisis in France, Milet (2005), shows that "frames of perception," and particularly different narrative presentations, make certain risks more visible at certain moments.

36 For an analysis and comparison of the methods of recording deaths in France, England, and the USA, see the book edited by Carine Vassy et al. (2010).

37 The concept of noise in reception theory developed by Eco (1976) is based on what is known as the watergate model, a device for transmitting information about the filling of a pool in order to trigger the opening of a sluice gate to empty it once the water reaches a certain level.

38 This controversy is one of the those analyzed in my book on South Africa (2007, pp. 112-117). It was reported in the *Sunday Times*, the main weekly Sunday newspaper.

39 The Interior Ministry's response appeared in *The Citizen* daily newspaper on 11 July 2000. This discussion of the weakness of the data under apartheid is based on an article by J. L. Botha and Debbie Bradshaw (1985).

40 Written under the aegis of the Medical Research Council, the study by Dorrington et al. (2001) had a foreword by Makgoba, the director of the MRC, who had spoken to the presidential panel the year before.

41 In his course at the Collège de France, Supiot (2015) develops the idea of a slippage of government toward governance by numbers, promoted by a technocracy convinced that the impersonal nature of numbers guarantees liberation from politics – a liberal dream under whose sway communism also fell.

42 Foucault (2014 [2012], pp. 20–21) is certainly no positivist. What interests him is not "under what conditions ... there can be true statements"; he "investigates the forms of veridiction, the different forms of truth-telling." He takes a step to the side, from truth to veridiction.

Epistemic Boundaries

1 Canguilhem (2012, pp. 68, 134) gives a categorically negative response to this question: "In pathology the first word historically speaking and the last word logically speaking comes back to clinical practice. Clinical practice is not and will never be a science."

2 In the "critique" section of his entry on "normal" in his classic *Vocabulaire* (1993, p. 689), Lalande insists: "A very equivocal term that lends itself to much confusion, for it may designate a fact that can be observed scientifically or a value attributed to that fact by the speaker, on the basis of a judgment he has made about it. Philosophical discussion frequently shifts between one meaning and the other."

3 Foucault (1978 [1976]: 139–141) defines two "poles" of "power over life": an "anatomo-politics of the human body" and a "biopolitics of the population." The latter is centered "on the species body, the body imbued with the mechan-

ics of life and serving as the basis of the biological processes: propagation, births and mortality, the level of health, life expectancy, with all the conditions that can cause these to vary," their supervision being "effected through an entire series of interventions and regulatory controls." In this original version, biopolitics is thus viewed critically as "an indispensable element in the development of capitalism," since these are "methods of power that can increase forces, capacities, life in general without making them more difficult to subjugate."

4 Hacking (1998, p. 1) argues that these transient mental illnesses "provoke banal debates about whether they are 'real' or 'socially constructed'. We need richer tools with which to think than reality or social construction."

5 Statistics on the number of Iraqi deaths, both military and civilian, vary widely from one source to another, and are particularly unreliable because the two sides in the conflict sought, for different reasons, to minimize them. Those cited here were formulated by the Pentagon (Heidenrich 1993).

6 Among the substantial medical literature on the subject, there is a useful meta-analysis by Alexis Maule et al. (2018). The authors assess twenty-one studies conducted mainly during the 1990s, among a total of 129,000 soldiers. The synthesis of these studies shows the frequency of a wide range of symptoms, the most common of which are fatigue, irritability, joint pain, headaches, and problems with memory, concentration, and sleep.

7 Anthropology establishes a clear distinction between these two terms, which Leon Eisenberg (1977) summarizes thus: "Patients suffer 'illnesses'; doctors diagnose and treat 'diseases'. Illnesses are experiences of discontinuities in states of being and perceived role performances. Diseases, in the scientific paradigm of modern medicine, are abnormalities in the function and/or structure of body organs and systems." Some clinicians have adopted this distinction themselves.

8 In one example of denial not only of the use of chemical substances, but even that there was any exposure to them, an article by military experts James Riddle, Mark Brown, Tyler Smith, et al. in *Military Medicine* (2003) asserts that the symptoms veterans reported were of psychological origin, linked to the false belief that chemical weapons had been used.

9 At the end of their discussion of the syndromes observed during the course of the main wars in which the USA has been involved, Kenneth Hyams et al. (1996) conclude that the only real point they have in common is the attention they drew and the studies they generated.

10 Sociological studies like that by Thomas Shriver (2001), and anthropological surveys like that by Susie Kilshaw (2004), are based mainly on interviews with veterans. Shriver's study focuses on their relationship with the administration, and Kilshaw's on their experience as patients.

11 Most experts took the view that Gulf War syndrome was not a genuine pathology. This is the case of the two authors quoted in this paragraph (Sartin 2000, p. 816; Durodié 2006, p. 694).

12 The very full literature review by Roberta White et al. (2016) is based on the report of her research committee that was created in 1998 but not convened until 2002.

13 White et al.'s article in *Cortex* (2016) summarizes the report published a year earlier by the official committee. The authors categorically affirm the origin of the symptoms presented by Gulf War veterans: "This disorder was caused by toxicant exposures, individually or in combination, that occurred in the GW theater."

14 However, the Veterans Department expressed reservations in this respect: "We prefer not to use the term 'Gulf War syndrome' when referring to medically unexplained symptoms reported by Gulf War veterans ... because symptoms vary widely" ("Gulf War Veterans' Medically Unexplained Illnesses," PublicHealth.VA.gov).

15 The definition and description of chronic multisymptom illness were presented by Kenji Fukuda et al. (1998). The twelve studies conducted between 2000 and 2012, on US and British veterans, which were synthesized by the Research Advisory Committee on Gulf War Veterans' Illnesses, give rates of prevalence between 29% and 65% using Fukuda's criteria. Most of these studies included a control group of soldiers who had not been deployed in the Persian Gulf, in whom the frequency of the clinical picture was 25–50% of that found in their colleagues who had been sent to the war. See *Gulf War Illness and the Health of Gulf War Veterans: Research Update and Recommendations, 2009–2013*, Washington, DC: US Government Printing Office, May 2014 (available at VA.gov).

16 There are reviews of the medical literature on fibromyalgia by Daniel Clauw (2014) and on multiple chemical hypersensitivity by Sabrina Rossi and Alessio Pitidis (2018). Fibromyalgia, which combines diffuse pain with intense fatigue, and which physicians attribute to an anomaly in the pain threshold, is the second most frequent reason for rheumatology consultations. Multiple chemical hypersensitivity is a polymorphous condition that sufferers attribute to chemicals in the environment such as pesticides. Etiologically fibromyalgia is likened to chronic fatigue, since it is attributed to fragile mental health, while multiple chemical hypersensitivity is similar to Gulf War syndrome in that toxicant exposure is the presumed cause.

17 The "Myalgic Encephalomyelitis/Chronic Fatigue Syndrome in Gulf War Veterans" page on PublicHealth.VA.gov notes that these two pathologies, together with fibromyalgia, are more frequently observed in South-West Asia veterans.

18 In a study of individuals suffering from Gulf War syndrome, chronic fatigue syndrome, and multiple chemical hypersensitivity, Debra Swoboda (2006) emphasizes the difficulties these patients encountered in constructing the "medical and cultural legitimacy of these emerging diseases."

19 Between July and November 1955, 292 members of staff became ill, of whom 255 were hospitalized with "encephalomyelitis" ("An outbreak of encephalomyelitis in the Royal Free Hospital Group, London, in 1955," *British Medical Journal*, 19 October 1957; available at NCBI.NLM.NIH.gov).

20 The members of this group (Holmes et al. 1988) identified chronic fatigue as a "syndrome," that is a set of symptoms, without making any judgment as to its etiology.

21 The case was widely reported in the regional and national press ("160 victims at Lake Tahoe: Chronic flu-like illness a medical mystery story," LATimes.com, 7 June 1986; "Fatigue 'virus' has experts more baffled and skeptical than ever," NYTimes.com, 28 July 1987). The Centers for Disease Control (the title did not yet include the word "prevention") conducted a study in the village where the epidemic was supposed to have occurred, but the results were inconclusive, since the levels of Epstein–Barr virus antibodies were no higher than in healthy subjects ("Chronic fatigue possibly related to Epstein–Barr virus – Nevada," CDC.gov, 30 May 1986).

22 James Jones and Stephen Straus (1987) discuss sporadicity, arguing against the idea of an epidemic.

23 According to historian Edward Shorter (1993), neurasthenia cannot be entirely aligned with chronic fatigue, if only because not all neurasthenics suffered from fatigue: indeed, Shorter states that only a minority did so.

24 In his book on the "neurasthenic nation," historian David Schuster (2011) shows that symptoms that were not new were newly taken to indicate the harmful effects of modernity in the United States.

25 The broad outlines of this history of infection are described by Stephen Straus (1991).

26 This retrovirus was found in peripheral blood mononuclear cells of 67% of patients compared to only 3.7% of healthy subjects, making it a serious contender for the etiology of the syndrome (Lombardi et al. 2009).

27 A specialist who has published widely on this subject, Wessely (1997) does not hide his irritation with both the proliferation of poorly defined syndromes and the insistence of unrecognized patients.

28 Ware (1992), an anthropologist, underscores the dilemma facing patients between not having their illness recognized and having it recognized as psychosomatic.

29 The Chief Medical Officer stated that ME/CFS is a "genuine disease" and that "patients should not be dismissed as malingerers" ("A short history of myalgic encephalomyelitis," MESupport.co.uk). The Centers for Disease Control and Prevention state on their website: "Myalgic encephalomyelitis/chronic fatigue syndrome is a serious, long-term illness that affects many body systems" ("Myalgic Encephalomyelitis/Chronic Fatigue Syndrome," CDC.gov).

30 The authors of the report (Institute of Medicine 2015) argued that it was essential to recognize the disease in the dual sense of confirming its existence and having the capacity to diagnose it.

31 These data, representing fifty-three cases per 100,000 inhabitants, are from Santé publique France [Public Health France], the French national health agency ("Borréliose de Lyme," SantePubliqueFrance.fr). More detailed statistics were published in a special issue of the *Bulletin épidémiologique hebdomadaire* [*Weekly Bulletin of Epidemiology*] on 19 June 2018.

32 A review of current knowledge on "chronic Lyme disease," which the authors place in inverted commas, was conducted by the Ad Hoc International Lyme Disease Group under the aegis of the Centers for Disease Control and Prevention. This review notes that the disease "is the latest in a series of syndromes that has been postulated in an attempt to attribute medically unexplained symptoms to particular infections. Other examples that have now lost credibility are 'chronic candida syndrome' and 'chronic Epstein–Barr virus infection'" (Feder et al. 2007, p. 1428).

33 Geneviève Massard-Guilbaud (2019, p. 129), who states that she suffers from chronic Lyme disease, analyzes the French controversy around the condition, and concludes with an appeal to physicians to "recognize the true value of both the voices of patients and the methods of social science."

34 The position of the National Institute of Allergy and Infectious Diseases is presented on its website, where chronic Lyme disease is placed in inverted commas ("Chronic Lyme disease," NIAID.NIH.gov). That of the Haute Autorité de santé is presented in its good practice guidelines ("Borréliose de Lyme et autres maladies vectorielles à tiques," June 2018, available at HAS-sante.fr). The

Haute Autorité de santé is an independent scientific body set up by the government to improve standards of health care.

35 The *Diagnostic and Statistical Manual of Mental Disorders* (*DSM*) is the classification of mental illness formulated in the USA but used widely throughout the world. In 2013, the fifth version was drawn up by the American Psychiatric Association on the basis of thousands of contributions and hundreds of reports ("*DSM* history," Psychiatry.org).

36 Young's (1995) research combines a history of PTSD with an ethnography of its application in the world of psychiatry, particularly in the context of care for veterans.

37 Our work combined a genealogy of trauma with three case studies conducted in the contexts of disaster, a conflict situation, and asylum, thus shifting the issue of trauma from the medical to the social arena, with its political and moral stakes (Fassin and Rechtman 2009).

38 The literature focuses mainly on the toxic substances used by allied – that is, essentially US – troops in Iraq (Ammash 2002), and cautiously offers general evidence of their potential risks, particularly of the effects of depleted uranium on congenital malformations (Hindin et al. 2005). An editorial in *The Lancet Oncology* noted in 2001: "NATO military personnel have all gone home; they do not have to live near burnt-out tanks and are not continually exposed to contamination in the air and water around them" with a metal of which "the main isotope has a half-life of 4.5 billion years." But where, the authors ask, are the ten-year follow-up studies of its effects? ("Mixed messages about depleted uranium," *The Lancet Oncology*, 2 February 2001).

Conspiracy Theories

1 Judith Rainhorn (2019) uses the term "legal poison" in her account of the workers' campaign to secure the ban in 1909, and the negotiation of the law in the French parliament.

2 The lead industry's marketing campaign was centered on the association of lead with modernity, boasting of a "scientific revolution that was transforming the very way Americans saw the world," as Markowitz and Rosner show (2013 [2002], pp. 64–65, 137).

3 Benjamin Ross, for example (2016, pp. 49–50), describes how in 1937 a Missouri congressional representative who owned orchards where lead-bearing insecticides were used on the fruit, and was Chair of the House Budget Committee, succeeded in getting a law passed that halted a Food and Drug Administration study of lead toxicity: 5,000 laboratory rats were killed without the experiment being able to be completed. On the advice of a lobbyist, the money thus saved was passed to the Public Health Service, where a researcher devised an experimental protocol that avoided establishing the dangers of lead by creating a toxicity study that took into account only apple pickers who were working, and leaving out those who had had to give up this work precisely because of complications. See also Ross and Amter (2010).

4 "Conspiracy" was the term used by the State of Rhode Island in its legal action against the lead industry, a charge that the judge upheld (Markowitz and Rosner 2013 [2002], p. 304). On the strategies used by the tobacco industry to deny the risks of smoking, see Allan Brandt (2012). On those used by the

asbestos industry to conceal asbestos toxicity, see Jock McCulloch (2006). Robert Proctor's book on "cancer wars" (1995) also analyses these two cases. Naomi Oreskes and Erik Conway (2010) draw a parallel between the "merchants of doubt" around global warming and their predecessors on the subjects of tobacco, acid rain, the hole in the ozone layer, and DDT. What characterizes these strategies, and others that conceal the risks of certain substances to public health, is the veritable conspiracy of silence woven by industry, with the help of governments and researchers.

5 With regard to the consequences of pollution caused by diesel engines, it has been shown that the addition of just one fraudulently certified vehicle per thousand leads to an increase of 1.9% in low birth weight and of 8% in acute childhood asthma ("VW emissions cheating scandal increased children's pollution exposure," ScientificAmerican.com, 17 July 2019). With regard to the consequences of asbestos exposure, the harmful effects of which have been known since the 1970s, but which was only banned in France in 1997, it is estimated that 35,000 people died between 1965 and 1995, but that between 50,000 and 100,000 further deaths are to be expected up to 2025, according to a French Senate report ("Le drame de l'amiante en France: Comprendre, mieux réparer, en tirer des leçons pour l'avenir," Senat.fr, 26 October 2005).

6 Anthropologist George Marcus (1999) led a research program that produced a book titled *Paranoia within Reason*.

7 A study conducted in the United States five years after the events (Stempel et al. 2007) shows that the most widespread conspiracy theory (36% of those interviewed) was that the federal government had assisted or allowed the attacks to happen in order to justify intervening in the Middle East. The second most popular was the belief that the collapse of the Twin Towers was facilitated by explosives secretly placed in the buildings (16%); then came the idea that the Pentagon was destroyed not by a plane but by a missile launched by the military (12%). These theories gained more credence among people who got their information from non-mainstream media, had low levels of education, or belonged to ethnic or racial minorities or to disadvantaged groups.

8 For an analysis of some of the theories currently flourishing in the United States, and a discussion of how they are circulated, see Cosentino (2020).

9 On 17 August 2020, US President Donald Trump, responding to a journalist's question about the conspiracy website QAnon, expressed his sympathy for "these people who love our country." A few days earlier he had declared his support for an openly racist, Islamophobic, and anti-Semitic Republican candidate for Congress, who was also an enthusiastic supporter of QAnon ("Trump says QAnon followers are people who 'love our country'," NYTimes.com, 19 August 2020). On the persistence of the myth of ritual murders by Jews, known as the "blood libel," see Tokarska-Bakir (2010).

10 The survey "on conspiracy theory," published in January 2018 by polling company Ifop, was commissioned by the Jean-Jaurès Foundation and Conspiracy Watch, which defines itself as a conspiracy theory observatory (survey available at Ifop.com). Its results made the front page of, among others, *Le Monde*, which headed its 7 January article "Conspiracy theories well established among French population"; *Le Figaro*, also on 7 January, with "79% of French people believe in at least one 'conspiracy theory'"; and *Libération*, on 8 January, with "The French are conspiracy theorists." Frédéric Lordon (2017) criticizes this "conspiracy theory of the anti-conspiracy theorists": "The

Notes to pp. 82–6

obsessive condemnation of conspiracy theories is therefore largely the conspiracy-driven guilty conscience of the dominant projected onto the dominated." It should be added that the campaign against conspiracy theories has become a standby for some of the media and a money-earner for some "experts."

11 The most rigorous study of "moral panics" is that by Stanley Cohen (2002 [1972]), who reveals the complexity of the issues involved both in moral panics (which create or inflate facts) and in labeling perceptions as moral panic (which minimizes or even denies the reality of these facts). This theory has been applied to conspiracy theories by Jack Bratich (2008), who seeks to understand the forms of dissent that are expressed through these theories and the regimes of truth that are manifested in the condemnation of them.

12 According to Popper (2012 [1945], p. 306), a conspiracy theory is "the view that an explanation of a social phenomenon consists in the discovery of the men or groups who are interested in the occurrence of this phenomenon. This view ... arises ... from the mistaken theory that, whatever happens in society – especially happenings such as war, unemployment, poverty, shortages ... – is the result of direct design by some powerful individuals and groups. This theory is widely held; it is older even than historicism ... In its modern form it is, like modern historicism ... a typical result of the secularization of a religious superstition."

13 See Latour (2004, p. 225). For a critique of his argument, I refer to my article (2017) and to Tom Mills's article (2018), which also offers a critique of actor-network theory.

14 On this theoretical distinction and its intellectual sources, see David Owen's useful article (2002).

15 In June 2015 *Le Monde diplomatique* newspaper assembled, under the title "A convenient vilification," a series of quotations from public intellectual Alain Finkelkraut, philosopher Pierre-André Taguieff, and journalist Philippe Val, all known for their reactionary ideas, that amalgamated critical theory with conspiracy theories, often with reference to Bourdieu and his school (article available at Monde-diplomatique.fr).

16 In Ricœur's (1965) view, Marx, Nietzsche, and Freud are thinkers of liberation and emancipation.

17 As Keeley shows (1999), this is a typical situation where there is both a conspiracy (that of terrorist Timothy McVeigh and his accomplices) and a conspiracy theory (of those who think that McVeigh was manipulated by political forces that obviously wished to preserve the secret of their conspiracy).

18 After all, Pigden (1995) notes: "history is littered with conspiracies, successful and otherwise."

19 According to Clarke (2002), conspiracy theories are usually benign. He cites the belief that the US military is concealing the existence of extraterrestrials, or that Elvis Presley faked his own death. He might perhaps take a different view in a context where these theories influence elections.

20 On 13 July 2020, the *Washington Post* reported an escalation in the production of false statements by Donald Trump, since the first 10,000 took him 827 days, while the next 10,000 took only 440 days ("President Trump has made more than 20,000 false or misleading claims," WashingtonPost.com, 13 July 2020).

21 According to Muirhead and Rosenblum (2019), Trump and his allies do not bother to back up their arguments with either theory or evidence, or even establish links between the various targets of their criticism.

22 Douglas et al. (2019) present a synthesis of current knowledge on the causes, modes of dissemination and consequences of conspiracy theories.

23 Sunstein and Vermeule (2009) go beyond analysis, proposing solutions for countering conspiracy theories and suggesting that the best way of proceeding is "cognitive infiltration of extremist groups" in order to monitor them, collate information toward potential later lawsuits, and disseminate arguments against the theories that hold sway there. This strategy has for obvious reasons been criticized for feeding conspiracy theories.

24 Hofstadter (1964) argues that the main difference between conspiracy theories of the nineteenth and twentieth centuries is that adherents of the latter, particularly on the right, felt dispossessed.

25 The ambiguities and indeed contradictions of the theme of transparency, which has become a common trope in public discourse, are analyzed by Todd Sanders and Harry West (2003).

26 The hidden economies the Comaroffs (1999) focus on relate to the proliferation of accusations of witchcraft, zombie stories, and ritual murders in South Africa, which they interpret as a manifestation of the social consequences of neoliberalism.

27 As Ginzburg (2004, pp. 91–92) notes, the charge against Jews echoed a previous episode seventeen years earlier, when a rumor circulated throughout France, and beyond, that "lepers or, in other versions, lepers encouraged by Jews, or even lepers encouraged by Jews themselves encouraged by the Muslim kings in Granada and Tunis, had hatched a plot to poison Christians spared by the disease," resulting in violence against lepers and Jews perpetrated not only by the general public but also by political and religious authorities.

28 Admittedly, adds Piquemal (1959, pp. 28, 45), the poor were statistically worse affected; he observes the "'genocidal' intentions attributed to the ruling classes" who were believed to have commissioned "shady" individuals to poison water and food.

29 As Epstein remarks (2014a, 2014b), the epidemic not only reawakened racist discourses around Africa and its travails, but also helped to weaken the economy of the countries affected.

30 Anne-Claire Defossez and I have developed an analysis of these programs in "Une liaison dangereuse" (1992).

31 On the *levantamiento indígena*, see the piece I wrote with Anne-Claire Defossez (1990), and Leon Zamosc's article (1994) which situates the uprising in a broader context.

32 The public health services' immediate explanation for the spread of the epidemic was the crabs the Warao fish for and eat. The blaming of this food and the ban on consuming it were experienced as an unjust and discriminatory measure devised to conceal deeper reasons involving "the state, global capitalism and international politics" (Briggs 2004, p. 164).

33 The challenge was reported in "Medical Notes" in the *Boston Medical and Surgical Journal* (vol. 163/25, 1910, p. 961), under the title "Dr. Osler's challenge to the anti-vaccinationists."

34 The article questioning the MMR vaccine was published in *The Lancet*, one of the world's most highly respected medical journals, which subsequently withdrew it. But as Olivia Benecke and Sarah Elizabeth DeYoung show (2019), while this article had damaging consequences, the factors that contributed to rejection of the vaccination in the United States were more sociological,

manifesting a challenge to medical power and a desire to take back control over health issues among the privileged classes, as well as a failure to comply among low-income families.

35 The article that cast suspicion on the polio vaccine was published in a journal issued by the Institut Pasteur. The history of the Nigerian boycott is recounted by Ayodele Samuel Jegede (2007). However, the population's distrust of the vaccine does not seem to be due purely to the spread of a conspiracy theory, since, according to Elisha Renne (2006), who conducted a study in Kaduna state, those interviewed complained that the focus was on a rare disease when measles and malaria were of much greater concern, and on this basis criticized top-down programs that focused purely on one health problem rather than developing horizontal programs that would allow for an integrated approach.

36 The account of this manipulation appears in an article by Saeed Shah ("CIA organised fake vaccination drive to get Osama Bin Laden's family DNA," *Guardian*, 11 July 2011).

37 The AIDS epidemic in South Africa, the conspiracy theories to which it has given rise, and the real conspiracies it has helped to expose are analyzed in detail in my book *When Bodies Remember* (2007).

38 On the plague epidemic, see Maynard Swanson (1977); on syphilis, see Karen Jochelson (2001); on tuberculosis, see Randall Packard (1989).

39 In a speech given at the inaugural Z. K. Matthews lecture, honoring the first Black South African to obtain a bachelor's degree, on 12 October 2001, Mbeki vented virulent criticism of racist prejudices about Africans' sexuality (extracts from the speech can be accessed at OMalley.NelsonMandela. org). Gilles Bibeau (1991) studies these prejudices within the scientific literature.

40 Virginia Van der Vliet (2001) analyzes the first years of AIDS in South Africa, including the stigmatization of the black population and the genocidal fantasies of the white supremacists.

41 The history of this conspiracy, the evidence of which takes up an entire section of the Truth and Reconciliation Commission's weighty report, is detailed by Marléne Burger and Chandré Gould (2002).

42 This quotation is drawn from an essay by Geertz first delivered as a distinguished lecture at an annual meeting of the American Anthropological Association (1984, p. 275). I have similarly argued in my Eric Wolf Lecture (2021) that conspiracy theories should be taken seriously for their heuristic openings on repressed aspects of societies.

Ethical Crises

1 In addition to Markowitz and Rosner's work (2013 [2002]), the most important historical study of lead poisoning in the United States, see also Richard Rabin's earliest article (1989).

2 The history of the Flint water crisis is the subject of many accounts, including one in the *Guardian*, "'Nothing to worry about: The water is fine': How Flint poisoned its people" (3 July 2018) and chronologies, particularly on the CNN website, with "Flint Water Crisis Fast Facts" (4 March 2016). The academic articles cited below add further detail.

3 The documentary, which Moore directed, wrote, and starred in, recounts the decline of the automobile industry in the city of Flint through the story of his failed attempt to meet with the CEO of General Motors.

4 The problem of what is known as "municipal fiscal distress" is not new. Indeed, it became increasingly serious during the 1990s owing to the decrease in contributions from the states concerned, and particularly from the federal state, to city budgets, placing major cities like New York and Philadelphia in a situation of bankruptcy (Cahill and James 1992). The situation was aggravated by the 2008 crisis, as Eric Scorsone shows in a research paper from 2014 ("Municipal fiscal emergency laws: Background and guide to state-based approaches," available at Mercatus.org).

5 The results obtained by Mark Edwards and researchers from Virginia Tech were immediately published on a specially created website ("Our sampling of 252 homes demonstrates a high lead in water risk: Flint should be failing to meet the EPA lead and copper rule," FlintWaterStudy.org, 8 September 2015). Data from the study conducted by Mona Hanna-Attisha et al. (2016) were published in the USA's most prestigious health journal.

6 In David Bellinger's words (2016), "the burden of childhood lead poisoning has always weighed most heavily on populations that are politically and economically disenfranchised."

7 The Michigan Civil Rights Commission report can be accessed at Michigan.gov (*The Flint Water Crisis: Systemic Racism Through the Lens of Flint*, February 2017). For the spatial study of lead poisoning, see Mona Hanna-Attisha et al. (2016).

8 See Mills (2017) and López (2013). In their studies of the Flint Water Crisis, Malini Ranganathan (2016) and Peter Hammer (2019) use the terms "racial liberalism" and "strategic racism" respectively.

9 In their study of the residents' campaign, Amy Krings et al. (2019) emphasize the strategic alliance between residents and researchers, who lent the campaign their scientific legitimacy.

10 See Bailly's dictionary of reference (1930 [1895]).

11 Koselleck's (2006 [1972]) article on crisis was first published in German in a chapter of an eight-volume history of concepts in Germany. The quotation that follows is from page 358.

12 See Furetière's classical *Dictionnaire universel* (1727 [1690]).

13 This is the published form of the William James Lectures delivered by Austin at Harvard (1962, p. 13).

14 The historical and epidemiological data on the epidemic of opioid addiction are taken from a number of scientific and journalistic sources. Reviews can be found in Kolodny et al. (2015) and Jones et al. (2018). The reports published by the Centers for Disease Control and Prevention ("Understanding the epidemic," CDC.gov) and the *New York Times*'s Upshot e-newsletter ("Drug deaths in America are rising faster than ever," 5 June 2017) are also useful.

15 It should be noted that this shocking figure followed a significant reduction in the prescription of these drugs throughout the 2010s, in the context of a prescription behavior surveillance program (Strickler et al. 2020). This indicates that the rate of mortality was probably higher during the preceding decade.

16 For a synthesis of research on the war on drugs and the social consequences of criminalizing the use and sale of drugs in the USA, see Provine (2011). For data on the racial composition of the prison population, see Nellis (2016).

17 As Stephen Bernard et al. show (2018), the role of government agencies and scientific associations was crucial in the production of the epidemic of opioid addiction.
18 The study by Nana Wilson et al. (2020) shows that the number of deaths from opioid overdose fell slightly between 2017 and 2018, but that the rate of overdose deaths from synthetic opioids was rising.
19 Case and Deaton's study was widely reported by the media, including National Public Radio ("In reversal, death rates rise for middle-aged whites," NPR.org, 2 November 2015).
20 Woolf and Schoomaker's study (2019) shows that the fall in life expectancy was highest in New England and the Ohio valley. Changes in overdose rates in specific racial groups have been studied by Kumiko Lippold et al. (2019).
21 This phrase was used by Sonia Mendoza et al. (2018), who conducted a study in New York where they interviewed prescribers and pharmacists and observed their practices in two public health centers. The racial dimension of the epidemic is also discussed by Helena Hansen and Julie Netherland (2016).
22 Ironically, this invidious law, which was supported by both Democrats and Republicans and voted for by the majority of Black members of Congress, was proposed by a young senator by the name of Joe Biden ("How an early Biden crime bill created the sentencing disparity for crack and cocaine trafficking," WashingtonPost.com, 28 July 2019).
23 The concept of racial capitalism was proposed by political scientist Cedric Robinson (1983). It describes the process whereby an individual or a group draws economic or social value from the racial identity of another individual or group. It was revisited, and critiqued, some decades later, by legal scholar Nancy Leong (2013).
24 Isabelle Baszanger (1995) traces the history of the recognition and management of pain in contemporary medicine. As it were, the dark side of legitimate relief of useless suffering, the US version of this history, involving a greedy and unscrupulous pharmaceutical industry, offers a very different picture with its hundreds of thousands of overdose deaths (Van Zee 2009).
25 When Frachon's book *Mediator 150 mg: combien de morts?* [*Mediator 150 mg: How Many Deaths?*] (2010) was published, the Servier laboratory won a temporary injunction to remove the subtitle. This decision was overturned on appeal a year later.
26 The charge of "deception" was not upheld because the statute of limitations had passed. The court decision noted "fraud on a considerable and unprecedented scale, to which thousands of patients fell victim" ("Procès du Mediator: le mensonge de Servier reconnu, les parties civiles partagées sur le jugement," LeMonde.fr, 30 March 2021).
27 Earlier clinical trials conducted in West Africa, including one by François Dabis et al. (1999), had focused on zidovudine taken for several weeks before and one week after birth, and showed a fall in transmission at 45 days from 22% to 15%. The innovation in the clinical trial carried out by Laura Guay et al. (1999) was to give nevirapine only at the moment of birth.
28 As Angell notes in her editorial (1997), "[an] essential ethical condition for a randomized clinical trial comparing two treatments for a disease is that there be no good reason for thinking one is better than the other." Comparison with a placebo is only justified when there is no evidence for the efficacy of the other treatment. This was not the case with zidovudine and other antiretrovirals,

whose efficacy had been demonstrated in trials of prevention of mother-child virus transmission conducted in Western countries. There was therefore no reason to give placebos to African women.

29 The title of this 2004 report, *Antiretroviral Drugs for Treating Pregnant Women and Preventing HIV Infections in Children*, emphasizes the shift in perspective: the focus is no longer on preventing transmission of the virus from mother to child but on treating pregnant women and preventing infection of newborns (report available at WHO.int).

Precarious Exiles

1 The seven-volume collection *Realms of Memory* edited by Pierre Nora (1996) contains no entry on colonization or the colonial empire as one of France's "realms of memory." Despite seeing himself as the author who drew immigration out of the shadows of its realm of non-memory in the 1980s, with his book *The French Melting Pot* (1996), Gérard Noiriel nevertheless passed over the link between his subject of research and colonial history. Finally, as Sarah Mazouz and I showed (2007), naturalization ceremonies, which are usually held in prefectures, follow a nationally set program, the centerpiece being a speech in which the state's representative reminds the audience of the difference between naturalized citizens and those amazingly called "native French." The ceremony concludes with a slideshow that traces, to the soundtrack of Ravel's *Bolero*, the traditional history of France, from the Gauls to the Fifth Republic, without mentioning the colonial history of which the newly naturalized citizens are often a product.

2 Sampson and Winter's study (2016) covers the period between 1995 and 2013.

3 The New York study was conducted by Parisa Tehranifar et al. (2008), and that for Michigan by Stan Kaplowitz et al. (2016). The two studies testify to a reorientation of studies of childhood lead poisoning to include immigrants.

4 Inquiry about these products should be included, with testing of the blood lead level, in the medical examination to which immigrants and refugees are subjected on arrival ("Screening for lead during the domestic medical examination for newly arrived refugees," CDC.gov).

5 Walker's presidential address (published in 2018) was set in the specific context following Donald Trump's announcement of a ban on nationals from seven countries where the main religion is Islam from entering the United States. Notwithstanding the security argument advanced, no citizen from any of these countries had participated in an act of terrorism in the United States: Iran, Iraq, Syria, Libya, Sudan, Yemen, and Somalia (others were added subsequently).

6 The history of the 1832 cholera epidemic in Canada is recounted by Geoffrey Bilson (1980), who shows how the disease transformed immigration practices.

7 The history of public health in New York city is analyzed by John Duffy (1968), who devotes an entire chapter to mass immigration in the second half of the nineteenth century.

8 Although the proportion of rejections on medical grounds was high, the total number of refused entries on these grounds at Ellis Island remained small, as Howard Markel and Alexandra Minna Stern show (1999).

9 British tuberculosis patients were encouraged to emigrate to New Zealand and Australia to treat their disease in a more favorable environment. They received a mixed welcome, as Linda Bryder notes (1996): on the one hand, there was fear of contagion, but, on the other, there was a need to populate these lands that were sparsely populated apart from the Aboriginal and Maori populations, where white residents felt threatened by the "yellow peril."

10 The limitations of the medical inspection of immigrants are revealed, as Becky Taylor notes (2016), in the fact that a businessman suffering from a sexually transmitted disease had more chance of entering than a third-class passenger presenting only lice: economic logic prevailed over medical logic.

11 Marie-Odile Safon's very useful bibliography on "migrant health," drawn up for the documentation center at the Institute for Research and Documentation on Health Economics (IRDES, Institut de recherche et documentation en économie de la santé) comprises 298 pages of annotated references for the field in France alone. This gives a sense of the importance of this domain today (bibliography accessible at Irdes.fr).

12 Words are important. The term "migrant," which is the main term used in both French and English, suggests a sort of perpetual nomadism, and loses some of its power through the falsely neutral application of it, because it is often used to distinguish between those who have left their country for economic reasons and those who have done so for broadly political reasons (who are called "refugees"). The term "exile," which organizations advocating for foreigners' rights tend to prefer, emphasizes the forced nature of the departure, whatever the reason. In what follows, I distinguish between the terms "recent immigrant," which refers to those seen by the authorities or medicine as recently arrived, and "person of immigrant origin," which implies an already established fact – as it were, a fait accompli. All these choices are of course conventions with no absolute meaning, but I feel it is useful to clarify them.

13 For a detailed analysis of the role of social hygiene in the definition of the "immigration health problem," see De Luca Barrusse (2012); on Doctor René Martial, a key figure in the slippage from solidarism to racial science, see Benoît Larbiou (2005).

14 Invoking the "higher interest of the Nation," Bernard (1925, pp. 770, 772, 786–787) calls on public hygiene to "claim the place demanded of it by the twofold concern of public health and the future of the race."

15 Velmet's argument (2020, p. 1) is that the relationship between the Institut Pasteur and the empire was reciprocal: the Pasteur Institutes transformed the empire, and the empire transformed Pasteurian science.

16 At the end of his pæan to the work of the Pasteur Institute, Pasteur Vallery-Radot (1939) notes: "A great research institute like the Institut Pasteur could not neglect the study of tropical diseases."

17 Keller's intellectual project (2007, p. 3) is to contextualize colonial psychiatry, and indeed more broadly the intersection between madness and religion, in the imaginary and politics of the French colonization of Algeria.

18 These quotations are drawn from "Notes de psychiatrie musulmane," which Porot (1918, pp. 378, 380, 383) published at the end of the war, after claiming to have seen, he says, many "native" patients.

19 Racialized, and often racist, stereotypes of mentally ill people in North Africa did not originate with Porot and the Algiers School, as Robert Berthelier shows (2007). He cites in particular Moreau de Tours's influential *Recherches*

sur les aliénés, en Orient [*Research on the Insane, in the Orient*], which dates from 1843.

20 At the end of *The Wretched of the Earth* (1967), Fanon presents a series of case studies of patients suffering from "reactionary psychoses," and speaks of the prevalence of behavioral and mental disorders both "among those who carry out the 'pacification'" and "among the 'pacified' population," for "the truth is that colonization, in its essence" is "a great supplier for psychiatric hospitals."

21 René Collignon (2006) presents a comparative analysis of the Algiers and Dakar Schools.

22 Carothers' career was unusual, as McCulloch (1995) shows: a physician who became a psychiatrist "on the job," he played an important role in establishing both a pseudo-scientific psychopathology of Africans and an official account of the Mau Mau rebellion.

23 Two essays, published twelve years apart, analyze these two versions (Fassin 1999 and 2011).

24 As noted by Namratha Kandula et al. (2004) in a review of the literature.

25 For Germany, see the study by Oliver Razum et al. (1998), and for Sweden, that by Magnus Helgesson et al. (2019). There is a substantial literature on the United States (Markides and Rote 2015).

26 These figures date from 1999–2001 (Singh and Hiatt 2006). White, Hispanic, and Black immigrants have a life expectancy of 75.6, 79, and 75.6 years, respectively. US-born people in the same three groups have a life expectancy of 74.8, 75.2 and 67.5 years, respectively.

27 These data come from the federal Department of Health and Human Services ("United States Life Tables, 2017," *National Vital Statistics Reports*, 68/7, 2019, available at CDC.gov). The comparison between Hispanics born in the United States and those born elsewhere is based on earlier figures (Singh and Siahpush 2002).

28 In order to account for the lower mortality of Moroccan immigrants to France and Turkish migrants to Germany, when compared to those born in these countries (Khlat and Darmon 2003).

29 The phenomenon of selection has been noted in various contexts, for example in Indonesia by Yao Lu (2008).

30 Cassio Turra and Irma Elo's study (2008) explores the impact of various biases of the "Hispanic mortality advantage" on Social Security data, and found the "salmon bias" to be minimal, as few subjects return to their country to die. However, Alberto Palloni and Elizabeth Arias (2004) show that the return effect wholly explains this advantage for Mexicans, who are closest to the United States, but not for other Hispanics.

31 In an analysis of the National Longitudinal Mortality study Ana Abraído-Lanza et al. (1999) show that neither the process of selection nor the "salmon effect" explains the advantage of Hispanic migrants.

32 The study by Marwân-al-Qays Bousmah et al. (2019), which focuses on foreigners in Europe, relates the more rapid deterioration in health among immigrants from poor countries to the fact that they are given "3D jobs (dirty, dangerous and demeaning)." A Canadian study by Marcelo Urquia et al. (2012) also shows a convergence between pregnant women in terms of complications during pregnancy and premature birth.

33 The indicators chosen in the study by Matthew Wallace et al. (2019) were mortality and length of stay in the country. For France, there is also a very

rich report edited by Myriam Khlat, entitled "Santé et recours aux soins des migrants en France" ["Health and use of healthcare services among migrants in France"] in the *Bulletin épidémiologique hebdomadaire* of 17 January 2012.

34 The initial hypothesis in Tod Hamilton and Robert Hummer's study (2011) was that there might be health differences between immigrants depending on whether they came from countries where they were in a discriminated minority or countries where they were in the majority. Their results did not validate this hypothesis.

35 Sally Moyce and Marc Schenker (2018) offer a substantial review of the literature.

36 The study by Elena Ronda Pérez et al. (2012) forms part of the fourth European Working Conditions Survey.

37 Christen Byler and Courtland Robinson's study (2018) drew on the US Census of Fatal Occupational Injuries.

38 A fairly complete synthesis with regard to Europe appears in the World Health Organization report edited by Soorej Jose Puthoopparambil and Paolo Parente (2018).

39 The study on diseases was carried out by Pascal Chaud et al. (2017) for Santé publique France [Public Health France]; that on violence by Malika Bouhenia et al. (2017) for Épicentre and Médecins sans frontières. It is quite remarkable that almost the same proportion of refugees reported having suffered violence as in Libya.

40 The Human Rights Watch report is available online ("'Like Living in Hell': Police abuse against child and adult migrants in Calais," HRW.org, 26 July 2017).

41 While they note that these studies are cross-sectional, limiting the potential for identifying relations of causality, Martha von Werthern et al. (2018) argue that the convergence of the results makes them more robust.

42 Written in Farsi in the form of thousands of text messages secretly sent from the prison where he was detained, Boochani's book (2018) tells of the humiliation, the degradation, the indignity, the despair, and the cynicism detainees experience daily. The island of Manus is part of Papua New Guinea, but under an agreement with the Australian government a detention center for those attempting to enter Australia without papers has been established there. This includes those seeking asylum, who make up the majority of the detainees. The island forms part of the program known, ironically or antonymically, as the "Pacific Solution."

43 The quotation from the High Commissioner for Refugees is drawn from a 2014 report called *Beyond Detention*, which proposes a strategy for ending this practice by states (available at UNHCR.org).

44 With regard to immigrant/emigrants' trajectories, Sayad (2004, p. 29) writes: "If ... they are to be fully explained, differences noted at the point of arrival must be related both to living and working conditions in France, and to the differences that initially – i.e., prior to and independently of emigration – already distinguished the emigrant or group of emigrants."

45 In *Life: A Critical User's Manual* (2018a), I proposed a theoretical analysis of the forms of life of these forced nomads who, depending on the place and time, but also the stage of their existence, may be called immigrants, refugees, asylum seekers, or undocumented foreigners.

46 The meta-analysis covered all of the usable studies published during the first two decades of the twenty-first century, analyzing the statistically confirmed relationships between state policies and exiles' health (Juárez et al. 2019).

Carceral Ordeals

1 See for example the articles by Jessica Reyes (2015) and Paul Stretesky and Michael Lynch (2004), as examples of prospective and ecological research respectively.
2 In Rick Nevin's view (2000), 90% of the variation in rates of violent crime from the early 1960s to 1998 can be traced to earlier changes in level of exposure to lead.
3 The "case-control" study conducted in Pittsburgh by Hubert Needleman et al. (2002) found the same associations between bone lead level and criminal convictions among Blacks and whites. The study by Amber Beckley et al. (2018) relates to a sample of residents of the city of Dunedin followed from the age of 11 to 38.
4 Rick Nevin's (2007) international study covers Canada, the United Kingdom, France, Italy, Germany, Finland, Australia, and New Zealand.
5 Feigenbaum and Muller's (2016, p. 77) study compares homicide rates in cities where the pipes in the public water supply system were or were not composed of lead between 1921 and 1936. The interest of this historical study is that lead poisoning levels were very high at that time, making it easier to demonstrate differences in crime rates.
6 For an analysis of the punitive development of contemporary societies, see my book *The Will to Punish* (2018b), which focuses in particular on the justification and distribution of punishment.
7 In two studies, one on the police (2013) and one on prisons (2016), I showed that the social distribution of criminal acts is not sufficient to account for the social distribution of the prison population, and the fact that low-income men of color are overrepresented in penal institutions is not due purely to their committing more crimes. Violations of the law are punished differently depending on the social position of the perpetrators. To cite just one example, in France during the 2000s convictions for drug use, predominantly marijuana, tripled, while convictions for breach of economic and financial legislation fell by 20%. During this period epidemiological studies show that the level of drug consumption remained the same, while the level of white-collar crime recorded by the police increased. This discrepancy between crimes and convictions was in fact due to a policy of harsher repression of drug users, on the one hand, and decriminalization of economic and financial crime, on the other. Furthermore, repression of possession of marijuana for personal use did not impact everyone in the same way, and the police focused their activity on young people from low-income neighborhoods while sparing those from wealthier areas, despite the fact that studies revealed similar levels of consumption across all social categories. Finally, when sanctions were issued, they were not executed in the same way: a young person from the projects who was sentenced to twelve months' imprisonment for possession of a certain quantity of marijuana would be subject to a committal order and immediately jailed, while a politician sentenced to five years' imprisonment for corruption would be required to serve,

in principle, only two years in jail, enabling the sentencing judge to propose an adjustment, and therefore would avoid incarceration. The penal population, and still more the prison population, thus reflects not criminality, but the way it is punished, and more particularly the way society decides who is to be punished and who is not.

8 As Foucault brilliantly exposes in *Madness and Civilization* (1989 [1961]) and *Discipline and Punish* (1979 [1975]).

9 In their history of the treatment of the insane since the Renaissance, Claude Quétel and Pierre Morel (1979) reveal the diversity of remedies used and point out that internment was not the rule.

10 Written in the early nineteenth century for the Ministry of the Interior, Esquirol's report (1819, pp. 14–19) shows how far the reforms introduced twenty years earlier by his mentor Philippe Pinel were from being implemented, with a few exceptions that he mentions, in Bicêtre and Salpêtrière, where Pinel had worked.

11 In Foucault's view (1989 [1961], pp. 65–75), madmen were treated no differently from animals, who were chained and exhibited, and the association of the two allowed the insane to be distinguished from the reasonable man.

12 Pieter Spierenburg (1995) offers a history of forms of punishment, including imprisonment, in the early modern period. Contrary to Foucault, Spierenburg argues that executions, the most horribly spectacular of which was that of Damiens, were the exception.

13 On the history of places of internment before the "birth of the prison," see Christian Carlier's brief history (2009), and the useful chronology he and Marc Renneville compiled (2007).

14 The *Rapport sur les prisons* [*Report on Prisons*] (1868, pp. 478–479), read to the Académie royale des sciences and submitted to Necker, the Controller General of Finances, in 1780, was prepared by Duhamel du Monceau, De Montigny, Le Roy, Tenon, and Lavoisier, but edited by Lavoisier.

15 A few decades later, in the first issue of the *Annales d'hygiène publique et de médecine légale* [*Annals of Public Hygiene and Forensic Medicine*], Louis-René Villermé (1829, p. 40) revealed the excess mortality in these various establishments, which he attributed to "the poor running of prisons," to "the current state of penury, of destitution of inmates," and to the "privations and sufferings they have borne prior to imprisonment."

16 According to Foucault (1979 [1975], p. 89), the late eighteenth century was a period of redistribution of illegalities, with illegalities of rights (fraud) being reserved for the bourgeoisie, and illegalities of property (theft) assigned to the lower classes.

17 In their history of the Bethlem Royal Hospital, Jonathan Andrews et al. (1997) note that it is probably the oldest mental institution in Europe.

18 Comparing English prisons of the eighteenth and nineteenth centuries, Randall McGowen (1998) notes that the former were characterized by disorder and chaos, while order and silence reigned in the latter.

19 One section of Pinel's (1809 [1801]) *Treatise* explored his "*traitement moral*," while Samuel Tuke (1813) devoted a chapter of his *Description* to the "moral treatment" promoted by his father William.

20 Beccaria's (2009 [1764]) book was translated into French in 1765 and into English the following year, ensuring immediate dissemination through the European continent. Howard's (1792 [1777]) report on prisons remains a refer-

ence: published just before the French Revolution, it presents both detailed observation and a reformist vision.

21 Rothman's (2008) book is a pioneering historical study of asylums and prisons in the United States, originally published in 1971, ten years after Goffman's *Asylums*, and four years before Foucault's *Discipline and Punish*.

22 In the introduction to the second edition of their report, Beaumont and Tocqueville (1833, p. 22; 1845 [1831], pp. 5, 7, 109, 114, 122) assert that the aim of the prison system is to "render better the criminals that society has temporarily removed from its heart, or at least to prevent them becoming more wicked in their prison," adding peremptorily that "the means to achieve this double end are silence and isolation." What they discovered "in America" became axiomatic for them.

23 In his chapter on Philadelphia, devoted almost entirely to the prison, Dickens (1842, p. 236) writes: "The system here is rigid, strict, and hopeless solitary confinement. I believe it, in its effects, to be cruel and wrong."

24 These figures are drawn from articles by France Meslé and Jacques Vallin (1981) for the statistics on mental health, and by Marie-Danièle Barré (1986) for those on prisons.

25 These figures are drawn respectively from the analyses by John Hunter et al. (1986) (mental health statistics), and by Margaret Werner Cahalan and Lee Anne Parsons (1986) (prison statistics).

26 These figures are drawn from articles by France Meslé and Jacques Vallin (1981) and François Chapireau (2007) (mental health statistics), and Marie-Danièle Barré (1986), supplemented by monthly Ministry of Justice statistics (prison statistics).

27 In the case of the United States, Harcourt (2006) shows that in 1923, 92% of in-patients at psychiatric hospitals were white, while today Blacks and Hispanics, although in the minority in the country as a whole, make up 60% of the prison population. With regard to France, my research (2016) in a short-stay prison (which I demonstrated was close to the national average in terms of several proxies, or variables of similar significance), showed that ethnic and racial minorities, primarily Blacks and Arabs, made up more than three-quarters of the prison population, while half of those interned were unemployed and half stated they had no profession.

28 The first of these studies, conducted by Émilie Fauchille et al. (2016) uses a standardized form to gather information on state of health. The second, conducted by Laurent Plancke et al. (2017) uses an internationally validated protocol, the Mini-International Neuropsychiatric Interview (MINI).

29 The study by Falissard et al. (2006) used four indicators: diagnosis by at least one psychiatrist, a diagnosis shared by two psychiatrists assessing separately, diagnosis established by consensus between them, and diagnosis from the MINI questionnaire.

30 Caroline Lafaye et al. (2016) analyzed changes in the legislation and the practices of judges. The proportion of judgments recognizing diminished responsibility halved between 1985 and 2014.

31 Magali Coldefy's (2005) survey offers a good analysis of the mental health provision in prisons, but is based only on the statements made by services, not on testimony from prisoners.

32 In Doris James and Lauren Glaze's (2006) study, prisoners presenting mental disorders had committed violent crimes, had been incarcerated multiple times,

and were dependent on drugs more often than other prisoners. They were more often homeless, and more often survivors of sexual abuse. Since their admission they had more often been injured in fights and were more often responsible for attacks.

33 Of the twelve countries in which studies were carried out, Seena Fazel and John Danesh (2002) note that three were not in the West – in Dubai, Kuwait, and Nigeria – but were based on small samples.

34 See Nikolaj Nielsen's article "Prison suicide rates in France highest in Europe" (EUobserver.com, 2 April 2019). The methodological problems of such international comparisons are discussed by Bruno Aubusson de Cavarlay (2009).

35 I discuss the notion of the punitive moment in my book *The Will to Punish* (2018b).

36 These statistics are drawn from studies by Angélique Hazard (2008) and Géraldine Duthé et al. (2009, 2014) commissioned by the Ministry of Justice.

37 Christopher Mumola's study (2005) shows that suicide rates fell sharply in both state prisons and local jails during the 1980s and 1990s. The study by Fatos Kaba et al. (2014) relates to almost 250,000 prisoners in local jails in New York City, calculating that although only 7.3% of prisoners had experienced solitary confinement, 53% of those who had self-harmed and 45% of those who had committed suicide had endured it.

38 Lisa Guenther's study (2013) is essentially philosophical, taking up Orlando Patterson's concept of "social death" coined in relation to enslavement, while Lorna Rhodes's study (2004) is based on several years of observation and interviews in various maximum security prisons in Washington state.

39 For comparisons of suicide rates in France and the United States, see the article by Fazel et al. (2017). For statistics and consequences of solitary confinement, which is unlimited in the United States, see David Cloud et al. (2015). France limits solitary confinement to thirty days, which is still one of the highest maximum durations in Europe. For an analysis of the opposition between physical death and social death in prison, see my contribution to the volume *Vies invisibles, morts indicibles* (2022b).

Readings of the Pandemic

1 Entitled "Le monde est un grand asile" ["The world is a great asylum"], Foucault's text was published in the now defunct Brazilian weekly *Manchete* (2001, vol. 1, p. 1302). The final paragraph, in which Foucault develops his idea of journalism and the present, seems suspended, quite disconnected from the rest of the text.

2 In the early 1980s, Foucault, together with Veyne and Wahl, edited a series published by Seuil entitled "Des travaux" ["On works"]. They gave this definition of the term: "Work: that which can introduce a significant difference into the field of knowledge, at the cost of some effort on the part of the author and the reader, and with the potential reward of some pleasure, in other words access to another face of truth."

3 In the second of his *Untimely Meditations*, "On the uses and disadvantages of history for life," Nietzsche (1997 [1873], pp. 59–60) inveighs against the dominant idea of his time: "We need history ... for the sake of life and action, not so as to turn comfortably away from life and action." The French translation

of the title, *Considérations inactuelles*, emphasizes the "non-contemporary" aspect of the concept.

4 The data that follow are drawn from multiple sources, particularly articles from the *New York Times* and the *Washington Post* as regards the United States, and *Le Monde* as regards France. Detailed timelines, including day-by-day statistics, were drawn up by David Leonhardt ("A complete list of Trump's attempts to play down coronavirus," NYTimes.com, 15 March 2020).

5 Editor-in-chief of *The Lancet*, one of the top medical journals worldwide, Horton (2020) considers the global response to the pandemic is "the greatest science policy failure in a generation."

6 In his study, Lakoff (2017, pp. 7, 167) offers "neither a heroic account of visionary planning by enlightened health authorities, nor a sinister story of the securitization of disease by an ever-expansive governmental apparatus." It focuses rather on "the assemblage of disparate elements – adapted from fields such as civil defense, emergency management, and international public health – by well-meaning experts and officials and of response failures that have typically led, in turn, to reforms that seek to strengthen or refocus the apparatus." The Covid pandemic reveals a reversal of this logic, since lessons were not drawn from previous failures, and the reforms even moved in the opposite direction.

7 A team of journalists from the *New York Times* conducted an in-depth study into these alerts ("Before virus outbreak, a cascade of warnings went unheeded," NYTimes.com, 19 March 2020).

8 The mask story is the subject of a very detailed article by Arnaud Mercier (2020). The disbanding of ÉPRUS has been analyzed by Claude Le Pen ("'En période de crise, l'État pense qu'il fait mieux que tout le monde,'" Politix.fr, 8 April 2020). The budget data are taken from the Senate report on ÉPRUS (see "L'établissement de préparation et de réponse aux urgences sanitaires: Comment investir dans la sécurité sanitaire de nos concitoyens?" Senat.fr, 15 July 2015).

9 In the view of Callon and Lascoumes (2020), the French government's weak and tardy reaction reveals not so much a forgetting of the principle of precaution but, rather, the triumph of the "preachers of anti-precaution."

10 It is remarkable that, as Caduff shows (2015), the discourse around the H1N1 epidemic that was later judged to have been catastrophist foreshadowed the reality of the Covid pandemic, in that it spoke of an infection with millions of victims that would lead to the interruption of all economic activity – a premonition that was not taken seriously at the time.

11 An investigation led by the *Washington Post* revealed how a month was lost in making tests available ("Inside the coronavirus testing failure: Alarm and dismay among the scientists who sought to help," WashingtonPost.com, 3 April 2020).

12 A detailed analysis of the available data on diagnostic tests in France and Germany appeared in the "CheckNews" column in *Libération* ("Covid-19: l'Allemagne effectue-t-elle vraiment 500 000 tests par semaine?" Liberation.fr, 3 April 2020).

13 The 2020 budget required that hospitals cut spending by 800 million euros. The plan, proposed in response to a strike by hospital staff, allocated 200 million euros, still leaving 600 million euros of cuts to be made. See the France Culture interview with André Grimaldi on 13 March 2020: according to the French physician, "health must not be subject to the laws of the market." The

healthcare system figures cited are drawn from *Health at a Glance*, produced by the OECD at the end of 2019 (available at OECD.org). See also the article by Philippe François and Sandrine Gorreri, who put the issue of the number of hospital beds in perspective ("Crise sanitaire: Tout ne se résume pas au nombre de lits d'hôpitaux," iFRAP.org, 25 April 2020).

14 The shortages of medication reported from early April 2020 on are analyzed in an article by Irène Lacamp in *Sciences et Avenir* ("Covid-19: Des tensions d'approvisionnement se font sentir pour certains médicaments," SciencesEtAvenir.fr, 3 April 2020).

15 For China's share of France's trade deficit, see the analysis by Camille Bortolini and Estelle Jacques for the French Treasury ("Les relations commerciales entre la France et la Chine en 2018," Tresor.Economie.gouv.fr, 4 April 2019). For an analysis of the United States' trade deficit with China, which was at the root of Donald Trump's aggressive policy toward the country, see the report drawn up for the Brookings Institution by Ryan Hass and Abraham Denmark, who quote estimates of 300,000 jobs lost and 316 billion dollars lost to the US economy owing to taxes levied on both sides ("More pain than gain: How the US-China trade war hurt America," Brookings.edu, 7 August 2020).

16 On 22 March 2021, among these four countries France was the one with by far the highest weekly death rate from Covid: 3.88 per million inhabitants, compared to 2.96 in the United States, 2.23 in Germany and 0.07 in South Korea (see "Coronavirus (COVID-19) deaths," OurWorldInData.org). The proportion of people who had received the first dose of vaccine in France was a quarter of that in the United States.

17 According to Kristian Andersen et al. (2020), two hypotheses can be formulated: either the mutation that gave rise to SARS-CoV-2 occurred in an animal host, and in this case there is a subsequent risk of it re-emerging, or it took place in a human, making this highly unlikely. The visit by seventeen Chinese researchers and seventeen international colleagues was reported and discussed in *Nature* ("'Major stones unturned': Covid origin search must continue after WHO report, say scientists," Nature.com, 10 February 2021).

18 For a detailed analysis, see the website of the International Civil Aviation Organization, which is a UN agency ("The world of air transport in 2018," ICAO.int).

19 On the first weeks of the epidemic and the coverage of it, see Fernando Bermejo's detailed analysis for the MediaCloud website ("Information pandemic: Initial explorations of COVID-19 coverage," MediaCloud.org, 22 March 2020). Taking the figure of 100 cases diagnosed as a benchmark, the time taken after this for the pandemic to take up 50% of news coverage was one day in Italy, eight days in the United Kingdom, ten days in the United States and Spain, and fourteen days in France and Germany.

20 Among the many discussions, see the commentaries by semiologist Cécile Alday in *Libération* ("Métaphore de Macron sur la guerre: 'Cela exonère le pouvoir de ses responsabilités'," Liberation.fr, 30 March 2020) and journalist Gaïdz Minassian in *Le Monde* ("Covid-19, ce que cache la rhétorique guerrière," LeMonde.fr, 8 April 2020).

21 Many incidents of racist language and acts against people of East Asian origin were reported in the United States, and the massacre of eight people, six of them young women of Asian origin, in three spas in Atlanta was attributed to this anti-Asian racism ("Spit on, yelled at, attacked: Chinese-Americans fear for

their safety," NYTimes.com, 23 March 2020; "8 dead in Atlanta spa shootings, with fears of anti-Asian bias," NYTimes.com, 17 March 2021). At the same time, manifestations of anti-Chinese xenophobia were so prevalent in France that activist organization SOS Racisme created an awareness-raising campaign ("Coronavirus: SOS Racisme lance une campagne contre les préjugés anti-asiatique," LeParisien.fr, 24 February 2020). The deportation of Nigerians from China prompted protests from the Nigerian government ("Africans in China: 'We face coronavirus discrimination'," BBC.com, 17 April 2020).

22 These figures are based on data from 15 April 2020. As of this date, the United States cited 633,630 cases and 28,214 deaths; France had 106,206 cases and 17,167 deaths; Germany 127,000 cases and 3,254 deaths.

23 In the conclusion of his article, Didier (2020) writes: "Figures and affects go hand in hand, they are at the heart of the crisis. And yet there has been little discussion of them."

24 The Centers for Disease Control and Prevention regularly published these forecasts ("Previous Covid-19 forecasts: Deaths," CDC.gov). The different simulations, including variations of that used by Neil Ferguson at Imperial College London, are discussed by journalist David Adam in *Nature* ("Special report: The simulations driving the world's response to Covid-19," Nature. com, 2 April 2020).

25 Didier Raoult's study was published in the *International Journal of Antimicrobial Agents*, whose editorial committee includes two members of his team and co-authors of the article (Gautret et al. 2020).

26 The poll on belief in hydroxychloroquine appeared in the daily newspaper *Le Parisien* ("Covid-19: 59% des Français croient à l'efficacité de la chloroquine," LeParisien.fr, 5 April 2020).

27 On the changing discourse of Donald Trump, from enthusiasm to reservations, see Kenya Evelyn's article in the *Guardian* ("Trump stops hyping hydroxychloroquine after study shows no benefit," TheGuardian.com, 22 April 2020).

28 This study, showing an excess mortality among US Army veterans treated with the drug, was by Joseph Magagnoli et al. (2020).

29 Damien Leloup and Lucie Soullier argued in *Le Monde* that Didier Raoult had become "the face of conspiracy theories" ("Coronavirus: comment le professeur Didier Raoult est devenu une figure centrale des théories complotistes," LeMonde.fr, 28 March 2020).

30 The Fox News journalists offered neither evidence nor direct testimony, instead extensively quoting the president and his acolytes who suggested that the virus might have been created by humans ("Sources believe coronavirus outbreak originated in Wuhan lab as part of China's efforts to compete with US," FoxNews.com, 15 April 2020). By this point, researchers were categorically certain that the virus's genome bore no resemblance to other known viruses, but that there was a high degree of similarity with two viruses found in bats and pangolins ("No, the coronavirus wasn't made in a lab. A genetic analysis shows it's from nature," ScienceNews.org, 26 March 2020).

31 The 26-minute video *Plandemic: The Hidden Agenda Behind Covid-19*, is unsophisticated, based essentially on an interview with a researcher with a scandalous scientific past ("How the 'Plandemic' movie and its falsehoods spread widely online," NYTimes.com, 20 May 2020). The 163-minute film *Hold-Up: Retour sur un Chaos* [*Hold-Up: A Look Back at Chaos*], is more subtly constructed, moving gradually from the actual lies of the French government to the idea of a

world conspiracy, accompanied by archive clips and interviews with well-known scientific figures ("Les contre-vérités de 'Hold-up', documentaire à succès qui prétend dévoiler la face cachée de l'épidémie," LeMonde.fr, 12 November 2020). The first received 2 million "likes" on Facebook in one week; the second was viewed 400,000 times on YouTube within forty-eight hours.

32 In the view of Guido Calabresi and Philip Bobbitt (1978), the question is, first, what level of resources should be allocated to a given problem, and, second, how they should be distributed. They use the example of dialysis machines for patients with kidney failure.

33 According to Stefano Fagiuoli et al. (2020), the number of intensive care beds and personnel was increased throughout the period, making it possible to care for all the patients who needed intensive care, but those considered less seriously ill had to remain at home, where some died.

34 See the interviews with senior staff in elderly care homes, conducted by Étienne Girard and Laurent Valdiguié ("'Des personnes âgées auraient probablement pu être sauvées': Le refus d'hospitalisation de résidents d'Ehpad, dernier tabou du Covid," Marianne.net, 15 May 2020).

35 For information on policies relating to discrimination or protection of migrants, refugees, and asylum seekers in the context of coronavirus, see the "Covid-19 Global Immigration Detention Platform" at GlobalDetentionProject.org.

36 The Council of State (Conseil d'état), to which advocacy organizations appealed, upheld the refusal to close the detention centers. See Pascal Riche's article in *L'Obs* ("Malgré le coronavirus, les centres de rétention pour étrangers ne seront pas fermés," NouvelObs.com, 27 March 2020). See also my article on these migrants, detained but not deportable (2020b). The OEE is an activist organization opposing routine detention of undocumented foreigners. The DDD is a publicly appointed independent official responsible for ensuring respect of citizens' and human rights.

37 On 24 March 2020, 732 people were evacuated from the largest unofficial exile camp, at Aubervilliers in the Seine-Saint-Denis department. Among these, the charity Médecins sans frontières identified twenty-five suspected cases of the virus, of whom only five could be tested because of the shortage of tests in the healthcare services ("Mise à l'abri des migrants: 'Les gymnases ne sont pas des lieux appropriés'," LeMonde.fr, 1 April 2020).

38 For a description of the Moria camp, where no case had yet been identified as of late April, see the website InfoMigrants ("Lesbos: dans le camp de Moria, 'le coronavirus a entraîné le chaos, le stress est énorme'," InfoMigrants.net, 25 March 2020).

39 Statistics on overcrowding in French prisons can be found in the data published each quarter ("Mesure de l'incarcération, au 1er Janvier 2020," Justice. gouv.fr). Articles from all over the world on coronavirus and prisons are collated on the World Prison Brief website ("International news and guidance on Covid-19 and prisons: 13 March–30 November," PrisonStudies.org, 18 March 2020).

40 Data on the fall in the French prison population are taken from an article in *Le Parisien* ("Coronavirus: Il y a plus de places de prison que de détenus, une situation 'sans précédent'," LeParisien.fr, 29 April 2020), supplemented by a series of interviews with a Ministry of Justice advisor, officers of the DAP, Direction de l'administration pénitentiare [Directorate of Prison Administration], prison directors, and prisoners during May and June 2020.

41 The figures for release of prisoners are drawn from an article by Katelyn Newman in *USA Today* ("For prisoners released due to COVID-19, a different world awaits," USnews.com, 15 April 2020). Detailed analysis of the data from Ohio's remarkable transparency initiative is presented in the table "Covid-19 Inmate Testing" on DRC.Ohio.gov.

42 This inaugural lecture (2020a) was delivered at the Collège de France on 16 January 2020.

43 At the end of his analysis of the impact of the state of emergency on basic freedoms, Vincent Sizaire (2020) concludes: "Given the extent of the infringement of freedom, it is essential that the legal framework be strictly defined. But the text adopted gave no specification as to the content of these measures, their duration, ways of appealing them, or of the rights of persons subjected to them."

44 See, for the United States, "En 2020, les États-Unis ont traversé la pire récession depuis 1946" (LeMonde.fr, 28 January 2021), and for France, "Le PIB a plongé de 8,3% en 2020" (LesEchos.fr, 29 January 2021).

45 This parallel between 1938 and 2018 is not a systematic comparison, but rather points to signs in the events of 1938 that could help to think the present. As Foessel (2019, p. 22) writes: "My exploration of 1938 left me convinced not of the weakness of French democracy, but rather that at the time France was only weakly democratic." In other words, it is not democracy itself that is at issue, but rather the way it is quietly rolled back.

46 "Job protection schemes," as redundancy programs were oxymoronically called, proliferated, in some cases with no connection to the pandemic, for example at Nokia, as Francine Aizicovici reported in *Le Monde* ("Le nouveau coronavirus, une aubaine pour les sociétés qui veulent licencier," LeMonde.fr, 13 August 2020).

47 See especially the article by Harvard historian of medicine David Jones (2020). According to the Centers for Disease Control and Prevention, the number of people infected with the H1N1 Spanish flu virus in 1918–19 was around 500 million, and there were approximately 50 million deaths (see "1918 Pandemic (H1N1) Virus," CDC.gov, 20 March 2019).

48 According to François Héran's estimates, of those young men who reached the age of 20 in 1914, 22% died at the front ("Comment évaluer le nombre de morts de la première guerre mondiale?" LeMonde.fr, 10 November 2018).

49 The phrase was uttered in a television interview on 12 May 1996: "The price is worth it," Albright declared (extract available at YouTube.com).

50 The International Organization for Migration's "Missing Migrants Project" keeps the somber tally of these deaths at sea – a tally that is clearly incomplete (MissingMigrants.IOM.int).

51 I have developed this concept in my work since the 1990s, and discussed it most recently in *Life: A Critical User's Manual* (2018a).

52 See Lois Beckett's article in the *Guardian* on Patrick's comments on Fox News ("Older people would rather die than let Covid-19 harm US economy – Texas official," TheGuardian.com, 24 March 2020).

53 See Nicolas Truong's interview for *Le Monde*, where Agamben returned to his argument first published in the Italian daily newspaper *Il Manifesto* ("Giorgio Agamben: 'L'épidémie montre clairement que l'état d'exception est devenu la condition normale.'" LeMonde.fr, 24 March 2020). This interview continues the line of Agamben's long-term research (Agamben 1998).

54 It is worth noting that when counties participated in projects to expand Medicaid, the medical assistance provided to people on low incomes, the incidence of infection fell by one-third (Liao and DeMaio 2021). With regard to life expectancy at birth, the gap was as much as 7.2 years between Black men and white men (Arias et al. 2021). See "The fullest look yet at the racial inequity of coronavirus" (NYTimes.com, 5 July 2020); "A grim measure of Covid's toll: Life expectancy drops sharply in US" (NYTimes.com, 18 February 2021).

55 As noted in the report by the National Institute for Demographic Research (Ined, Institut national d'études démographiques), in France data on racial categories are not available ("Surmortalité due à la Covid-19 en Seine-Saint-Denis," Ined.fr, 25 June 2020). See also the report by the Île-de-France Regional Health Observatory (Orsif, Observatoire régional de la santé d'Île-de-France) ("La surmortalité durant l'épidémie de Covid-19 dans les départements franciliens," ORS-IDF.org, 16 April 2020).

56 According to Case and Deaton (2020), from the late 1990s this excess mortality related mainly to white middle-aged men and women with a low level of education, but Steven Woolf and Heidi Schoomaker's analysis of a more recent period (2019) shows that, over the 2010s, mortality in adulthood rose in all racial groups, and mainly impacted the lowest-income groups.

57 The increase in inequality in the United States from the 1980s on has been demonstrated by Thomas Piketty (2017).

58 The causes of this gap in mortality are complex, since poor health can be a cause of unemployment and unemployment is damaging to health, as Annie Mesrine (2000) explains.

59 Honneth (1997) bases his reflection on recognition on Hegel's work.

60 With regard to the unemployed, Robert Castel (1995) talks of disaffiliation, in other words, the loss of the social bond.

61 According to Benjamin (1996, p. 251), "The proposition that existence stands higher than a just existence is false and ignominious, if existence is to mean nothing other than mere life."

References

Abdelghafour, Nassima, 2017. "Randomized controlled experiments to end poverty? A sociotechnical analysis," *Anthropologie et développement*, 46–47, pp. 235–262.

Abenhaïm, Lucien, 2003. *Canicules: La santé publique en question*. Paris: Fayard.

Abraído-Lanza, Ana, Dohrenwend, Bruce, Ng-Mak, Daisy, and Turner, Blake, 1999. "The Latino mortality paradox: A test of the 'salmon bias' and healthy migrant hypotheses," *American Journal of Public Health*, 89/10, pp. 1543–1548.

Adams, Vincanne, 2016. "Metrics of the global sovereign: Numbers and stories in global health," in Vincanne Adams (ed.), *Metrics: What Counts in Global Health*. Durham, NC: Duke University Press, pp. 19–54.

Agamben, Giorgio, 1998. *Homo Sacer: Sovereign Power and Bare Life*, trans. Daniel Heller-Roazen. Stanford, CA: Stanford University Press.

Aiken, Alexander M., Davey, Calum, Hargreaves, James R., and Hayes, Richard J., 2015. "Re-analysis of health and educational impacts of a school-based deworming programme in Western Kenya: A pure replication," *International Journal of Epidemiology*, 44/5, pp. 1572–1580.

Ammash, Huda S., 2002. "Toxic pollution, the Gulf War, and sanctions: The Impact on the environment and health in Iraq," in Anthony Arnove (ed.), *Iraq Under Siege: The Deadly Impact of Sanctions and War*. Cambridge, MA: South End Press, pp. 205–214.

Andersen, Kristian G., Rambaut, Andrew, Lipkin, W. Ian, et al., 2020. "The proximal origin of SARS-COV-2," *Nature Medicine*, 26/4, pp. 450–452.

Andrews, Jonathan, Briggs, Asa, Porter, Roy, et al., 1997. *The History of Bethlem*. Abingdon: Routledge.

Angell, Marcia, 1997. "The ethics of clinical research in the Third World," *The New England Journal of Medicine*, 337/12, pp. 847–849.

Arias, Elizabeth, Tejada-Vera, Betzaida, and Ahmed, Farida, 2021. "Provisional life expectancy estimates for January through June 2020," *Vital Statistics Rapid Release*, US Department of Health and Human Services, Report no. 10, February.

Aubusson de Cavarlay, Bruno, 2009. "Note sur la sursuicidité carcérale en Europe: Du choix des indicateurs," *Champ pénal/Penal Field*, 6 (online).

Austin, John Langshaw, 1962. *How to Do Things with Words: The William James Lectures Delivered at Harvard University in 1955*. Oxford: Clarendon Press.

Bailly, Anatole, 1930 [1895]. *Dictionnaire grec-français*. Paris: Hachette.

Banerjee, Abhijit, and Duflo, Esther, 2011. *Poor Economics: A Radical Rethinking of the Way to Fight Global Poverty*. New York: Public Affairs.

Barré, Marie-Danièle, 1986. "130 années de statistique pénitentiaire en France," *Déviance et société*, 10/2, pp. 107–128.

Baszanger, Isabelle, 1995. *Douleur et médecine, la fin d'un oubli*. Paris: Seuil.

Bazin, Jean, 2008. *Des Clous dans la Joconde. L'anthropologie autrement*. Toulouse, Anacharsis.

Beaumont, Gustave de, and Tocqueville, Alexis de, 1833. *On the Penitentiary System in the United States and its Application in France*, trans. Francis Lieber. Philadelphia, PA: Carey, Lea and Blanchard.

Beaumont, Gustave de, and Tocqueville, Alexis de, 1845 [1831]. *Système pénitentiaire aux États-Unis et de son application en France*. Paris: Charles Gosselin.

Beccaria, Cesare, 2009 [1764]. *On Crime and Punishments*, trans. Graeme R. Newman and Pietro Marongiu. New Brunswick, NJ: Transaction Publishers.

Beckley, Amber L., Caspi, Avshalom, Broadbent, Jonathan, et al., 2018. "The association between childhood blood lead level and criminal offending," *Journal of the American Medical Association Pediatrics*, 172/2, pp. 166–173.

Bédécarrats, Florent, Guérin, Isabelle, and Roubaud, François, 2020. *Randomized Control Trials in the Field of Development: A Critical Perspective*. Oxford: Oxford University Press.

Bellinger, David C., 2016. "Lead contamination in Flint: An abject failure to protect public health," *The New England Journal of Medicine*, 374/12, pp. 1101–1103.

Benecke, Olivia, and DeYoung, Sarah Elizabeth, 2019. "Anti-vaccine decision-making and measles resurgence in the United States," *Global Pediatric Health*, 6 (online).

Benjamin, Walter, 1996. "A critique of violence," in *Selected Writings, 1: 1913–1926*. Cambridge, MA: Belknap Press.

Bernard, Léon, 1925. "Le problème sanitaire de l'immigration," *Revue d'hygiène et de médecine préventive*, 47, pp. 769–787.

Bernard, Stephen A., Cheminski, Raul R., Ives, Timothy J., et al., 2018. "Management of pain in the United States: A brief history and implications for the opioid epidemic," *Health Services Insights*, 11 (online).

Berney, Barbara, 1993. "Round and round it goes: The epidemiology of childhood lead poisoning," *The Milbank Quarterly*, 71/1, pp. 3–39.

Berthelier, Robert, 2007. "À la recherche de l'homme musulman," *Sud/Nord*, 22, pp. 127–146.

Bibeau, Gilles, 1991. "L'Afrique, terre imaginaire du sida. La subversion du discours scientifique par le jeu des fantasmes," *Anthropologie et sociétés*, 15/2–3, pp. 125–147.

Biehl, João, and Petryna, Adriana, 2013. "Global public health," in João Biehl and Adriana Petryna (eds.), *When People Come First. Critical Studies in Global Health*. Princeton: Princeton University Press, pp. 1–20.

Bilson, Geoffrey, 1980. *A Darkened House: Cholera in Nineteenth-Century Canada*. Toronto: University of Toronto Press.

Boochani, Behrouz, 2018. *No Friend but the Mountains: The True Story of an Illegally Imprisoned Refugee*. Sydney: Picador.

Botha, J. L., and Bradshaw, Debbie, 1985. "African vital statistics – a black hole?" *South African Medical Journal*, 67/24, pp. 977–981.

Bouhenia, Malika, Ben Farhat, Jihane, Coldiron, Matthew, et al., 2017. "Quantitative survey on health and violence endured by refugees during their journey and in Calais, France," *International Health*, 9/6, pp. 335–342.

Bourdillon, François, Fontaine, Alain, Luciolli, Esmeralda, and Nedellec, Vincent, 1990. *L'Intoxication par les peintures au plomb aux États-Unis et quelques recommandations pour la France*. Paris: Médecins sans frontières-Migrations santé.

Bousmah, Marwân-al-Qays, Combes, Jean-Baptiste Simon, and Abu-Zaineh, Mohammad, 2019. "Health differentials between citizens and immigrants in Europe: A heterogeneous convergence," *Health Policy*, 123/2, pp. 235–243.

Brandt, Allan M., 2012. "Inventing conflicts of interest: A history of tobacco industry tactics," *American Journal of Public Health*, 102/1, pp. 63–71.

Brard, Delphine, 2004. *La Fabrique médiatique de la canicule d'août 2003 comme problème public*. Master's thesis in political science. Paris: Université Paris 1 Panthéon-Sorbonne.

Bratich, Jack Z., 2008. *Conspiracy Panics: Political Rationality and Popular Culture*. Albany: State University of New York Press.

Briggs, Charles L., 2004. "Theorizing modernity conspiratorially: Science, scale, and the political economy of public discourses in explanation of a cholera epidemic," *American Ethnologist*, 31/2, pp. 164–187.

Brown, Lesley (ed.), 1993. *New Shorter Oxford English Dictionary*. Oxford: Oxford University Press.

Brownson, Ross C., Fielding, Jonathan E., and Maylahn, Christopher M., 2009. "Evidence-based public health: A fundamental concept for public health practice," *Annual Review of Public Health*, 30, pp. 175–201.

Bryder, Linda, 1996. "'A health resort for consumptives': Tuberculosis and immigration to New Zealand, 1880–1914," *Medical History*, 40/4, pp. 453–471.

Burger, Marléne, and Gould, Chandré, 2002. *Secrets and Lies: Wouter Basson and South Africa's Chemical and Biological Warfare Programme*. Cape Town: Struik Publishers.

Byers, R. K., 1959. "Lead poisoning: Review of the literature and report on 45 cases," *Pediatrics*, 23/3, pp. 585–603.

Byler, Christen G., and Robinson, W. Courtland, 2018. "Differences in patterns of mortality between foreign-born and native-born workers due to fatal occupational injury in the USA from 2003 to 2010," *Journal of Immigrant and Minority Health*, 20/1, pp. 26–32.

Caduff, Carlo, 2015. *The Pandemic Perhaps: Dramatic Events in a Public Culture of Danger*. Berkeley: University of California Press.

Cahalan, Margaret Werner, and Parsons, Lee Anne, 1986. *Historical Corrections Statistics in the United States 1850–1984*. Washington, DC: US Department of Justice.

Cahill, Anthony G., and James, Joseph A., 1992. "Responding to municipal fiscal distress: An emerging issue for state governments in the 1990s," *Public Administration Review*, 52/1, pp. 88–94.

Calabresi, Guido, and Bobbitt, Philip, 1978. *Tragic Choices: The Conflicts Society Confronts in the Allocation of Tragically Scarce Resources*. New York: Norton.

Callon, Michel, and Lascoumes, Pierre, 2020. "Covid-19 et néfaste oubli du principe de précaution," aoc.media, 27 March.

Canfield, Richard L., Henderson, Charles R., Cory-Slechta, Deborah A., et al., 2003. "Intellectual impairment in children with blood lead concentrations below 10 μg per deciliter," *The New England Journal of Medicine*, 348/16, pp. 1517–1526.

Canguilhem, Georges, 2012. *The Normal and the Pathological*, trans. Carolyn R. Fawcett. Dordrecht: Reidel.

Carlier, Christian, 2009. "Histoire des prisons et de l'administration pénitentiaire française de l'Ancien régime à nos jours," *Criminocorpus. Revue d'histoire de la justice, des crimes et des peines* (online).

Carlier, Christian, and Renneville, Marc, 2007. "Histoire des prisons en France. De l'Ancien Régime à la Restauration," *Criminocorpus. Revue d'histoire de la justice, des crimes et des peines* (online).

Case, Anne, and Deaton, Angus, 2015. "Rising morbidity and mortality in midlife among white non-Hispanic Americans in the 21st century," *Proceedings of the National Academy of Sciences*, 112/49, pp. 15078–15083.

Case, Anne, and Deaton, Angus, 2020. *Deaths of Despair and the Future of Capitalism*. Princeton, NJ: Princeton University Press.

Castel, Robert, 1995. *Les Métamorphoses de la question sociale. Une chronique du salariat*. Paris: Fayard.

Chapireau, François, 2007. "Le recours à l'hospitalisation psychiatrique au XXe siècle," *L'Information psychiatrique*, 83/7, pp. 563–570.

Chaud, Pascal, Haeghebaert, Sylvie, Leduc, Ghislain, et al., 2017. "Surveillance des maladies infectieuses dans les populations migrantes accueillies à Calais et à Grande-Synthe, novembre 2015–octobre 2016," *Bulletin épidémiologique hebdomadaire*, 19–20, pp. 374–381.

Clarke, Steve, 2002. "Conspiracy theories and conspiracy theorizing," *Philosophy of the Social Sciences*, 32/2, pp. 131–150.

Clauw, Daniel J., 2014. "Fibromyalgia: A clinical review," *Journal of the American Medical Association*, 311/15, pp. 1547–1555.

Cloud, David H., Drucker, Ernest, Browne, Angela, and Parsons, Jim, 2015. "Public health and solitary confinement in the United States," *American Journal of Public Health*, 105/1, pp. 18–26.

Cohen, Régis, 1987. "L'intoxication par le plomb chez l'enfant. Un problème toujours actuel," *Revue de pédiatrie*, 23/2, pp. 83–89.

Cohen, Stanley, 2002 [1972]. *Folk Devils and Moral Panics: The Creation of the Mods and Rockers*. Abingdon: Routledge.

Coldefy, Magali, 2005. "La prise en charge de la santé mentale des détenus en 2003," *Études et résultats*, 427, Drees, September.

Collignon, René, 2006. "La psychiatrie coloniale française en Algérie et au Sénégal. Esquisse d'une historisation comparative," *Revue Tiers Monde*, 187, pp. 527–546.

Comaroff, Jean, and Comaroff, John L., 1999. "Occult economies and the violence of abstraction: Notes from the South African postcolony," *American Ethnologist*, 26/2, pp. 279–303.

Cosentino, Gabriele, 2020. *Social Media and the Post-Truth World Order*. London: Palgrave.

Cueto, Marcos, 2004. "The origins of primary health care and selective primary health care," *American Journal of Public Health*, 94/11, pp. 1864–1874.

Dabis, François, Msellati, Philippe, Meda, Nicolas, et al., 1999. "6-month efficacy, tolerance, and acceptability of a short regimen of oral zidovudine to reduce vertical transmission of HIV in breastfed children in Côte d'Ivoire and Burkina Faso," *The Lancet*, 353/9155, pp. 766–792.

Daston, Lorraine, 1995. "The moral economy of science," *Osiris*, 10, pp. 2–24.

Davey, Calum, Aiken, Alexander M., Hargreaves, James R., and Hayes, Richard J., 2015. "Re-analysis of health and educational impacts of a school-based deworming programme in Western Kenya: A statistical replication of a cluster quasi-randomized stepped-wedge trial," *International Journal of Epidemiology*, 44/5, pp. 1581–1592.

De Luca Barrusse, Virginie, 2012. "L'invention du 'problème sanitaire de l'immigration' au cours des années 1920," *Revue d'histoire de la protection sociale*, 5, pp. 61–77.

Deaton, Angus, and Cartwright, Nancy, 2016. "Understanding and misunderstanding randomized controlled trials," NBER Working Paper Series, 22595, September.

Delour, Marcelle, and Squinazi, Fabien, 1989a. "Stratégie de dépistage du saturnisme infantile. Une intoxication endémique dans certaines couches de la population enfantine," *Revue du praticien*, 68, pp. 61–64.

Delour, Marcelle, and Squinazi, Fabien, 1989b. "Intoxication saturnine chronique du jeune enfant. Dépistage et prise en charge médico-sociale," *Revue de pédiatrie*, 25, pp. 38–47.

Demanze, Laurent, 2019. *Un nouvel âge de l'enquête. Portrait de l'écrivain contemporain en enquêteur*. Paris: José Corti.

Denno, Deborah, 2008. "Considering lead poisoning as a criminal defense," *Fordham Urban Law Journal*, 20/3, pp. 377–400.

Desrosières, Alain, 1993. *La Politique des grands nombres. Histoire de la raison statistique*. Paris: La Découverte.

Dickens, Charles, 1842. *American Notes for General Circulation*, vol. 1. London: Chapman & Hall.

Didier, Emmanuel, 2020. "Politique du nombre de morts," aoc.media, 16 avril.

Dorrington, Rob, Bourne, David, Bradshaw, Debbie, et al., 2001. *The Impact of HIV/ AIDS on Adult Mortality in South Africa*. Tygerberg: Medical Research Council.

Douglas, Karen M., Uscinski, Joseph E., Sutton, Robbie M., et al., 2019. "Understanding conspiracy theories," *Political Psychology*, 40/S1, pp. 3–35.

Duc, Michel, Kaminsky, Pierre, and Kayl, Pascale, 1986. "Le saturnisme hydrique. Expérience d'un service de médecine générale de 1974 à 1984," *Semaine des hôpitaux de Paris*, 62/39, pp. 3043–3052.

Duffy, John, 1968. *History of Public Health in New York City, 1625–1866*. New York: Russell Sage Foundation.

Durodié, Bill, 2006. "Risk and the social construction of 'Gulf War syndrome'," *Philosophical Transactions of the Royal Society B: Biological Sciences*, 361/1468, pp. 689–695.

Duthé, Géraldine, Hazard, Angélique, and Kensey, Annie, 2014. "Suicide des personnes écrouées en France: Évolution et facteurs de risque," *Population*, 69/4, pp. 519–549.

Duthé, Géraldine, Hazard, Angélique, Kensey, Annie, and Pan Ké Shon, Jean-Louis, 2009. "Suicide en prison: La France comparée à ses voisins européens," *Population et sociétés*, 462, INED, December.

Eco, Umberto, 1976. *A Theory of Semiotics*. Bloomington: Indiana University Press.

Eisenberg, Leon, 1977. "Disease and illness: Distinction between professional and popular ideas of sickness," *Culture, Medicine and Psychiatry*, 1/1, pp. 9–23.

Epstein, Helen, 2014a. "Liberia: The hidden truth about Ebola," *The New York Review of Books*, October 27.

Epstein, Helen, 2014b. "Ebola in Liberia: An epidemic of rumors," *The New York Review of Books*, December 18.

Esquirol, Étienne, 1819. *Des Établissements des aliénés en France et des moyens d'améliorer le sort de ces infortunés*. Paris: Imprimerie de Madame Huzard.

Evans-Pritchard, E. E., 1940. *The Nuer: A Description of the Modes of Livelihood and Political Institutions of a Nilotic People*. Oxford: Clarendon Press.

Expertise Collective, 1999. *Plomb dans l'environnement. Quels risques pour la santé?* Paris: Inserm.

Fagiuoli, Stefano, Lorini, Fernando Luca, and Remuzzi, Giuseppe, 2020. "Adaptations and lessons in the province of Bergamo," *The New England Journal of Medicine*, 382/21, e71.

Falissard, Bruno, Loze, Jean-Yves, Gasquet, Isabelle, et al., 2006. "Prevalence of mental disorders in French prisons for men," *BMC Psychiatry*, 6/33.

Fanon, Frantz, 1967. *The Wretched of the Earth*, trans. Constance Farrington. Harmondsworth: Penguin.

Fassin, Didier, 1996. *L'Espace politique de la santé. Essai de généalogie*. Paris: PUF.

Fassin, Didier, 1999. "L'ethnopsychiatrie et ses réseaux. Une influence qui grandit," *Genèses*, 35, pp. 146–171.

Fassin, Didier, 2001. "Culturalism as ideology," in Carla Makhlouf Obermeyer (ed.), *Cross-Cultural Perspectives on Reproductive Health*. Oxford: Oxford University Press, pp. 300–317.

Fassin, Didier, 2002. "L'invention française de la discrimination," *Revue française de science politique*, 52/4, pp. 403–423.

Fassin, Didier, 2003. "Naissance de la santé publique. Deux descriptions de saturnisme infantile à Paris (1987–1989)," *Genèses*, 53, pp. 139–152.

Fassin, Didier, 2007. *When Bodies Remember: Experience and Politics of AIDS in South Africa*, trans. Amy Jacobs and Gabrielle Varro. Berkeley: University of California Press.

Fassin, Didier, 2008. *Faire de la santé publique*, 2nd rev. edn. Rennes: Éditions de l'École des hautes études en santé publique.

Fassin, Didier, 2009. "Les économies morales revisitées. Étude critique suivie de quelques propositions," *Annales. Histoire, Sciences Sociales*, 64/6, pp. 1237–1266.

Fassin, Didier, 2011. "Ethnopsychiatry and the postcolonial encounter: A French psychopolitics of otherness," in Warwick Anderson, Richard C. Keller, and Deborah Jenson (eds.), *Unconscious Dominions: Psychoanalysis, Colonial Trauma, and Global Sovereignties*. Durham, NC: Duke University Press, pp. 223–245.

Fassin, Didier, 2013. *Enforcing Order: An Ethnography of Urban Policing*, trans. Rachel Gomme. Cambridge: Polity.

Fassin, Didier, 2016. *Prison Worlds: An Ethnography of the Carceral Condition*, trans. Rachel Gomme. Cambridge: Polity.

Fassin, Didier, 2017. "The endurance of critique," *Anthropological Theory*, 17/1, pp. 4–29.

Fassin, Didier, 2018a. *Life: A Critical User's Manual*. Cambridge: Polity.

Fassin, Didier, 2018b. *The Will to Punish*. New York: Oxford University Press.

Fassin, Didier, 2020a. *De l'Inégalité des vies*. Paris: Collège de France-Fayard.

Fassin, Didier, 2020b. "Hazardous confinement during the Covid-19 pandemic: The fate of migrants detained yet non-deportable," *Journal of Human Rights*, 19/5, pp. 613–623.

Fassin, Didier, 2021. "Of plots and men: The heuristics of conspiracy theories," *Current Anthropology*, 62/2, pp. 128–137.

Fassin, Didier, 2022a. "The moral economy of life in the pandemic," in Didier Fassin and Marion Fourcade (eds.), *Pandemic Exposures: Economy and Society in the Time of Coronavirus*. Chicago, IL: Hau Books, pp. 155–176.

Fassin, Didier, 2022b. "Morts physiques et morts sociales dans le monde carcéral," in Didier Fassin, *Vies invisibles, morts indicibles*. Paris: Collège de France Éditions, pp. 111–128.

Fassin, Didier, and Defossez, Anne-Claire, 1990. "La colère des Indiens d'Équateur," *Le Monde diplomatique*, August.

Fassin, Didier, and Defossez, Anne-Claire, 1992. "Une liaison dangereuse. Sciences sociales et santé publique dans les programmes de réduction de la mortalité maternelle en Équateur," *Cahiers des sciences humaines*, 28/1, pp. 23–36.

Fassin, Didier, and Fassin, Éric (eds.), 2006. *De la question sociale à la question raciale? Représenter la société française*. Paris: La Découverte.

Fassin, Didier, and Mazouz, Sarah, 2007. "Qu'est-ce que devenir français? La naturalisation comme rite d'institution républicain," *Revue française de sociologie*, 48/4, pp. 723–750.

Fassin, Didier, and Naudé, Anne-Jeanne, 2004. "Plumbism reinvented: Childhood lead poisoning in France, 1985–1990," *American Journal of Public Health*, 94/11, pp. 1854–1863.

Fassin, Didier, and Rechtman, Richard, 2009. *The Empire of Trauma: An Inquiry into the Condition of Victimhood*, trans. Rachel Gomme. Princeton, NJ: Princeton University Press.

Fauchille, Émilie, Thienpont, Céline, Sannier, Olivier, et al., 2016. "Description de l'état de santé et des caractéristiques sociales des personnes entrées en détention en Picardie en 2013," *Bulletin épidémiologique hebdomadaire*, 18–19, pp. 344–349.

Favret-Saada, Jeanne, 2015 [1977]. *The Anti-Witch*, trans. Matthew Carey. Chicago, IL: University of Chicago Press.

Fazel, Seena, and Danesh, John, 2002. "Serious mental disorder in 23,000 prisoners: A systematic review of 62 surveys," *The Lancet*, 359/9306, pp. 545–550.

Fazel, Seena, Ramesh, Taanvi, and Hawton, Keith, 2017. "Suicide in prisons: An international study of prevalence and contributing factors," *The Lancet Psychiatry*, 4/12, pp. 946–952.

Feder, Henry M., Johnson, Barbara J. B., O'Connell, Susan, et al., 2007. "A critical appraisal of 'chronic Lyme disease'," *The New England Journal of Medicine*, 357/14, pp. 1422–1430.

Fee, Elizabeth, 1990. "Public health in practice: An early confrontation with the 'silent epidemic' of childhood lead paint poisoning," *Journal of the History of Medicine and Allied Sciences*, 45/4, pp. 570–606.

Feigenbaum, James J., and Muller, Christopher, 2016. "Lead exposure and violent crime in the early twentieth century," *Explorations in Economic History*, 62/C, pp. 51–86.

Foessel, Michaël, 2019. *Récidive. 1938*. Paris: PUF.

Fontaine, Alain, Xu, Qian, Brodain, Marc, et al., 1992. "Dépistage du saturnisme infantile à Paris," *Bulletin épidémiologique hebdomadaire*, 2, pp. 5–7.

Fontanet, Arnaud, 2019. *L'Épidémiologie ou la science de l'estimation du risque en santé publique*. Paris: Collège de France-Fayard.

Foucault, Michel, 1978 [1976]. *The History of Sexuality*. Vol. 1: *The Will to Knowledge*, trans. Robert Hurley. London: Penguin.

Foucault, Michel, 1979 [1975]. *Discipline and Punish: The Birth of the Prison*, trans. Alan Sheridan. New York: Vintage.

Foucault, Michel, 1987 [1963]. *The Birth of the Clinic: An Archaeology of Medical Perception*, trans. Alan Sheridan. London: Routledge.

Foucault, Michel, 1988. "The concern for truth," in *Michel Foucault: Politics, Philosophy, Culture. Interviews and Other Writings, 1977–1984*, trans. Alan Sheridan. London: Routledge, pp. 255–267.

Foucault, Michel, 1989 [1961]. *Madness and Civilization: The History of Insanity in the Age of Reason*, trans. Richard Howard. London: Routledge.

Foucault, Michel, 2001. *Dits et écrits*. Vol. 1: *1954–1975*; Vol. 2: *1976–1988*. Paris: Gallimard.

Foucault, Michel, 2008 [2004]. *The Birth of Biopolitics: Lectures at the Collège de France 1978–1979*, trans. Graham Burchell. Basingstoke: Palgrave Macmillan.

Foucault, Michel, 2014 [2012]. *Wrong-Doing, Truth-Telling: The Function of Avowal in Justice*, trans. Stephen W. Sawyer. Chicago, IL: University of Chicago Press.

Fourcade, Marion, Ollion, Étienne, and Algan, Yann, 2015. "The superiority of economists," *Journal of Economic Perspectives*, 29/1, pp. 89–114.

Frachon, Irène, 2010. *Mediator 150mg: Combien de morts?* Brest: Dialogues.

Fukuda, Keiji, Nisenbaum, Rosane, Stewart, Geraldine, et al., 1998. "Chronic multisymptom illness affecting Air Force veterans of the Gulf War," *Journal of the American Medical Association*, 280/11, pp. 981–988.

Furetière, Antoine, 1727 [1690]. *Dictionnaire universel contenant généralement tous les mots françois, tant vieux que modernes*. La Haye: Pierre Husson.

Gaffiot, Félix, 1934. *Dictionnaire latin-français*. Paris: Hachette.

Gautret, Philippe, Lagier, Jean-Christophe, Parola, Philippe, et al., 2020. "Hydroxychloroquine and azithromycin as a treatment of Covid-19: Results of an open-label non-randomized clinical trial," *International Journal of Antimicrobial Agents*, 56/1 (online).

Geertz, Clifford, 1984. "Anti anti-relativism," *American Anthropologist*, New Series, 86/2, pp. 263–278.

Ginzburg, Carlo, 2004. "Tactiques et pratiques de l'historien. Le problème du témoignage: preuve, vérité, histoire," *Tracés*, 7, pp. 91–109 (translation of a lecture delivered in 1990).

Goffman, Erving, 1961. *Asylums. Essays on the Social Situation of Mental Patients and Other Inmates*. Garden City, NY: Anchor Books, Doubleday & Company, Inc.

Guay, Laura A., Musoke, Philippa, Fleming, Thomas, et al., 1999. "Intrapartum and neonatal single-dose nevirapine compared with zidovudine for prevention of mother-to-child transmission of HIV-1 in Kampala, Uganda," *The Lancet*, 354/9181, pp. 795–802.

Guenther, Lisa, 2013. *Solitary Confinement: Social Death and Its Afterlives*. Minneapolis: Minnesota University Press.

Hacking, Ian, 1990. *The Taming of Chance*. Cambridge: Cambridge University Press.

Hacking, Ian, 1998. *Mad Travelers: Reflections on the Reality of Transient Mental Illnesses*. Charlottesville: University Press of Virginia.

Hamilton, Tod G., and Hummer, Robert A., 2011. "Immigration and the health of US Black adults: Does country of origin matter?" *Social Science & Medicine*, 73/10, pp. 1551–1560.

Hammer, Peter J., 2019. "The Flint water crisis, the Karegnondi Water Authority, and strategic-structural racism," *Critical Sociology*, 45/1, pp. 103–119.

Hanna-Attisha, Mona, LaChance, Jenny, Sadler, Richard C., and Schnepp, Allison

C., 2016. "Elevated blood lead levels in children associated with the Flint drinking water crisis: A spatial analysis of risk and public health response," *American Journal of Public Health*, 106/2, pp. 283–290.

Hansen, Helena, and Netherland, Julie, 2016. "Is the prescription opioid epidemic a white problem?" *American Journal of Public Health*, 106/12, pp. 2127–2129.

Harant, Hervé, and Delage, Alix, 1984. *L'Épidémiologie*. Paris: PUF.

Harcourt, Bernard E., 2006. "From the asylum to the prison: Rethinking the incarceration revolution," *Texas Law Review*, 84/7, pp. 1751–1786.

Hazard, Angélique, 2008. "Baisse des suicides en prison depuis 2002," *Cahiers d'études pénitentiaires et criminologiques*, 22, May.

Heidenrich, John G., 1993. "The Gulf War: How many Iraqis died?" *Foreign Policy*, 90, pp. 108–125.

Helgesson, Magnus, Johansson, Bo, Nordquist, Tobias, et al., 2019. "Healthy migrant effect in the Swedish context: A register-based, longitudinal cohort study," *British Medical Journal Open*, 9/3, e026972.

Hémon, Denis, and Jougla, Éric, 2003. *Estimation de la surmortalité et principales caractéristiques épidémiologiques*. Report submitted to the Minister of Health. Paris: Inserm.

Hindin, Rita, Brugge, Doug, and Panikkar, Bindu, 2005. "Teratogenicity of depleted uranium aerosols: A review from an epidemiological perspective," *Environmental Health*, 4, art. 17.

Hofstadter, Richard, 1964. "The paranoid style in American politics," *Harper's Magazine*, November, pp. 77–86.

Holmes, Gary P., Kaplan, Jonathan E., Gantz, Nelson M., et al., 1988. "Chronic fatigue syndrome: A working case definition," *Annals of Internal Medicine*, 108/3, pp. 387–389.

Honneth, Axel, 1997. "Recognition and moral obligation," *Social Research*, 64/1, pp. 16–35.

Horton, Richard, 2020. *The Covid-19 Catastrophe. What's Gone Wrong and How to Stop It Happening Again*. Cambridge: Polity.

Howard, John, 1792 [1777]. *The State of the Prisons in England and Wales, with Preliminary Observations, and an Account of Some Foreign Prisons and Hospitals*, 4th edn. London: Johnson, Dilly & Cadell.

Hunter, John M., Shannon, Gary W., and Sambrook, Stephanie L., 1986. "Rings of madness: Service areas of 19th-century asylums in North America," *Social Science & Medicine*, 23/10, pp. 1033–1050.

Hyams, Kenneth C., Wignall, F. Stephen, and Roswell, Robert, 1996. "War syndromes and their evaluation: From the US Civil War to the Persian Gulf War," *Annals of Internal Medicine*, 125/5, pp. 398–405.

Institute of Medicine, 2015. *Beyond Myalgic Encephalomyelitis/Chronic Fatigue Syndrome. Redefining an Illness*. Washington, DC: The National Academies Press.

James, Doris J., and Glaze, Lauren E., 2006. "Mental health problems of prison and jail inmates," Bureau of Justice Statistics Special Report, US Department of Justice, September.

Jegede, Ayodele Samuel, 2007. "What led to the Nigerian boycott of the polio vaccination campaign," *PLOS Medicine*, 4/3, e73.

Jochelson, Karen, 2001. *The Colour of Disease: Syphilis and Racism in South Africa, 1880–1950*. Basingstoke: Palgrave.

Jones, David S., 2020. "History in crisis: Lessons for Covid-19," *The New England Journal of Medicine*, 382/18, pp. 1681–1683.

240   *References*

Jones, James F., and Straus, Stephen E., 1987. "Chronic Epstein–Barr virus infection," *Annual Review of Medicine*, 38, pp. 195–209.

Jones, Mark R., Viswanath, Omar, Peck, Jacquelin, et al., 2018. "A brief history of the opioid epidemic and strategies for pain medicine," *Pain and Therapy*, 7/1, pp. 13–21.

Juárez, Sol Pîa, Honkaniemi, Helena, Dunlavy, Andrea C., et al., 2019. "Effects of non-health-targeted policies on migrant health: A systematic review and meta-analysis," *The Lancet Global Health*, 7/4, e420–435.

Kaba, Fatos, Lewis, Andrea, Glowa-Kollisch, Sara, et al., 2014. "Solitary confinement and risk of self-harm among jail inmates," *American Journal of Public Health*, 104/3, pp. 442–447.

Kandula, Namratha R., Kersey, Margaret, and Lurie, Nicole, 2004. "Assuring the health of immigrants: What the leading indicators tell us," *Annual Review of Public Health*, 25, pp. 357–376.

Kaplowitz, Stan A., Perlstadt, Harry, Dziura, James D., and Post, Lori A., 2016. "Behavioral and environmental explanations of elevated blood lead levels in immigrant children and children of immigrants," *Journal of Immigrant and Minority Health*, 18/5, pp. 979–986.

Keeley, Brian L., 1999. "Of conspiracy theories," *The Journal of Philosophy*, 96/3, pp. 109–126.

Keller, Richard C., 2007. *Colonial Madness: Psychiatry in French North Africa*. Chicago, IL: University of Chicago Press.

Keller, Richard C., 2015. *Fatal Isolation: The Devastating Paris Heat Wave of 2003*. Chicago, IL: University of Chicago Press.

Khlat, Myriam, and Darmon, Nicole, 2003. "Is there a Mediterranean migrants mortality paradox in Europe?" *International Journal of Epidemiology*, 32/6, pp. 1115–1118.

Kilshaw, Susie M., 2004. "Friendly fire: The construction of the Gulf War syndrome narratives," *Anthropology & Medicine*, 11/2, pp. 149–160.

King, Gary, 2014. "Restructuring the social sciences: Reflections from Harvard's Institute for Quantitative Social Science," *Political Science & Politics*, 47/1, pp. 165–172.

Kolodny, Andrew, Courtwright, David T., Hwang, Catherine S., et al., 2015. "The prescription opioid and heroin crisis: A public health approach to an epidemic of addiction," *Annual Journal of Public Health*, 36, pp. 559–574.

Koselleck, Reinhart, 2006 [1972]. "Crisis," *Journal of the History of Ideas*, 67/2, pp. 357–400.

Krings, Amy, Kornberg, Dana, and Lane, Erin, 2019. "Organizing under austerity: How residents' concerns became the Flint Water Crisis," *Critical Sociology*, 45/4–5, pp. 583–593.

Lafaye, Caroline, Lancelevée, Camille, and Protais, Caroline, 2016. *L'Irresponsabilité pénale au prisme des représentations sociales de la folie et de la responsabilité des personnes souffrant de troubles mentaux*. Paris: Mission de recherche Droit et Justice.

Lakoff, Andrew, 2017. *Unprepared: Global Health in a Time of Emergency*. Berkeley, CA: University of California Press.

Lalande, André, 1993 [1926]. *Vocabulaire technique et critique de la philosophie*. Paris: PUF.

Larbiou, Benoît, 2005. "René Martial, 1873–1955. De l'hygiénisme à la raciologie, une trajectoire possible," *Genèses*, 60, pp. 98–120.

Latour, Bruno, 2004. "Why has critique run out of steam? From matters of fact to matters of concern," *Critical Inquiry*, 30/2, pp. 225–248.

Lavoisier, Antoine Laurent, 1868. *Rapport sur les prisons fait à l'Académie royale des sciences* et *Observations sur les prisons actuelles de la Conciergerie*, in *Œuvres de Lavoisier*, 3. Paris: Imprimerie impériale, pp. 465–485.

Leong, Nancy, 2013. "Racial capitalism," *Harvard Law Review*, 126/8, pp. 2151–2226.

Lévi-Strauss, Claude, 2011 [1955]. *Tristes Tropiques*, trans. John Weightman and Doreen Weightman. Harmondsworth: Penguin.

Liao, Tim F., and De Maio, Fernando, 2021. "Association of social and economic inequality with coronavirus disease 2019 incidence and mortality across US counties," *Journal of the American Medical Association*, 4/1, e2034578.

Lippold, Kumiko M., Jones, Christopher M., Olsen, Emily O'Malley, and Giroir, Brette P., 2019. "Racial-ethnic and age group differences in opioid and synthetic opioid involved overdose deaths among adults aged >18 years in metropolitan areas: United States, 2015–2017," *Morbidity and Mortality Weekly Report*, 68/43, pp. 967–973.

Lock, Margaret, 2013. *The Alzheimer Conundrum: Entanglements of Dementia and Aging*. Princeton, NJ: Princeton University Press.

Lombardi, Vincent C., Ruscetti, Francis W., Das Gupta, Jaydip, et al., 2009. "Detection of an infectious retrovirus, XMRV, in blood cells of patients with chronic fatigue syndrome," *Science*, 326/5952, pp. 585–589.

López, Ian Haney, 2013. *Dog Whistle Politics: Strategic Racism, Fake Populism, and the Dividing of America*. Oxford: Oxford University Press.

Lordon, Frédéric, 2017. "Le complotisme de l'anticomplotisme," *Le Monde diplomatique*, October.

Lu, Yao, 2008. "Test of the 'healthy migrant hypothesis': A longitudinal analysis of health selectivity of internal migration in Indonesia," *Social Science & Medicine*, 67/8, pp. 1331–1339.

Magagnoli, Joseph, Narendran, Siddharth, Pereira, Felipe, et al., 2020. "Outcomes of hydroxychloroquine usage in United States veterans hospitalized with Covid-19," MedRxiv.org, 23 April.

Marcus, George E., 1999. "The paranoid style now. Introduction," in George E. Marcus (ed.), *Paranoia within Reason: A Casebook on Conspiracy as Explanation*. Chicago, IL: University of Chicago Press, pp. 1–11.

Markel, Howard, and Stern, Alexandra Minna, 1999. "Which face? Whose nation? Immigration, public health and the construction of disease in America's ports and borders, 1891–1928," *American Behavioral Scientist*, 42/9, pp. 1314–1331.

Markides, Kyriakos S., and Rote, Sunshine, 2015. "Immigrant health paradox," in Robert A. Scott and Stephen M. Kosslyn (eds.), *Emerging Trends in the Social and Behavioral Sciences*. Hoboken, NJ: Wiley (online).

Markowitz, Gerald, and Rosner, David, 2013 [2002]. *Deceit and Denial: The Deadly Politics of Industrial Pollution*. Berkeley: University of California Press.

Massard-Guilbaud, Geneviève, 2019. "'Maladie de Lyme'. Quand des médecins refusent de soigner," *Écologie et politique*, 58, pp. 107–128.

Maule, Alexis L., Janulewicz, Patricia A., Sullivan, Kimberly A., et al., 2018. "Meta-analysis of self-reported health symptoms in 1990–1991 Gulf War and Gulf War-era veterans," *British Medical Journal Open*, 8/2, e016086.

Mazouz, Sarah, 2020. *Race*. Paris: Anamosa.

McCulloch, Jock, 1995. *Colonial Psychiatry and the "African Mind."* Cambridge: Cambridge University Press.

McCulloch, Jock, 2006. "Saving the asbestos industry, 1960–2006," *Public Health Reports*, 121/5, pp. 609–614.

McGowen, Randall, 1998. "The well-ordered prison. England 1780–1865," in Norval Morris and David J. Rothman (eds.), *The Oxford History of the Prison: The Practice of Punishment in Western Society*. Oxford: Oxford University Press, pp. 71–99.

Mendoza, Sonia, Rivera, Alyssa Stephanie, and Hansen, Helena Bjerring, 2018. "Re-racialization of addiction and the redistribution of blame in the white opioid epidemic," *Medical Anthropology Quarterly*, 33/2, pp. 242–262.

Mercier, Arnaud, 2020. "La France en pénurie de masques: Aux origines des décisions d'état," TheConversation.com, 22 March.

Meslé, France, and Vallin, Jacques, 1981. "La population des établissements psychiatriques: évolution de la morbidité ou changement de stratégie médicale?" *Population*, 36/6, pp. 1035–1068.

Mesrine, Annie, 2000. "La surmortalité des chômeurs: un effet catalyseur du chômage? ," *Économie et statistique*, 334, pp. 33–48.

Miguel, Edward, and Kremer, Michael, 2004. "Worms: Identifying impacts on education and health in the presence of treatment externalities," *Econometrica*, 72/1, pp. 159–217.

Milet, Marc, 2005. "Cadres de perception et luttes d'imputation dans la gestion de crise: l'exemple de la 'canicule' d'août 2003," *Revue française de science politique*, 55/4, pp. 573–605.

Mills, Charles W., 2017. *Black Rights/White Wrongs: The Critique of Racial Liberalism*. Oxford: Oxford University Press.

Mills, Tom, 2018. "What has become of critique? Reassembling sociology after Latour," *The British Journal of Sociology*, 69/2, pp. 286–305.

Monso, Olivier, and Saint Pol, Thibaut de, 2006. "L'origine géographique des individus dans les recensements de la population en France," *Courrier des statistiques*, 117–119, pp. 33–42.

Moyce, Sally C., and Schenker, Marc, 2018. "Migrant workers and their occupational health and safety," *Annual Review of Public Health*, 39, pp. 351–365.

Muirhead, Russell, and Rosenblum, Nancy L., 2019. *A Lot of People Are Saying: The New Conspiracism and the Assault on Democracy*. Princeton, NJ: Princeton University Press.

Muller, Seán Mfundza, Chelwa, Grieve, and Hoffmann, Nimi, 2019. "How randomized trials became big in development economics," TheConversation.com, 9 December.

Mumola, Christopher J., 2005. "Suicide and homicide in state prisons and local jails," *Bureau of Justice Statistics Special Report*, US Department of Justice, August.

Musil, Robert, 1996 [1955]. *The Man Without Qualities*, trans. Sophie Wilkins and Burton Pike. New York: Vintage.

Naudé, Anne-Jeanne, and Fassin, Didier, 2004. *Une Politique urbaine de santé publique. Les débuts de la lutte contre le saturnisme infantile en France*. Research report. Paris: Cresp.

Needleman, Herbert L., 1990. "The future challenge of lead toxicity," *Environmental Health Perspectives*, 89, pp. 85–89.

Needleman, Herbert L., and Bellinger, David, 1991. "The health effects of low-level exposure to lead," *Annual Review of Public Health*, 12, pp. 111–140.

Needleman, Herbert L., Gunnoe, Charles, Leviton, Alan, et al., 1979. "Deficits in psychologic and classroom performance of children with elevated dentine lead levels," *The New England Journal of Medicine*, 300/13, pp. 689–695.

Needleman, Herbert L., McFarland, Christine, Ness, Roberta B., et al., 2002. "Bone lead levels in adjudicated delinquents: A case control study," *Neurotoxicology and Teratology*, 24/6, pp. 711–717.

Nellis, Ashley, 2016. *The Color of Justice: Racial and Ethnic Disparity in State Prisons*. Washington, DC: The Sentencing Project.

Nevin, Rick, 2000. "How lead exposure relates to temporal changes in IQ, violent crime and unwed pregnancy," *Environmental Research*, 83/1, pp. 1–22.

Nevin, Rick, 2007. "Understanding international crime trends: The legacy of pre-school lead exposure," *Environmental Research*, 104/3, pp. 315–336.

Nietzsche, Friedrich, 1997 [1873]. *Untimely Meditations*, trans. R. J. Hollingdale. Cambridge: Cambridge University Press.

Noiriel, Gérard, 1996. *The French Melting Pot: Immigration, Citizenship, and National Identity*, trans. Geoffroy de Laforcade. Minneapolis: University of Minnesota Press.

Nora, Pierre (ed.), 1996. *Realms of Memory: The Construction of the French Past*, trans. Arthur Goldhammer. New York: Columbia University Press.

O'Neill, Michel, 1983. "Les départements de santé communautaire," *Recherches sociographiques*, 24/2, pp. 171–201.

Oni-Orisan, Adeola, 2016. "The obligation to count: The politics of monitoring maternal mortality in Nigeria," in Vincanne Adams (ed.), *Metrics: What Counts in Global Health*. Durham, NC: Duke University Press, pp. 82–101.

Oreskes, Naomi, and Conway, Erik M., 2010. *Merchants of Doubt: How a Handful of Scientists Obscured the Truth on Issues from Tobacco Smoke to Global Warming*. New York: Bloomsbury Press.

Owen, David, 2002. "Criticism and captivity: On genealogy and critical theory," *European Journal of Philosophy*, 10/2, pp. 216–230.

Packard, Randall M., 1989. *White Plague, Black Labor: Tuberculosis and the Political Economy of Health and Disease in South Africa*. Berkeley: University of California Press.

Palloni, Alberto, and Arias, Elizabeth, 2004. "Paradox lost: Explaining the Hispanic adult mortality advantage," *Demography*, 41/3, pp. 385–415.

Pasteur Vallery-Radot, Louis, 1939. "Le bilan de l'effort français. L'institut Pasteur," *Revue des Deux Mondes*, 50/3, pp. 604–625.

Pigden, Charles, 1995. "Popper revisited, or What is wrong with conspiracy theories?" *Philosophy of the Social Sciences*, 25/1, pp. 3–34.

Piketty, Thomas, 2017. *Capital in the Twenty-First Century*, trans. Arthur Goldhammer. Cambridge, MA: Belknap Press.

Pinch, Trevor J., 1992. "Opening black boxes: Science, technology and society," *Social Studies of Science*, 22/3, pp. 487–510.

Pinel, Philippe, 1809 [1801]. *Traité médico-philosophique sur l'aliénation mentale*. Paris: Brosson.

Piquemal, Jacques, 1959. "Le choléra de 1832 en France et la pensée médicale," *Thalès*, 10, pp. 27–73.

Plancke, Laurent, Sy, Aminata, Fovet, Thomas, et al., 2017. *La Santé mentale des personnes entrant en détention dans le Nord et le Pas-de-Calais*. Lille: F2RSM Psy.

Pluye, Pierre, and Hong, Quan Nha, 2014. "Combining the power of stories and the power of numbers: Mixed methods research and mixed studies reviews," *Annual Review of Public Health*, 35, pp. 29–45.

Popper, Karl, 2012 [1945]. *The Open Society and Its Enemies*. London: Routledge.

Porot, Antoine, 1918. "Notes de psychiatrie musulmane," *Annales médico-psychologiques*, 74/9, pp. 377–384.

Porter, Dorothy, 1999. *Health, Civilization and the State: A History of Public Health from Ancient to Modern Times*. London: Routledge.

Proctor, Robert N., 1995. *Cancer Wars: How Politics Shapes What We Know and Don't Know about Cancer*. New York: Basic Books.

Provine, Doris Marie, 2011. "Race and inequality in the war on drugs," *Annual Review of Law and the Social Science*, 7, pp. 41–60.

Puthooparambil, Soorej Jose, and Parente, Paolo, 2018. *Report on the Health of Refugees and Migrants in the WHO European Region*. Copenhagen: World Health Organization.

Quétel, Claude, and Morel, Pierre, 1979. *Les Fous et leurs médecines: De la Renaissance au XXe siècle*. Paris: Hachette.

Rabin, Richard, 1989. "Warnings unheeded: A history of child lead poisoning," *American Journal of Public Health*, 79/12, pp. 1668–1674.

Rainhorn, Judith, 2019. *Blanc de plomb. Histoire d'un poison légal*. Paris: Presses de Sciences Po.

Ranganathan, Malini, 2016. "Thinking with Flint: Racial liberalism and the roots of an American water tragedy," *Capitalism. Nature. Socialism*, 27/3, pp. 17–33.

Razum, Oliver, Zeeb, Hajo, Akgün, H. Seval, et al., 1998. "Low overall mortality of Turkish residents in Germany persists and extends into a second generation: Merely a healthy migrant effect?" *Tropical Medicine and International Health*, 3/4, pp. 297–303.

Renne, Elisha, 2006. "Perspectives on polio and immunization in northern Nigeria," *Social Science & Medicine*, 63, pp. 1857–1869.

Rey, Alain, 1998. *Dictionnaire historique de la langue française*, 2nd edn. Paris: Le Robert.

Reyes, Jessica W., 2015. "Lead exposure and behavior: Effects on anti-social and risky behavior among children and adolescents," *Economic Inquiry*, 53/3, pp. 1580–1605.

Rezkallah, Nadia, and Epelboin, Alain, 1997. *Chroniques du saturnisme infantile, 1989–1994*. Paris: L'Harmattan.

Rhodes, Lorna A., 2004. *Total Confinement: Madness and Reason in the Maximum Security Prison*. Berkeley: University of California Press.

Ricœur, Paul, 1965. *De l'Interprétation. Essai sur Freud*. Paris: Seuil.

Riddle, James R., Brown, Mark, Smith, Tyler, et al., 2003. "Chemical warfare and the Gulf War: A review of the impact on Gulf veterans' health," *Military Medicine*, 168/8, pp. 606–613.

Robine, Jean-Marie, Cheung, Siu Lan K., Le Roy, Sophie, et al., 2007. "Death toll exceeded 70,000 in Europe during the summer of 2003," *Comptes rendus biologies*, 331/2, pp. 171–178.

Robinson, Cedric J., 1983. *Black Marxism: The Making of the Black Radical Tradition*. London: Zed Press.

Ronda Pérez, Elena, Benavides, Fernando G., Levecque, Katia, et al., 2012. "Differences in working conditions and employment arrangements among migrant and non-migrant workers in Europe," *Ethnicity & Health*, 17/6, pp. 563–577.

Rosen, George, 1958. *A History of Public Health*. New York: MD Publications.

Ross, Benjamin, 2016. "Science in the service of untruth: A century of lead poisoning," *Dissent*, 4 February, pp. 49–52.

Ross, Benjamin, and Amter, Steven, 2010. *The Polluters: The Making of Our Chemically Altered Environment*. Oxford: Oxford University Press.

Rossi, Sabrina, and Pitidis, Alessio, 2018. "Multiple chemical sensitivity: Review of the state of the art in epidemiology, diagnosis and future perspectives," *Journal of Occupational and Environmental Medicine*, 60/2, pp. 138–146.

Rothman, David J., 2008 [1971]. *The Discovery of Asylum: Social Order and Disorder in the New Republic*. New Brunswick, NJ: Aldine Transaction.

Russell, Bertrand, 1950. "Logical positivism," *Revue internationale de philosophie*, 4/11, pp. 3–19.

Sackett, David L., Rosenberg, William M. C., Gray, J. A. Muir, et al., 1996. "Evidence based medicine: What it is and what it isn't," *British Medical Journal*, 312, pp. 71–72.

Sampson, Robert J., and Winter, Alix S., 2016. "The racial ecology of lead poisoning: Toxic inequality in Chicago neighborhoods, 1995–2013," *Du Bois Review*, 13/2, pp. 261–283.

Sanders, Todd, and West, Harry G., 2003. "Power revealed and concealed in the new world order," in Todd Sanders and Harry G. West (eds.), *Transparency and Conspiracy: Ethnographies of Suspicion in the New World Order*. Durham, NC: Duke University Press, pp. 1–37.

Sartin, Jeffrey S., 2000. "Gulf War illnesses: Causes and controversies," *Mayo Clinic Proceedings*, 75/8, pp. 811–819.

Sayad, Abdelmalek, 2004. *The Suffering of the Immigrant*, trans. David Macey. Cambridge: Polity.

Schuster, David G., 2011. *The Neurasthenic Nation: America's Search for Health, Happiness and Comfort, 1869–1920*. New Brunswick, NJ: Rutgers University Press.

Shorter, Edward, 1993. "Chronic fatigue in historical perspective," in Gregory R. Bock and Julie Whelan (eds.), *Chronic Fatigue Syndrome*. Chichester: John Wiley & Sons, pp. 6–22.

Shriver, Thomas E., 2001. "Environmental hazards and veterans' framing of Gulf War Illness," *Sociological Inquiry*, 71/4, pp. 403–420.

Simon, Patrick, 2014. "La question des statistiques ethniques en France," in Marie Poinsot (ed.), *Migrations et mutations de la société française. L'état des savoirs*. Paris: La Découverte, pp. 297–306.

Singh, Gopal K., and Hiatt, Robert A., 2006. "Trends and disparities in socioeconomic and behavioral characteristics, life expectancy, and cause-specific mortality of native-born and foreign-born populations in the United States, 1979–2003," *International Journal of Epidemiology*, 35/4, pp. 903–919.

Singh, Gopal K., and Siahpush, Mohammad, 2002. "Ethnic-immigrant differentials in health behaviors, morbidity, and cause-specific mortality in the United States: An analysis of two national data bases," *Human Biology*, 74/1, pp. 83–109.

Sizaire, Vincent, 2020. "L'état d'urgence sanitaire menace-t-il les libertés fondamentales?" TheConversation.com, 6 April.

Spierenburg, Pieter, 1995. "The body and the state: Early modern Europe," in Norval Morris and David J. Rothman (eds.), *The Oxford History of the Prison: The Practice of Punishment in Western Society*. Oxford: Oxford University Press, pp. 43–70.

Steinmetz, George (ed.), 2005. *The Politics of Method in the Human Sciences: Positivism and Its Epistemological Others*. Durham, NC: Duke University Press.

Stempel, Carl, Hargrove, Thomas, and Stempel, Guido H., 2007. "Media use, social structure and belief in 9/11 conspiracy theories," *Journalism & Mass Communication Quarterly*, 84/2, pp. 353–372.

Straus, Stephen E., 1991. "History of chronic fatigue syndrome," *Reviews of Infectious Diseases*, 13/S1, pp. 52–57.

Strauss, Anselm, 1978. "A social worlds perspective," *Studies in Symbolic Interaction*, 1, pp. 119–128.

Stretesky, Paul B., and Lynch, Michael J., 2004. "The relationship between lead and crime," *Journal of Health and Social Behavior*, 45/2, pp. 214–229.

Strickler, Gail K., Kreiner, Peter W., Halpin, John F., et al., 2020. "Opioid prescribing behaviors: Prescription Behavior Surveillance System, 11 states, 2010–2016," *Morbidity and Mortality Weekly Report*, 69/1, pp. 1–14.

Sunstein, Cass R., and Vermeule, Adrian, 2009. "Conspiracy theories: Causes and cures," *The Journal of Political Philosophy*, 17/2, pp. 202–227.

Supiot, Alain, 2015. *La Gouvernance par les nombres. Cours au Collège de France, 2012–2014*. Paris: Fayard.

Swanson, Maynard W., 1977. "The sanitation syndrome: Bubonic plague and urban native policy in the Cape Colony, 1900–1909," *Journal of African History*, 18/3, pp. 387–410.

Swoboda, Debra A., 2006. "The social construction of contested illness legitimacy: A grounded theory analysis," *Qualitative Research in Psychology*, 3/3, pp. 233–251.

Taylor, Becky, 2016. "Immigration, statecraft and public health: The 1920 Aliens Order, medical examinations and the limitations of the state in England," *Social History of Medicine*, 29/3, pp. 512–533.

Tehranifar, Parisa, Leighton, Jessica, Auchincloss, Amy H., et al., 2008. "Immigration and risk of childhood lead poisoning: Findings from a case-control study of New York City children," *American Journal of Public Health*, 98/1, pp. 92–97.

Thompson, E. P., 1971. "The moral economy of the English crowd in the eighteenth century," *Past & Present*, 50/1, pp. 76–136.

Tokarska-Bakir, Joanna, 2010. "Des racines mythiques de l'antisémitisme: Le meurtre rituel juif," *Ethnologie française*, 40/2, pp. 305–313.

Tratner, Isabelle, 2003. "La lutte contre le saturnisme infantile: Quels progrès en vingt ans?" *Médecine/Sciences*, 19/8–9, pp. 873–877.

Tuke, Samuel, 1813. *Description of the Retreat, an Institution Near York, for Insane Persons of the Society of Friends*. Philadelphia, PA: Isaac Pierce.

Turra, Cassio M., and Elo, Irma T., 2008. "The impact of salmon bias on the Hispanic mortality advantage," *Population Research and Policy Review*, 27/5, pp. 515–530.

Urquia, Marcelo L., O'Campo, Patricia J., and Heaman, Maureen I., 2012. "Revisiting the immigrant paradox in reproductive health: The role of duration and ethnicity," *Social Science & Medicine*, 74/10, pp. 1610–1621.

Vallée, Jean-François, 2004. "L'étrangeté sans qualités: le cas de Robert Musil," *Tangence*, 76, pp. 25–49.

Van der Vliet, Virginia, 2001. "AIDS: Losing 'the new struggle'?" *Daedalus*, 130/1, pp. 151–184.

Van Zee, Aer, 2009. "The promotion and marketing of Oxycontin: Commercial triumph, public health tragedy," *American Journal of Public Health*, 99/2, pp. 221–227.

Vassy, Carine, Keller, Richard C., and Dingwall, Robert (eds.), 2010. *Enregistrer les morts, identifier les surmortalités. Une comparaison Angleterre, États-Unis et France*. Rennes: Presses de l'École des hautes études en santé publique.

Velmet, Aro, 2020. *Pasteur's Empire: Bacteriology and Politics in France, Its Colonies, and the World*. Oxford: Oxford University Press.

Villermé, Louis-René, 1829. "Mémoire sur la mortalité dans les prisons," *Annales d'hygiène publique et de médecine légale*, 1/1, pp. 1–100.

Walker, Patricia Frye, 2018. "Presidential address. Migration medicine: Notes on a young science," *American Journal of Tropical Medicine and Hygiene*, 99/4, pp. 820–826.

Wallace, Matthew, Khlat, Myriam, and Guillot, Michel, 2019. "Mortality advantage among migrants according to the duration of stay in France, 2004–2014," *BMC Public Health*, 19, art. 327.

Walsh, Julia A., and Warren, Kenneth S., 1979. "Selective primary health care: An interim strategy for disease control in developing countries," *The New England Journal of Medicine*, 301/18, pp. 967–974.

Ware, Norma C., 1992. "Suffering and the social construction of illness: The delegitimation of illness experience in chronic fatigue syndrome," *Medical Anthropology Quarterly*, 6/4, pp. 347–361.

Werthern, Martha von, Robjant, Katy, Chui, Zoe, et al., 2018. "The impact of immigration detention on mental health: A systematic review," *BMC Psychiatry*, 18, art. 382.

Wessely, Simon, 1997. "Chronic fatigue syndrome: A 20th-century illness?" *Scandinavian Journal of Work and Environmental Health*, 23/S3, pp. 17–34.

White, Roberta F., Steele, Lea, O'Callaghan, James P., et al., 2016. "Recent research on Gulf War illness and other health problems in veterans of the 1991 Gulf War: Effect of toxicant exposures during deployment," *Cortex*, 74, pp. 449–475.

Wilson, Nana, Kariisa, Mbabazi, Seth, Puja, et al., 2020. "Drug and opioid-involved overdose deaths: United States, 2017–2018," *Morbidity and Mortality Weekly Report*, 69/11, pp. 290–297.

Winslow, Charles-Edward A., 1920. "The untilled fields of public health," *Science*, 51/1306, pp. 23–33.

Woolf, Steven H., and Schoomaker, Heidi, 2019. "Life expectancy and mortality rates in the United States, 1959–2017," *Journal of the American Medical Association*, 322/20, pp. 1996–2016.

Young, Allan, 1995. *The Harmony of Illusions: Inventing Post-Traumatic Stress Disorder*. Princeton, NJ: Princeton University Press.

Zamosc, Leon, 1994. "Agrarian protest and the Indian movement in the Ecuadorian highlands," *Latin American Research Review*, 29/3, pp. 37–68.

Index